New Directions in Barrett's Esophagus

Editor

NICHOLAS J. SHAHEEN

GASTROINTESTINAL ENDOSCOPY CLINICS OF NORTH AMERICA

www.giendo.theclinics.com

Consulting Editor
CHARLES J. LIGHTDALE

July 2017 • Volume 27 • Number 3

ELSEVIER

1600 John F. Kennedy Boulevard • Suite 1800 • Philadelphia, Pennsylvania, 19103-2899

http://www.theclinics.com

GASTROINTESTINAL ENDOSCOPY CLINICS OF NORTH AMERICA Volume 27, Number 3 July 2017 ISSN 1052-5157, ISBN-13: 978-0-323-53132-0

Editor: Kerry Holland

Developmental Editor: Donald Mumford

Gastrointestinal Endoscopy Clinics of North America (ISSN 1052-5157) is published quarterly by Elsevier Inc., 360 Park Avenue South, New York, NY 10010-1710. Months of issue are January, April, July, and October. Business and Editorial Offices: 1600 John F. Kennedy Blvd., Suite 1800, Philadelphia, PA, 19103-2899. Periodicals postage paid at New York, NY and additional mailing offices. Subscription prices are $342.00 per year for US individuals, $560.00 per year for US institutions, $100.00 per year for US students and residents, $377.00 per year for Canadian individuals, $662.00 per year for Canadian institutions, $474.00 per year for international individuals, $662.00 per year for international institutions, and $245.00 per year for Canadian and foreign students/residents. To receive student/resident rate, orders must be accompanied by name of affiliated institution, date of term, and the *signature* of program/residency coordinator on institution letterhead. Orders will be billed at individual rate until proof of status is received. Foreign air speed delivery is included in all *Clinics* subscription prices. All prices are subject to change without notice. **POSTMASTER:** Send address change to *Gastrointestinal Endoscopy Clinics of North America*, Elsevier Health Sciences Division, Subscription Customer Service, 3251 Riverport Lane, Maryland Heights, MO 63043. **Customer Service: 1-800-654-2452 (US). From outside the United States, call 1-314-447-8871. Fax: 1-314-447-8029. E-mail: JournalsCustomerService-usa@elsevier.com (for print support) or JournalsOnlineSupport-usa@elsevier.com (for online support)**.

Reprints. For copies of 100 or more, of articles in this publication, please contact the Commercial Reprints Department, Elsevier Inc., 360 Park Avenue South, New York, NY 10010-1710. Tel. 212-633-3874; Fax: 212-633-3820; E-mail: reprints@elsevier.com.

Gastrointestinal Endoscopy Clinics of North America is covered in *Excerpta Medica, MEDLINE/PubMed (Index Medicus), and MEDLINE/MEDLARS.*

Contributors

CONSULTING EDITOR

CHARLES J. LIGHTDALE, MD
Professor of Medicine, Division of Digestive and Liver Diseases, Columbia University Medical Center, New York, New York

EDITOR

NICHOLAS J. SHAHEEN, MD, MPH
Professor of Medicine, University of North Carolina, Chapel Hill, North Carolina

AUTHORS

KAMAR BELGHAZI, MD
Department of Gastroenterology and Hepatology, Academic Medical Center, Amsterdam, The Netherlands

JACQUES J.G.H.M. BERGMAN, MD, PhD
Department of Gastroenterology and Hepatology, Academic Medical Center, Amsterdam, The Netherlands

CHRISTOPHER H. BLEVINS, MD
Fellow, Division of Gastroenterology and Hepatology, Mayo Clinic Minnesota, Rochester, Minnesota

MARCIA IRENE CANTO, MD, MHS
Division of Gastroenterology and Hepatology, Johns Hopkins Medical Institutions, Johns Hopkins University School of Medicine, Baltimore, Maryland

DOUGLAS A. CORLEY, MD, PhD
Division of Research, Kaiser Permanente Northern California, Oakland, California; San Francisco Medical Center, Kaiser Permanente Northern California, San Francisco, California

KERRY B. DUNBAR, MD, PhD
Associate Professor, Division of Gastroenterology and Hepatology, Department of Medicine, Esophageal Diseases Center, Dallas VA Medical Center, VA North Texas Health Care System, University of Texas Southwestern Medical Center, Dallas, Texas

REBECCA C. FITZGERALD, MD
Professor of Cancer Prevention, MRC Cancer Unit, Hutchinson/MRC Research Centre, University of Cambridge, Cambridge, United Kingdom

GREGORY G. GINSBERG, MD
Division of Gastroenterology and Hepatology, Department of Medicine, University of Pennsylvania, Philadelphia, Pennsylvania

JOHN M. INADOMI, MD
Cyrus E. Rubin Chair and Head, Division of Gastroenterology, Department of Medicine, University of Washington School of Medicine, Seattle, Washington

PRASAD G. IYER, MD, MSc
Professor of Medicine, Division of Gastroenterology and Hepatology, Mayo Clinic Minnesota, Rochester, Minnesota

PUJAN KANDEL, MD
Department of Gastroenterology and Hepatology, Mayo Clinic Florida, Jacksonville, Florida

LEILA KIA, MD
Assistant Professor of Medicine, Division of Gastroenterology and Hepatology, Northwestern University Feinberg School of Medicine, Chicago, Illinois

SRINADH KOMANDURI, MD, MS
Associate Professor of Medicine, Division of Gastroenterology and Hepatology, Northwestern University Feinberg School of Medicine, Chicago, Illinois

GENE K. MA, MD
Division of Gastroenterology and Hepatology, Department of Medicine, University of Pennsylvania, Philadelphia, Pennsylvania

JUDITH OFFMAN, PhD
Epidemiologist, Centre for Cancer Prevention, Wolfson Institute of Preventive Medicine, Barts and The London School of Medicine and Dentistry, Queen Mary University of London, London, United Kingdom

ROOS E. POUW, MD, PhD
Department of Gastroenterology and Hepatology, Academic Medical Center, Amsterdam, The Netherlands

BASHAR J. QUMSEYA, MD, MPH
Clinical Assistant Professor of Medicine, Division of Gastroenterology and Hepatology, Florida State University, Tallahasee, Florida; Archbold Medical Group, Thomasville, Georgia

NINA SAXENA, MD
Division of Gastroenterology, Department of Medicine, University of Washington School of Medicine, Seattle, Washington

JENNIFER L. SCHNEIDER, MPH
Division of Research, Kaiser Permanente Northern California, Oakland, California

RHONDA F. SOUZA, MD, AGAF, FASGE
Center for Esophageal Diseases, Department of Medicine, Baylor University Medical Center and Center for Esophageal Research, Baylor Scott and White Research Institute, Dallas, Texas

KAVEL VISRODIA, MD
Division of Gastroenterology and Hepatology, Department of Internal Medicine, Mayo Clinic, Rochester, Minnesota

MICHAEL B. WALLACE, MD, MPH
Department of Gastroenterology and Hepatology, Mayo Clinic Florida, Jacksonville, Florida

KENNETH K. WANG, MD
Russ and Kathy Van Cleve Professor of Gastroenterology Research, Division of Gastroenterology and Hepatology, Department of Internal Medicine, Mayo Clinic, Rochester, Minnesota

THOMAS J. WATSON, MD, FACS
Professor of Surgery, Division of Thoracic and Esophageal Surgery, Regional Chief of Surgery, MedStar Washington, Georgetown University School of Medicine, Washington, DC

HERBERT C. WOLFSEN, MD
Professor of Medicine, Division of Gastroenterology and Hepatology, Mayo Clinic, Jacksonville, Florida

LIAM ZAKKO, MD
Division of Gastroenterology and Hepatology, Department of Internal Medicine, Mayo Clinic, Rochester, Minnesota

Contents

Foreword: Barrett's Esophagus and the Prevention of Esophageal Adenocarcinoma xiii

Charles J. Lightdale

Preface: New Directions in Barrett's Esophagus xv

Nicholas J. Shaheen

The Troublesome Epidemiology of Barrett's Esophagus and Esophageal Adenocarcinoma 353

Jennifer L. Schneider and Douglas A. Corley

Barrett's esophagus and esophageal adenocarcinoma diagnoses have increased markedly in recent decades. Recent research with patients diagnosed with Barrett's esophagus (the only known precursor for esophageal adenocarcinoma) and esophageal adenocarcinoma has identified several modifiable and nonmodifiable potential risk factors. Consistent risk factors for both disorders include increasing age, male sex, white non-Hispanic race/ethnicity, gastroesophageal reflux disease, lack of infection with Helicobacter pylori, smoking, abdominal obesity, and a Western diet. The authors present detailed discussions of these risk factors along with possible explanations for some apparent discrepancies and ideas for future study.

Who Deserves Endoscopic Screening for Esophageal Neoplasia? 365

Christopher H. Blevins and Prasad G. Iyer

Despite the availability of safe and effective endoscopic treatment of Barrett's esophagus (BE)–related dysplasia and neoplasia, the incidence and mortality from esophageal adenocarcinoma (EAC) have continued to increase. This likely stems from the large population of patients that develop EAC outside of a BE screening and surveillance program. Identification of BE with screening followed by enrollment in an appropriate surveillance/risk stratification program could be a strategy to address both the incidence of and mortality from EAC. This article summarizes the rationale and challenges for BE screening, the risk factors for BE, and the currently described BE risk assessment tools.

Alternatives to Traditional Per-Oral Endoscopy for Screening 379

Judith Offman and Rebecca C. Fitzgerald

Barrett's esophagus (BE) predisposes patients to esophageal adenocarcinoma. 3 to 6% of individuals with gastro-esophageal reflux disease are estimated to have BE but only 20 to 25% of BE patients are currently diagnosed. The current gold standard for diagnosis of BE is per-oral upper GI endoscopy. As this is not suitable for large-scale screening, a number of alternative methods are currently being investigated: transnasal and video capsule endoscopy, endomicroscopy, cell collection devices like the

dissection may also play a role in the treatment of neoplastic Barrett's esophagus. Treatment of early Barrett's neoplasia should be centralized and limited to expert centers with a high-volume load and sufficient expertise in the detection and treatment of esophageal neoplasia.

The Role of Endoscopic Ultrasound in the Management of Patients with Barrett's Esophagus and Superficial Neoplasia **471**

Bashar J. Qumseya and Herbert C. Wolfsen

Endoscopic ultrasound (EUS) is a minimally invasive advanced imaging procedure using high-frequency sound waves to produce detailed images of the esophageal wall with fine-needle aspiration to biopsy adjacent lymph nodes. The role of EUS is well established in patients with locally advanced Barrett esophagus neoplasia. The utility of EUS in the evaluation of Barrett esophagus patients is controversial. This is a review of the evidence using EUS in BE patients. The assessment is that EUS may be a powerful tool in managing patients with BE neoplasia.

Radiofrequency Ablation of Barrett's Esophagus: Patient Selection, Preparation, and Performance **481**

Gene K. Ma and Gregory G. Ginsberg

Radiofrequency ablation (RFA) is a safe and effective thermal ablative therapy for dysplastic Barrett's esophagus (BE) and, to a lesser extent, nondysplastic BE. Before the utilization of RFA, there must be an appropriate indication, assessment of potential contraindications, discussion of risks and benefits with patients, and careful endoscopic planning. The ease of performance of the procedure along with its efficacy and low rate of adverse events have established RFA as a reliable technique for endoscopic management of dysplastic BE.

Radiofrequency Ablation of Barrett's Esophagus: Efficacy, Complications, and Durability **491**

Kavel Visrodia, Liam Zakko, and Kenneth K. Wang

In the last decade, radiofrequency ablation in combination with endoscopic mucosal resection has simplified and improved the treatment of Barrett's esophagus. These treatments not only reduced the progression of dysplastic Barrett's esophagus to esophageal adenocarcinoma but also decreased treatment-related complications. More recent data from larger series with extended follow-up periods are emerging to refine expectations in patients treated with radiofrequency ablation. Although most patients achieve eradication of neoplasia and intestinal metaplasia, in the long-term a substantial portion of patients develop recurrent disease. This article provides an updated review of radiofrequency ablation efficacy, complications, and durability.

Cryotherapy for Barrett's Esophagus **503**

Marcia Irene Canto

Cryotherapy or cryoablation involves the freezing of tissues to destroy unwanted tissue or to control bleeding. Endoscopic cryotherapy has been developed for gastrointestinal application by through-the-scope noncontact delivery of compressed carbon dioxide gas or liquid nitrogen (cryospray) or contact balloon cryoablation. The mechanism of cryotherapy ablative effects includes immediate injury as well as coagulation necrosis occurring over several hours and days, unlike heat-based thermal ablation. This article reviews the basis, technique, safety, efficacy, and durability for the use of endoscopic cryotherapy in Barrett's esophagus and esophageal adenocarcinoma.

Care of the Postablation Patient: Surveillance, Acid Suppression, and Treatment of Recurrence **515**

Leila Kia and Srinadh Komanduri

Endoscopic eradication therapy is effective and durable for the treatment of Barrett's esophagus (BE), with low rates of recurrence of dysplasia but significant rates of recurrence of intestinal metaplasia. Identified risk factors for recurrence include age and length of BE before treatment and may also include presence of a large hiatal hernia, higher grade of dysplasia before treatment, and history of smoking. Current guidelines for surveillance following ablation are limited, with recommendations based on low-quality evidence and expert opinion. New modalities including optical coherence tomography and wide-area tissue sampling with computer-assisted analysis show promise as adjunctive surveillance modalities.

Esophagectomy for Superficial Esophageal Neoplasia **531**

Thomas J. Watson

Endoscopic therapies have become the standard of care for most cases of Barrett's esophagus with high-grade dysplasia or intramucosal adenocarcinoma. Despite a rapid and dramatic evolution in treatment paradigms, esophagectomy continues to occupy a place in the therapeutic armamentarium for superficial esophageal neoplasia. The managing physician must remain cognizant of the limitations of endoscopic approaches and consider surgical resection when they are exceeded. Esophagectomy, performed at experienced centers for appropriately selected patients with early-stage disease can be undertaken with the expectation of cure as well as low mortality, acceptable morbidity, and good long-term quality of life.

GASTROINTESTINAL ENDOSCOPY CLINICS OF NORTH AMERICA

FORTHCOMING ISSUES

October 2017
Progress in Endoscopic Ultrasonography
Frank Gress, *Editor*

January 2018
Eosinophilic Esophagitis
David A. Katzka, *Editor*

April 2018
Lumen-Apposing Stents
Jacques Van Dam, *Editor*

RECENT ISSUES

April 2017
Bariatric and Metabolic Endoscopy
Richard I. Rothstein, *Editor*

January 2017
Evaluation of the Small Bowel
Lauren B. Gerson, *Editor*

October 2016
Endoscopy in Inflammatory Bowel Disease
Maria T. Abreu, *Editor*

RELATED INTEREST

Gastroenterology Clinics of North America, June 2015, (Vol. 44, No. 2)
Barrett's Esophagus
Prasad G. Iyer and Navtej S. Buttar, *Editors*

Foreword

Barrett's Esophagus and the Prevention of Esophageal Adenocarcinoma

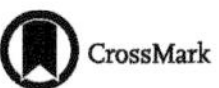

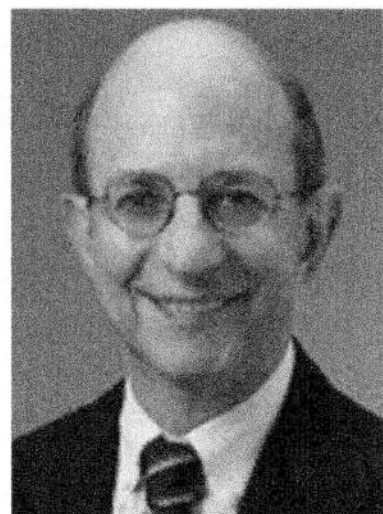

Charles J. Lightdale, MD
Consulting Editor

The incidence of esophageal adenocarcinoma has risen 10-fold in the United States since the 1970s and continues to rise at an alarming rate. While squamous cell cancer occurs at high rates in northern China and in areas of the developing world, adenocarcinoma is now the predominant form of esophageal cancer in the United States and other western countries. The major risk factor for esophageal adenocarcinoma is gastroesophageal reflux disease (GERD) and the subset of GERD patients with Barrett's esophagus, where the normal squamous mucosa is replaced by columnar tissue with intestinal metaplasia.

The past two decades have seen improvements in endoscopic diagnosis of Barrett's esophagus and in identification of dysplasia in Barrett's mucosa. At the same time, there has been remarkable progress in endoscopic therapies that can effectively and safely eradicate Barrett's tissue at high risk of progression to cancer. While this progress is impressive, there remain many questions and controversies in the management of Barrett's esophagus. These are presented and discussed in detail in this issue of *Gastrointestinal Endoscopy Clinics of North America* devoted to new directions in Barrett's esophagus. Dr Nicholas Shaheen, the editor for the issue, is widely recognized for his dynamic leadership in this area, and his research has had a major impact on how Barrett's patients are treated. He has selected an all-star international group of authors who present a comprehensive state-of-the art review with a look to the future.

The foundation of the issue is the first article on the epidemiology of Barrett's esophagus and esophageal adenocarcinoma. Since more than 90% of patients with esophageal adenocarcinoma present at the time of diagnosis with usually lethal advanced stage cancer and have never been diagnosed previously with Barrett's esophagus, the need to screen patients for Barrett's esophagus comes to the fore. The important

Gastrointest Endoscopy Clin N Am 27 (2017) xiii–xiv
http://dx.doi.org/10.1016/j.giec.2017.04.002
1052-5157/17/© 2017 Published by Elsevier Inc.

questions of who to screen and how to screen are discussed in following articles, including new nonendoscopic screening methods. Cost-effectiveness of screening and surveillance is covered as well as the place of advanced imaging methods and the role of biomarkers in cancer risk stratification in patients with Barrett's esophagus. The fine points of endoscopic mucosal resection and endoscopic submucosal dissection, the use of endoscopic ultrasonography for staging, the impact of radiofrequency ablation, and the emergence of cryoablation are other topics. How to follow and manage patients after complete eradication of dysplasia and intestinal metaplasia for possible recurrence and the role of surgery for esophageal adenocarcinoma are additional important subjects given detailed review.

Jam-packed with information on the management of Barrett's esophagus and the prevention of esophageal adenocarcinoma, this is a terrific issue of *Gastrointestinal Endoscopy Clinics of North America*. Don't miss it!

Charles J. Lightdale, MD
Department of Medicine
Columbia University Medical Center
161 Fort Washington Avenue
New York, NY 10032, USA

E-mail address:
CJL18@columbia.edu

Preface
New Directions in Barrett's Esophagus

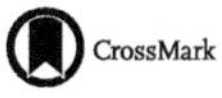

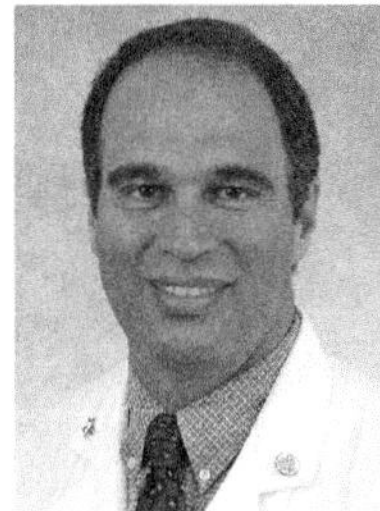

Nicholas J. Shaheen, MD, MPH
Editor

I am so pleased to introduce this issue of *Gastrointestinal Endoscopy Clinics of North America*, "New Directions in Barrett's Esophagus." In terms of the morbidity and mortality associated with it, as well as the resources expended on it, Barrett's esophagus (BE) and esophageal adenocarcinoma rank high in gastrointestinal (GI) maladies. Indeed, the question of how to manage the patient with chronic heartburn is probably second only to colorectal cancer screening as a public health concern in GI, and indications related to gastroesophageal reflux disease are routinely at or near the top the list for upper endoscopy. So it is both timely and highly relevant that we revisit the best practices with respect to care of this disease.

In addition, the past decade has finally brought some progress in the care of these patients on several fronts. Endoscopic imaging, endoscopic eradication therapy, and risk stratification in the disease have all seen welcome advances during this time, after a lengthy period with little change in the care of patients with BE.

This issue of *Gastrointestinal Endoscopy Clinics of North America* seeks to chronicle the progress made in BE as well as the plentiful challenges that remain. We have endeavored to assemble some of the most prolific researchers and outstanding teachers from across the globe, to give a textured and comprehensive view of the care of these patients. While the technical advances in BE continue to impress, I suspect that the cognitive challenges will be those that most consume your intellectual effort as you peruse this text. Indeed, very fundamental questions like who should be screened for BE and how, who should undergo intervention to prevent neoplasia, and how should those patients be managed after intervention, all remain largely unanswered, despite extensive efforts to address them. While the uncertainty regarding best management of these patients may be daunting, they also make this area an exciting and rapidly evolving area of inquiry, which I hope will continue to attract bright minds.

Gastrointest Endoscopy Clin N Am 27 (2017) xv–xvi
http://dx.doi.org/10.1016/j.giec.2017.04.001
1052-5157/17/© 2017 Published by Elsevier Inc.

I feel lucky to have as colleagues the renowned authors whose work forms the body of this issue, and I thank them for their efforts on this project. Thanks also to Kerry Holland, Nicole Congleton, and the staff at Elsevier for their tireless efforts in managing us to bring this issue together. I hope you enjoy reading the fruits of their labor, and that this work helps you better care for your patients.

Nicholas J. Shaheen, MD, MPH
University of North Carolina
Chapel Hill, NC 27599, USA

E-mail address:
nshaheen@med.unc.edu

The Troublesome Epidemiology of Barrett's Esophagus and Esophageal Adenocarcinoma

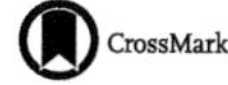

Jennifer L. Schneider, MPH[a,*], Douglas A. Corley, MD, PhD[a,b]

KEYWORDS

• Barrett's esophagus • Esophageal adenocarcinoma • Epidemiology

KEY POINTS

- The incidence and prevalence of esophageal adenocarcinoma and Barrett's esophagus, respectively, have increased markedly in recent decades, without conclusive explanation.
- There are marked differences in disease incidence by region, sex, and gender.
- The main risk factors for these disorders are abdominal obesity, smoking, gastroesophageal reflux disease, a Western diet, and the absence of *Helicobacter pylori* colonization.
- The demographic distributions of the risk factors generally do not match the distributions of disease incidence, creating confusion regarding the underlying explanation for what is causing the incidence increases, potential interventions, and the unusual demographic patterns.
- The differences found may, in part, be related to interactions between strong risk factors.

DISEASE DESCRIPTION

Esophageal adenocarcinoma is a highly fatal neoplasm of the esophagus, which has surpassed esophageal squamous cell carcinoma as the most common form of esophageal cancer in the United States. It most commonly occurs in the distal half of the esophagus and is frequently associated with Barrett's esophagus. Its location, in the esophageal area adjacent to the stomach, by itself supports a role for gastroesophageal reflux disease (GERD) in its cause. Barrett's esophagus is a metaplastic transformation of portions of the esophageal squamous cell lining to glandular mucosa. Barrett's esophagus is thought to result from an aberrant healing

Neither author has any financial conflicts of interest to disclose.
[a] Division of Research, Kaiser Permanente Northern California, 2000 Broadway, Oakland, CA 94612, USA; [b] San Francisco Medical Center, Kaiser Permanente Northern California, San Francisco, CA 94115, USA
* Corresponding author.
E-mail address: jennifer.l1.schneider@kp.org

Gastrointest Endoscopy Clin N Am 27 (2017) 353–364
http://dx.doi.org/10.1016/j.giec.2017.03.002
giendo.theclinics.com

response to esophageal mucosal injury, typically from GERD, although it has also been reported after other forms of esophageal mucosal injury, including caustic injection and therapeutic radiation exposure. Barrett's esophagus is associated with a markedly increased risk of esophageal adenocarcinoma, and most esophageal adenocarcinomas are presumed to arise from preexisting Barrett's esophagus. Thus, evaluating risk factors and demographic distributions for both Barrett's esophagus and esophageal adenocarcinoma may inform modifiable risk factors along the neoplastic continuum from normal esophagus to Barrett's esophagus to esophageal adenocarcinoma.

NATIONAL AND GLOBAL INCIDENCE OF ESOPHAGEAL ADENOCARCINOMA

The incidence rate of esophageal adenocarcinoma in the United States has increased at least 6-fold over the last 40 years and is projected to continue increasing (**Fig. 1**).[1,2] Several studies, using national cancer data from Surveillance, Epidemiology, and End Results (SEER) and international cancer registries, have demonstrated that the incidence of esophageal adenocarcinoma varies geographically, by race and by gender, as does the rate at which the incidence is increasing.[3,4]

Globally, the incidence increase of esophageal adenocarcinoma during this time period has been highest among non-Hispanic white men[5–7]; within this group, in the United States, the incidence increased from 1 to ~6/100,000 between 1977 and 2010.[2,6] The regions with the highest global incidence rates of esophageal adenocarcinoma were Northern and Western Europe, Northern America, and Oceania, and the lowest rates were in Sub-Saharan Africa (range 0.4–3.5 for men) (**Fig. 2**). The male-to-female ratio was 4.4 globally and was highest in developed countries (North America [8.5], Europe, and Oceania) and lowest in Africa (1.7). Based on data from the International Agency for Research on Cancer, the sex ratio of esophageal adenocarcinoma incidence remained relatively stable during the period of study, with a rising overall absolute incidence.[5,8] However, a rising absolute incidence, with a stable ratio, led to an even greater difference between men and women in the absolute numbers of cases because a doubling of the low incidence among women leads to fewer additional cases than a doubling of the higher incidence among men. As a result, in 2012, 88% of cases of esophageal adenocarcinoma diagnoses in the United States were among men.[8]

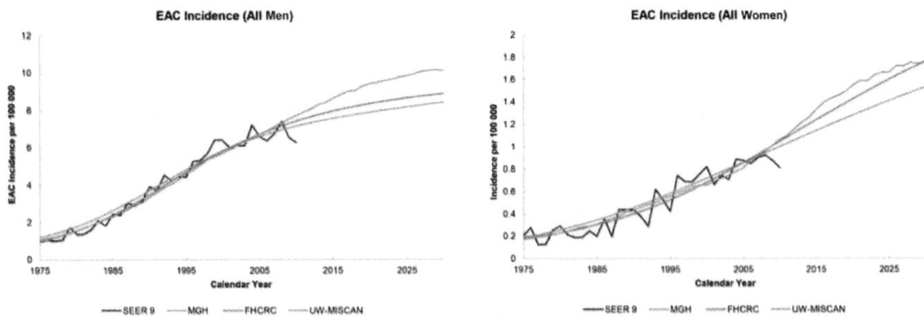

Fig. 1. Age-adjusted incidence of esophageal adenocarcinoma (EAC) among all men and women in the United States: SEER) database and projected incidence from 3 simulation models. FHCRC, Fred Hutchinson Cancer Research Center simulation model; MGH, Massachusetts General Hospital simulation model; SEER 9, actual incidence 1975-2010; UW-MISCAN, University of Washington/Erasmus University simulation model collaboration. (*Adapted from* Kong CY, Kroep S, Curtius K, et al. Exploring the recent trend in esophageal adenocarcinoma incidence and mortality using comparative simulation modeling. Cancer Epidemiol Biomarkers Prev 2014;23:997–1006.)

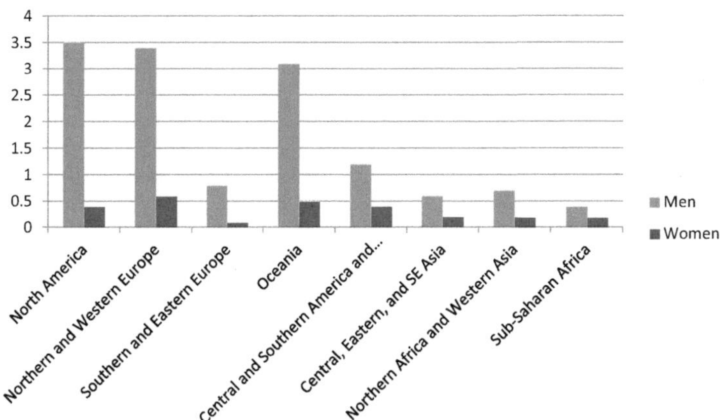

Fig. 2. Global incidence (per 100,000 person-years) esophageal adenocarcinoma, by region and gender, 2012. SE, Southeast. (*Adapted from* Arnold M, Soerjomataram I, Ferlay J, et al. Global incidence of oesophageal cancer by histological subtype in 2012. Gut 2015;64:381–7.)

Less is known about changes in the prevalence of Barrett's esophagus, the only known precursor for esophageal adenocarcinoma. The prevalence of Barrett's esophagus is estimated to be 1.6% to 3% in the US population, although estimates vary markedly and are difficult to estimate, because the condition does not cause any symptoms.[9] A large community-based study found a several-fold increase in the prevalence of persons diagnosed with Barrett's esophagus between 1994 and 2006, despite adjustment for the number of endoscopic examinations. It also found demographic differences in prevalence that generally paralleled those of esophageal adenocarcinoma. These similar demographic profiles between Barrett's esophagus and esophageal adenocarcinoma strongly suggest that risk factors acting early in the carcinogenic pathway, in the formation of Barrett's esophagus, may partially explain the unusual demographic patterns by gender and race/ethnicity.

RISK FACTORS OVERVIEW

Extensive recent research on risk factors for Barrett's esophagus and esophageal adenocarcinoma has shown substantial consensus on several modifiable and unmodifiable risk factors for both conditions (**Table 1**).

The epidemiology of esophageal adenocarcinoma is troubling, in part, because although the overall incidence in esophageal adenocarcinoma has been *increasing* for a few decades, many of the main risk factors are fixed (eg, demographics) or have been *decreasing* during this same time. Risk factors for Barrett's esophagus and esophageal adenocarcinoma include increasing age, male sex, white race, GERD, smoking, increased waist circumference, absence of prior infection with *Helicobacter pylori*, and Western diet.[10–27] The primary risk factors, some modifiable and others not, by race and sex when available, are outlined in **Table 1**.

Demographic Factors (Nonmodifiable Risk Factors: Race, Gender, and Geography)

Across racial groups, men have a consistently higher incidence of esophageal adenocarcinoma than women (see **Fig. 2**), and differences exist by race/ethnicity (**Fig. 3**). On the basis on national SEER registry data, it was found that white men have 8 times higher incidence esophageal adenocarcinoma than white women, twice the rate of Hispanic men, and 5 times the rate of black men. Among women, although much

Table 1
Summary of factors studied and their associations with Barrett's esophagus and esophageal adenocarcinoma

Risk Factors	**Barrett's Esophagus**	**Esophageal Adenocarcinoma**
Risk factor	Direction of Association	
Age	+	+
Sex	+ (male)	+ (male)
Race	+ (white)	+ (white)
GERD	+	+
H pylori	–	–
Smoking	+	+
Total alcohol intake	None	None
BMI	None	+
Waist circumference	+	+
Dietary factors		
Dietary fiber, vitamin C, diets high in fruits/vegetables/fish	–	–
Beta-carotene, vitamin A	?	–
Omega-3 fatty acids, polyunsaturated fat, vitamin E	–	?
High trans fats/red meat	+	+
Aspirin/Nonsteroidal anti-inflammatory drugs	?	–
Hormonal status	?	–

+, the presence of the risk factor increases likelihood of Barrett's esophagus/esophageal adenocarcinoma; –, presence of the risk factor decreases the likelihood of Barrett's esophagus/esophageal adenocarcinoma; ?, the relationship is unknown or inconsistent.

(*From* Schneider JL, Corley DA. A review of the epidemiology of Barrett's oesophagus and oesophageal adenocarcinoma. Best Pract Res Clin Gastroenterol 2015;29:35; with permission.)

lower absolute incidence rates are observed (0.2–0.6), white women have twice the rate of Hispanics women and 3 times the rate of black women.[4] Geographic variation in race- and gender-specific rates has also been observed, with rates of esophageal adenocarcinoma among white men ranging from 2.4 to 5.3/100,000 person-years among 11 SEER regions and among black men ranging from 0.0 to 3.1/100,000 person-years by region. Much less variation by geography has been reported for

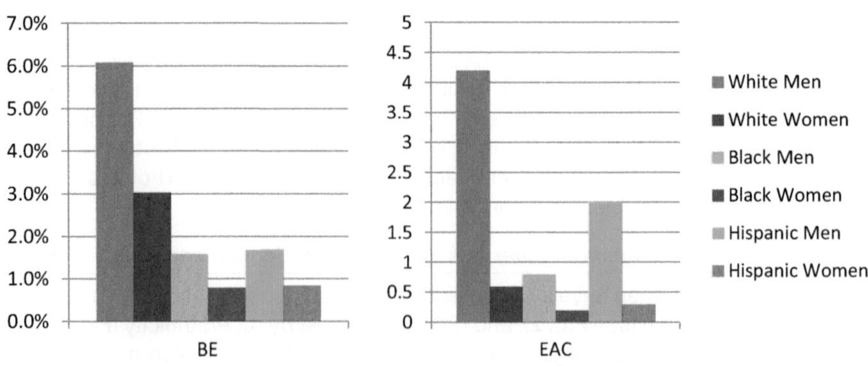

Fig. 3. Prevalence of Barrett's esophagus (%) and risk of esophageal adenocarcinoma (incidence rate/100,000), by race and gender.

women, likely because of lack of representative data and/or low counts.[3] Although white men have the overall highest incidence rate in the United States, some regions have incidence rates among black men that are higher than the incidence rate for white men in other regions.

If Barrett's esophagus is the primary precursor to esophageal adenocarcinoma, it would be expected that the 2 would have similar demographic distributions; this is generally the case. The demographic distributions of Barrett's esophagus are generally similar to those of esophageal adenocarcinoma, although the associations are weaker, with prevalence proportions of Barrett's esophagus being highest among whites (6.1%), and lower among blacks (1.6%) and Hispanics (1.7%), with a similar ratio of 2:1 for men:women across races[12] (see **Fig. 3**).

Obesity and Body Composition

Both body mass index (BMI) and abdominal obesity are known risk factors for esophageal adenocarcinoma.[24] In contrast, BMI is not independently associated with Barrett's esophagus[23] even among persons with GERD.[28] However, other measures of adiposity/body composition, such as abdominal obesity or waist circumference, are associated with Barrett's esophagus, even after adjustment for BMI. The association between abdominal obesity and Barrett's esophagus may, in part, be through GERD, although the visceral fat area, measured in a cohort of Japanese men and women, has been associated with increased reflux esophagitis, but not Barrett's esophagus.[29]

According to a national survey, the prevalence of obesity among adults in the United States increased from 30% in 1999 to 2000 to more than 36% by 2011 to 2014, with even more marked increases since the 1960s (**Fig. 4**).[30] If obesity alone was the predominant predictor for Barrett's esophagus or esophageal adenocarcinoma, it would be expected that the demographic groups with the highest prevalence of obesity to be at the highest risk and that the changes in risk factor prevalence over time would approximate the change in cancer incidence. However, in contrast to esophageal adenocarcinoma incidence, obesity prevalence has been generally *higher* among women and non-Hispanic blacks (compared with other races) (**Fig. 5**), particularly

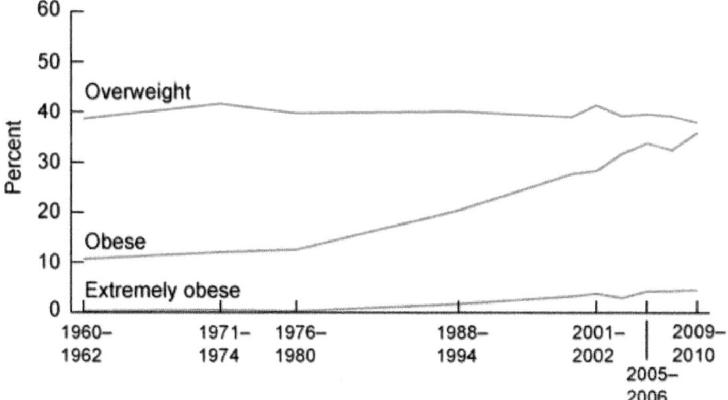

Fig. 4. Trends in overweight, obesity, and extreme obesity among men aged 20–74 years: United States, 1960–1962 through 2009–2010. (*From* Fryar C, Carroll MD, Ogden CL. Prevalence of overweight, obesity, and extreme obesity among adults: United States, trends 1960–1962 through 2009–2010. NCHS Publications and Information Products Health E-Stats. 2012. Available at: https://www.cdc.gov/nchs/data/hestat/obesity_adult_09_10/obesity_adult_09_10.htm. Accessed December 29, 2016; with permission.)

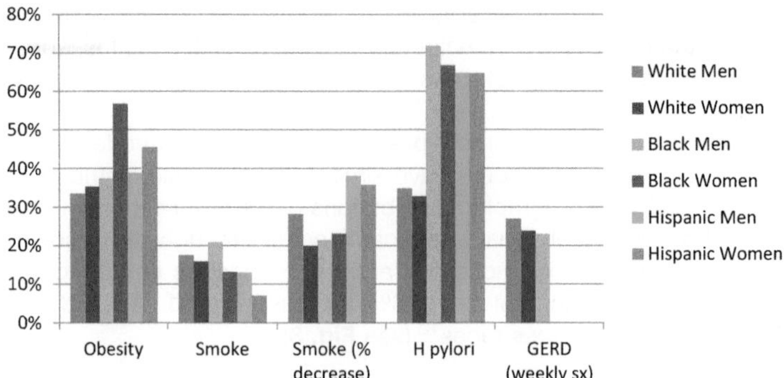

Fig. 5. Prevalence of risk factors for esophageal adenocarcinoma, by gender and race/ethnicity. Data for weekly GERD symptoms are not available for black women or Hispanic men/women. Sx, symptoms. (*Data from* Refs.[30,35,37,43,47])

black women, who are one of the lowest risk groups for esophageal adenocarcinoma and Barrett's esophagus. In addition, obesity has been increasing at a similar or even greater rate among demographic groups at low risk of esophageal adenocarcinoma (eg, women and blacks) as among those at high risk (non-Hispanic white and men) (**Fig. 6**A [men] and B [women]). These discrepancies leave the biological mechanism for obesity's carcinogenic effects poorly understood.

Several studies in recent years have evaluated the associations between adipokines (cell signaling proteins released by adipose tissue) and Barrett's esophagus/esophageal adenocarcinoma in an attempt to better understand the pathway between obesity and carcinogenesis; for example, adipokines might theoretically alter the likelihood that persons who have esophageal injury heal with esophageal metaplasia. In one case-control study, increasing adiponectin levels were associated with increased risk of Barrett's esophagus among patients with GERD, but not among persons without GERD. The association with adipokines in another study suggests that their associations with Barrett's esophagus may differ between men and women.[31,32] Higher ghrelin levels also appear to be associated with an increased risk of Barrett's esophagus, and leptin is associated with GERD symptoms, but inversely associated

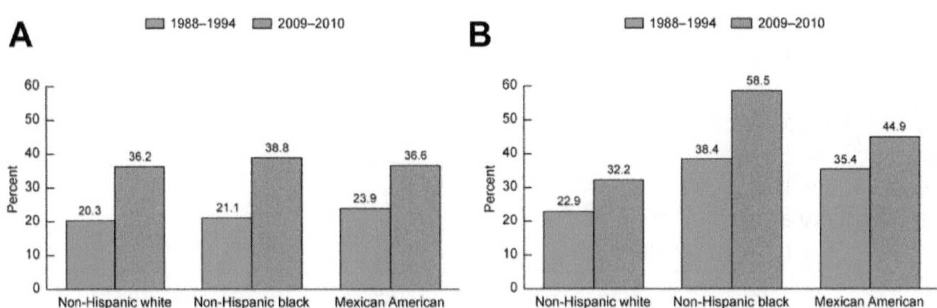

Fig. 6. (*A*) Prevalence of obesity among men aged 20 years and over, by race and ethnicity: United States, 1988–1994 and 2009–2010. (*B*) Prevalence of obesity among women aged 20 years and over, by race and ethnicity: United States, 1988–1994 and 2009–2010. (*From* Fryar C, Carroll MD, Ogden CL. Prevalence of overweight, obesity, and extreme obesity among adults: United States, trends 1960–1962 through 2009–2010. NCHS Publications and Information Products Health E-Stats. 2012. Available at: Https://www.cdc.gov/nchs/data/hestat/obesity_adult_09_10/obesity_adult_09_10.htm. Accessed December 29, 2016; with permission.)

with Barrett's esophagus among persons with GERD.[33] A systematic review reported that increased serum levels of both leptin and insulin are associated with an increased risk of Barrett's esophagus, but that no association existed between total serum levels of adiponectin or insulin and Barrett's esophagus.[34] Thus, the adipokine studies to date have demonstrated some inconsistent associations, and the mechanisms, if present, may be complex. Studies with larger numbers of women and non-whites are needed to evaluate if race/ethnicity differences in adipokines may partially explain the differences in cancer demographics.

Smoking

Smoking, another known risk factor for esophageal adenocarcinoma, has been declining in the United States for decades, with a reported 28% overall decline in national prevalence from 2005 to 2015[35]; however, this trend is opposite that of esophageal adenocarcinoma incidence. Both ever smoking and current smoking are associated with an increased risk of Barrett's esophagus (although not strong risk factors) and esophageal adenocarcinoma, and trends with increasing pack-years have also been reported.[16–18] Declines in smoking prevalence have been seen in all racial groups; although prevalence ranged from 7% to 18% for white, black, and Hispanic men and women (see **Fig. 5**), the highest smoking prevalence is reported for black men, a group at relatively low risk of esophageal adenocarcinoma. **Fig. 5** illustrates the percent declines in smoking prevalence (%) from 2005 to 2013, by race and gender for each risk group: smoking decreased the most among Hispanic men and women, although their baseline prevalence in 2005 was also lowest. In addition, smoking rates differ by age (current smoking more common among adults <65 years), poverty status (highest among those below poverty level), geographic region, and health insurance coverage (highest among those with Medicaid and the uninsured), which may confound relationships between smoking, race, and disease.[35,36]

Gastroesophageal Reflux Disease

GERD is a strong risk factor for esophageal adenocarcinoma and Barrett's esophagus; 10% of people with GERD will harbor Barrett's esophagus.[13–15] Both frequency and duration of GERD symptoms have been positively associated with esophageal adenocarcinoma risk. A cross-sectional survey with racial diversity, but only 8% Hispanics, reported that 29% of black participants and 28% of white participants experienced weekly heartburn and/or regurgitation.[37] Similar findings were reported from a meta-analysis of GERD symptoms, whereby the prevalence of at least monthly heartburn was relatively comparable for men (28%) and women (24%); another study that reported heartburn or regurgitation among white men and women had similar findings.[25,38] However, although GERD symptoms are fairly equally distributed among genders, the risks of erosive esophagitis, Barrett's esophagus, and esophageal adenocarcinoma are much higher among men. Predominance of disease among males suggests that symptoms may not predict the presence of esophageal injury. It is also possible, that, although point prevalence of GERD symptoms may be higher, men may have a longer duration or severity of symptoms, contributing to their higher cancer risk. Thus, although the demographic distributions of GERD symptoms do not match those of esophageal adenocarcinoma incidence, some GERD-related complications that likely predispose to Barrett's esophagus (ie, esophagitis) may be more similar.

Helicobacter pylori

A history of *H pylori* infection is strongly inversely associated with the risk of Barrett's esophagus and esophageal adenocarcinoma, with odds ratios of 0.46 (95%

confidence interval [CI]: 0.35, 0.60) and 0.57 (95% CI, 0.44–0.73), respectively.[26,27,39] *H pylori* is one of the most common human pathogens with a very high prevalence in some populations. It has been estimated that more than half of the world's population has been infected and that prevalence is consistently lower in developed countries, compared with developing countries.[40] Within countries, differences in prevalence can be observed by ethnic and social groups.[41] A US study among almost 500 asymptomatic adults found evidence of infection among 52% overall, with higher prevalence among black men (72%) and women (67%) than among white men (35%) and women (33%).[42] Comparable prevalence data for Hispanics are not readily available by gender but are overall similar to blacks.[41] The male-to-female ratio of infection has been similar among both white and blacks in some studies; however, a more recent meta-analysis suggested infection is more common among men, after adjustment for factors such as age and socioeconomic status(SES).[43] Age and SES have been consistently reported to be associated with infection, with the risk of infection increasing with age and lower SES.[33,41] Thus, the demographic distributions of *H pylori* versus those of Barrett's esophagus and esophageal adenocarcinoma are mixed: they parallel the disease risk by race/ethnicity, but not by gender. Higher frequencies of *H pylori* infection may partially explain the lower cancer risk among blacks, but it does not, for example, explain the marked gender difference, especially among non-Hispanic whites.

DISCUSSION: MAKING SENSE OF THE RISK FACTORS FOR BARRETT'S AND CANCER

The epidemiology of Barrett's esophagus and esophageal adenocarcinoma is troublesome: there are strong demographic trends, with increased risks among men and non-Hispanic whites, but most putative risk factors are fairly similarly distributed in the population or their distributions even run in the opposite direction of what would be expected. Most epidemiologic studies cannot directly answer this conundrum, because most risk factor analyses adjust for race or, because of low numbers, completely exclude non-whites. Thus, given that most cancers occur among non-Hispanic white men, these studies mainly answer the question, "what are the risk factors for esophageal adenocarcinoma among white non-Hispanic men?" They are unable to evaluate why the same factor may have very different associations, for example, among men versus women, or among non-Hispanic whites versus blacks. No single risk factor clearly explains the incidence discrepancies by race and sex. Although black and Hispanic women have the highest reported prevalence of overall obesity, for example, they also exhibit the lowest incidence of esophageal adenocarcinoma among all race/gender groups presented. Some have hypothesized that body composition and fat distribution, and not just overall obesity, may influence the associations between cancer risk, race, and gender. National Health and Nutrition Examination Survey data have shown that at the same BMI and height, the percentage fat, waist circumference, and total adiposity (or fat-free mass) differ across racial groups and is further altered by age and gender.[44] Black men, although more likely than white men to be obese by BMI cutoffs, have a different body composition with greater appendicular mass and lower central body mass, the latter of which has been associated with risk of Barrett's esophagus, independent of BMI.[24] The roles of adipokines and other hormones may also contribute to the sex-specific differences; these effects may differ by race and other nonmodifiable factors, although exploring these associations would require larger numbers of non-whites. Future analyses of the complex association between race, body composition, gender, and possibly dietary/lifestyle patterns may identify additional areas of focus for minimizing risk and/or identifying potentially high-risk subgroups.

For smoking, the temporal disparities between declining smoking prevalence and rising cancer incidence may in part be explained by where smoking acts in the carcinogenic pathway. If, for example, smoking mainly increased the risk of Barrett's esophagus, multidecade lag might be expected between changes in smoking rates and esophageal adenocarcinoma incidence trends. Nevertheless, the prevalence of smoking does not differ greatly by race; therefore, a lag effect may explain the discordant temporal trends, but it is unlikely to explain the variation in incidence for whites, blacks, and Hispanics. In summary, although smoking rates have decreased drastically in recent decades, across all racial groups, the delayed potential effects of smoking reduction in disease incidence cannot yet be fully measured or seen, although it may have an impact in the future.

The demographic distributions of *H pylori* infection and complicated GERD partially match those of Barrett's esophagus/esophageal adenocarcinoma, such as between higher-risk non-Hispanic whites and lower-risk blacks. *H pylori* infection is also more common among other low-risk demographic groups, including Hispanics and Asians. Thus, although its distribution does not explain differences by gender, it may partially explain differences by race/ethnicity, particularly given the strength of its association. Similarly, although symptomatic GERD is common among both black and white men, among patients with similar amounts of GERD symptoms, blacks may be less likely to develop esophagitis.[37] Even among patients with esophagitis, blacks may be less likely to develop Barrett's esophagus,[45,46] although these studies were retrospective and subject to selection biases. More detailed high-quality research in this area seems warranted, possibly looking at the severity of symptoms, frequency, and duration by race and other factors that may be contributing to the symptoms.

Future research should further explore the observed differences in rates of disease by geographic region, and the likely complex interactions of different risk factors. Risk factors likely cluster in some regions or demographic groups. For example, studying geographic and demographic clustering of the combined effects of low SES, obesity, smoking, and *H pylori* infection may help understand how these risk factors may interact for GERD, Barrett's esophagus, and esophageal adenocarcinoma. Studies like this may afford a better understanding of attributable risks and their influence on demographic distributions. There are several challenges to evaluating risk factors, demographics, Barrett's esophagus, and esophageal adenocarcinoma, particularly the likely decades-long lag time between development of Barrett's esophagus and its potential progression to esophageal adenocarcinoma. Thus, esophageal adenocarcinoma incidence at any point in time likely differs from the recent prevalence of risk factors. Studies of patients with Barrett's esophagus can partially address this concern, but given Barrett's esophagus is itself asymptomatic, its lag time to development in relation to risk factor exposures is also unknown and potentially unknowable. In addition, modest available data for Hispanic populations, and women in general, make comparisons difficult, and commonly used statistical methods for evaluating confounding and interaction are inadequate for explaining why risk factors may act differently in different groups. Better understanding of the underlying biological mechanisms for the development of GERD, esophagitis, and Barrett's esophagus would likely inform how these different risk factors act to increase the risk of esophageal adenocarcinoma. Ongoing studies of genetic risk factors, pathway studies, and gene-environment interactions offer perhaps the greatest potential for explaining the troubling epidemiology of Barrett's esophagus and esophageal adenocarcinoma.

REFERENCES

1. Simard EP, Ward EM, Siegel R, et al. Cancers with increasing incidence trends in the United States: 1999 through 2008. CA Cancer J Clin 2012;62:118–28.
2. Kong CY, Kroep S, Curtius K, et al. Exploring the recent trend in esophageal adenocarcinoma incidence and mortality using comparative simulation modeling. Cancer Epidemiol Biomarkers Prev 2014;23:997–1006.
3. Kubo A, Corley DA. Marked regional variation in adenocarcinomas of the esophagus and the gastric cardia in the United States. Cancer 2002;95:2096–102.
4. Kubo A, Corley DA. Marked multi-ethnic variation of esophageal and gastric cardia carcinomas within the United States. Am J Gastroenterol 2004;99:582–8.
5. Xie SH, Lagergren J. A global assessment of the male predominance in esophageal adenocarcinoma. Oncotarget 2016;7:38876–83.
6. Cook MB, Dawsey SM, Freedman ND, et al. Sex disparities in cancer incidence by period and age. Cancer Epidemiol Biomarkers Prev 2009;18:1174–82.
7. Lagergren J, Lagergren P. Recent developments in esophageal adenocarcinoma. CA Cancer J Clin 2013;63:232–48.
8. Arnold M, Soerjomataram I, Ferlay J, et al. Global incidence of oesophageal cancer by histological subtype in 2012. Gut 2015;64:381–7.
9. Gilbert EW, Luna RA, Harrison VL, et al. Barrett's esophagus: a review of the literature. J Gastrointest Surg 2011;15:708–18.
10. Corley DA, Kubo A, Levin TR, et al. Race, ethnicity, sex and temporal differences in Barrett's oesophagus diagnosis: a large community-based study, 1994-2006. Gut 2009;58:182–8.
11. Bhat S, Coleman HG, Yousef F, et al. Risk of malignant progression in Barrett's esophagus patients: results from a large population-based study. J Natl Cancer Inst 2011;103:1049–57.
12. Abrams JA, Fields S, Lightdale CJ, et al. Racial and ethnic disparities in the prevalence of Barrett's esophagus among patients who undergo upper endoscopy. Clin Gastroenterol Hepatol 2008;6:30–4.
13. Spechler SJ, Goyal RK. The columnar-lined esophagus, intestinal metaplasia, and Norman Barrett. Gastroenterology 1996;110:614–21.
14. McDougall NI, Johnston BT, Collins JS, et al. Three- to 4.5-year prospective study of prognostic indicators in gastro-oesophageal reflux disease. Scand J Gastroenterol 1998;33:1016–22.
15. Lagergren J, Bergstrom R, Lindgren A, et al. Symptomatic gastroesophageal reflux as a risk factor for esophageal adenocarcinoma. N Engl J Med 1999; 340:825–31.
16. Kubo A, Levin TR, Block G, et al. Cigarette smoking and the risk of Barrett's esophagus. Cancer Causes Control 2009;20:303–11.
17. Thrift AP, Kramer JR, Richardson PA, et al. No significant effects of smoking or alcohol consumption on risk of Barrett's esophagus. Dig Dis Sci 2014;59:108–16.
18. Cook MB, Shaheen NJ, Anderson LA, et al. Cigarette smoking increases risk of Barrett's esophagus: an analysis of the Barrett's and esophageal adenocarcinoma consortium. Gastroenterology 2012;142:744–53.
19. Hardikar S, Onstad L, Blount PL, et al. The role of tobacco, alcohol, and obesity in neoplastic progression to esophageal adenocarcinoma: a prospective study of Barrett's esophagus. PLoS One 2013;8:e52192.
20. Kubo A, Levin TR, Block G, et al. Dietary patterns and the risk of Barrett's esophagus. Am J Epidemiol 2008;167:839–46.

21. Kubo A, Corley DA, Jensen CD, et al. Dietary factors and the risks of oesophageal adenocarcinoma and Barrett's oesophagus. Nutr Res Rev 2010;23:230–46.
22. Hoyo C, Cook MB, Kamangar F, et al. Body mass index in relation to oesophageal and oesophagogastric junction adenocarcinomas: a pooled analysis from the International BEACON Consortium. Int J Epidemiol 2012;41:1706–18.
23. Corley DA, Kubo A, Levin TR, et al. Abdominal obesity and body mass index as risk factors for Barrett's esophagus. Gastroenterology 2007;133:34–41 [quiz: 311].
24. Kubo A, Cook MB, Shaheen NJ, et al. Sex-specific associations between body mass index, waist circumference and the risk of Barrett's oesophagus: a pooled analysis from the international BEACON consortium. Gut 2013;62(12):1684–91.
25. Moayyedi P, Axon AT. Review article: gastro-oesophageal reflux disease–the extent of the problem. Aliment Pharmacol Ther 2005;22(Suppl 1):11–9.
26. Fischbach LA, Nordenstedt H, Kramer JR, et al. The association between Barrett's esophagus and Helicobacter pylori infection: a meta-analysis. Helicobacter 2012;17:163–75.
27. Corley DA, Kubo A, Levin TR, et al. Helicobacter pylori and gastroesophageal reflux disease: a case-control study. Helicobacter 2008;13:352–60.
28. Cook MB, Greenwood DC, Hardie LJ, et al. A systematic review and meta-analysis of the risk of increasing adiposity on Barrett's esophagus. Am J Gastroenterol 2008;103:292–300.
29. Matsuzaki J, Suzuki H, Kobayakawa M, et al. Association of visceral fat area, smoking, and alcohol consumption with reflux esophagitis and Barrett's esophagus in Japan. PLoS One 2015;10:e0133865.
30. Ogden CL, Carroll MD, Fryar CD, et al. Prevalence of obesity among adults and youth: United States, 2011-2014. NCHS Data Brief 2015;1–8.
31. Almers LM, Graham JE, Havel PJ, et al. Adiponectin may modify the risk of Barrett's esophagus in patients with gastroesophageal reflux disease. Clin Gastroenterol Hepatol 2015;13:2256–64.e1-3.
32. Greer KB, Falk GW, Bednarchik B, et al. Associations of serum adiponectin and leptin with Barrett's esophagus. Clin Gastroenterol Hepatol 2015;13:2265–72.
33. Thomas SJ, Almers L, Schneider J, et al. Ghrelin and leptin have a complex relationship with risk of Barrett's esophagus. Dig Dis Sci 2016;61:70–9.
34. Chandar AK, Devanna S, Lu C, et al. Association of serum levels of adipokines and insulin with risk of Barrett's esophagus: a systematic review and meta-analysis. Clin Gastroenterol Hepatol 2015;13:2241–55.e1-4 [quiz: e179].
35. Jamal A, King BA, Neff LJ, et al. Current cigarette smoking among adults - United States, 2005-2015. MMWR Morb Mortal Wkly Rep 2016;65:1205–11.
36. Lagergren J, Andersson G, Talback M, et al. Marital status, education, and income in relation to the risk of esophageal and gastric cancer by histological type and site. Cancer 2016;122:207–12.
37. El-Serag HB, Petersen NJ, Carter J, et al. Gastroesophageal reflux among different racial groups in the United States. Gastroenterology 2004;126:1692–9.
38. Locke GR 3rd, Talley NJ, Fett SL, et al. Prevalence and clinical spectrum of gastroesophageal reflux: a population-based study in Olmsted County, Minnesota. Gastroenterology 1997;112:1448–56.
39. Nie S, Chen T, Yang X, et al. Association of Helicobacter pylori infection with esophageal adenocarcinoma and squamous cell carcinoma: a meta-analysis. Dis Esophagus 2014;27:645–53.
40. Khalifa MM, Sharaf RR, Aziz RK. Helicobacter pylori: a poor man's gut pathogen? Gut Pathog 2010;2:2.

41. Malaty HM, Evans DG, Evans DJ Jr, et al. Helicobacter pylori in Hispanics: comparison with blacks and whites of similar age and socioeconomic class. Gastroenterology 1992;103:813–6.
42. Graham DY, Malaty HM, Evans DG, et al. Epidemiology of Helicobacter pylori in an asymptomatic population in the United States. Effect of age, race, and socioeconomic status. Gastroenterology 1991;100:1495–501.
43. de Martel C, Parsonnet J. Helicobacter pylori infection and gender: a meta-analysis of population-based prevalence surveys. Dig Dis Sci 2006;51:2292–301.
44. Heymsfield SB, Peterson CM, Thomas DM, et al. Why are there race/ethnic differences in adult body mass index-adiposity relationships? A quantitative critical review. Obes Rev 2016;17:262–75.
45. Vega KJ, Chisholm S, Jamal MM. Comparison of reflux esophagitis and its complications between African Americans and non-Hispanic whites. World J Gastroenterol 2009;15:2878–81.
46. Alkaddour A, McGaw C, Hritani R, et al. African American ethnicity is not associated with development of Barrett's oesophagus after erosive oesophagitis. Dig Liver Dis 2015;47:853–6.
47. Ogden CL, Carroll MD, Kit BK, et al. Prevalence of childhood and adult obesity in the United States, 2011-2012. JAMA 2014;311:806–14.

Who Deserves Endoscopic Screening for Esophageal Neoplasia?

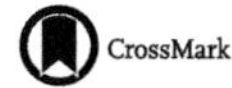

Christopher H. Blevins, MD, Prasad G. Iyer, MD, MSc*

KEYWORDS

• Barrett's esophagus • Screening • Esophageal adenocarcinoma • Endoscopy

KEY POINTS

- Barrett's esophagus (BE) is regarded as the precursor to most esophageal adenocarcinomas (EAC).
- EAC that is diagnosed while in a BE surveillance program (constituting <10% of all EAC) likely has better outcomes compared with EAC diagnosed after the onset of symptoms (constituting >90% of all cases).
- Most BE in the community remains undetected despite increasing endoscopy volumes, likely due to the absence of widespread targeted screening.
- Given the prevalence of BE in the population is likely less than 10%, many BE risk assessment scores have been proposed, using known risk factors for BE. Most have not been validated in independent cohorts, and threshold for recommending screening is not yet defined.
- Validation of these scores in independent populations, defining the threshold for proceeding with screening followed by their utilization for targeting those at risk may help in making BE/EAC screening more efficient and effective.

INTRODUCTION

Barrett's esophagus (BE) was first described more than 60 years ago as a change in the esophageal mucosa from a squamous-type to a columnar-type that was associated with esophageal ulcers.[1] Today, this largely asymptomatic change in the esophageal lining is regarded as the precursor lesion to most esophageal adenocarcinoma (EAC). Even after understanding this association for the last several decades, the incidence of EAC continues to increase with an estimated 6-fold increase since 1975.[2]

Disclosure Statement: No relevant disclosures (C.H. Blevins). Research funding from Exact Sciences, Intromedic Inc, and C2 Therapeutics (P.G. Iyer).
Division of Gastroenterology and Hepatology, Mayo Clinic Minnesota, 200 First Street Southwest, Rochester, MN 55905, USA
* Corresponding author.
E-mail address: Iyer.Prasad@mayo.edu

Gastrointest Endoscopy Clin N Am 27 (2017) 365–378
http://dx.doi.org/10.1016/j.giec.2017.02.006
giendo.theclinics.com

Once EAC is diagnosed after the onset of symptoms, the prognosis is grim with an estimated 20% survival at 5 years.[3] On the other hand, survival of early stage EA (T1a: mucosally confined) is far superior: greater than 80% at 5 years.[4,5] Given the rising incidence of this lethal cancer that has a known precursor lesion, there is mounting interest in finding a cost-effective, patient and provider acceptable, easily applicable and accurate means by which the population at risk for developing BE can be screened followed by enrollment in a surveillance program. However, this seemingly logical rationale has several limitations, which include the lack of an accurate risk assessment tool and a suitable widely applicable screening tool. This article reviews and summarizes the emerging data regarding the development and validation of BE risk assessment tools.

ACCURATELY DIAGNOSING THE PRECURSOR LESION

Before addressing screening, being able to define BE is critical. Although this metaplastic change in the esophageal mucosa was described several decades ago, an unambiguous and universally acceptable definition remains elusive. Diagnosing BE requires an endoscopic assessment and histologic evaluation. Under direct white-light endoscopy, the metaplastic columnar epithelium of BE is differentiated from the surrounding squamous epithelial lining by its salmon color appearance. In order to diagnose BE, columnar epithelium must be located at least 1 cm proximal to the gastroesophageal junction (GEJ), which is defined by all major gastrointestinal (GI) societies as being located at the top of the gastric folds.[6–9] This diagnostic criteria is supported by studies that have shown that intestinal metaplasia (IM) at the GEJ (<1 cm in length of esophageal columnar metaplasia) does not appear to increase the risk of developing EAC.[10,11] In addition, the interobserver agreement in documenting columnar segments less than 1 cm is low.[12]

Once endoscopically defined, metaplasia has to be histologically confirmed. There remains controversy regarding the type of metaplasia that qualifies as diagnostic for BE.[13] Currently, although almost all major GI societies accept that only intestinal-type epithelium with goblet cells (denoting the presence of IM) constitutes a diagnosis of BE, the British Society of Gastroenterology recommends that goblet cells need not be present to make the diagnosis, that is, any type of columnar metaplasia in the esophagus satisfies the diagnostic criteria for BE.

The British Society of Gastroenterology's recommendations are based on the argument that columnar metaplasia (irrespective of the presence of IM) increases the risk of developing EAC. Supporting data for this view come from a population study of 319 patients over a median of 12 years showing that they developed EAC at a similar rate as those with IM.[14] There are data to suggest that columnar mucosa without IM has similar DNA abnormalities as well as cytokeratin (CK7/CK20, which are markers of ductal and intestinal differentiation) and DAS-1 staining patterns as BE with IM.[15–18] However, these data are contradicted by a large population-based study of 8522 patients that showed the rate for developing EAC in the setting of IM was 0.38% per year when compared with those without IM, which progressed at a rate of 0.07% per year ($P<.001$).[19] There are also data to suggest that follow-up biopsies in those without IM at initial endoscopy may reveal IM in 29% of cases.[20]

Beyond just making the diagnosis of BE, challenges exist when attempting to determine the degree of dysplasia at the time of diagnosis. An accurate diagnosis is important, because dysplasia, despite limitations, remains the best available and clinically used marker for predicting cancer risk. Most challenging is being able to differentiate BE with low-grade dysplasia (LGD) from nondysplastic BE (NDBE).[21] Worryingly, in a study from the Netherlands, 147 patients were diagnosed with LGD dysplasia in the community, and 85% of them were downgraded to NDBE after review by 2 GI pathologists with significant experience in BE.[22]

BARRETT'S ESOPHAGUS SCREENING: RATIONALE AND CHALLENGES

Approximately 10,000 new cases of EAC are diagnosed every year in the United States.[2] Although this number is lower than that of other malignancies such as colon and lung cancer with active screening recommendations, this needs to be viewed in the context of persistently poor 5-year survival (less than 20%), exponentially rising incidence (600% over the last several decades), and high incidence of mortality ratios (0.55–0.66) associated with this lethal tumor.[2,3] In addition, the presence of a precancerous state (BE), which can be detected and followed endoscopically to detect the interval development of dysplasia or early carcinoma, renders screening for BE a potential strategy for EAC prevention. The last decade has seen incredible progress with the development of safe and effective endoscopic modalities (endoscopic resection and ablation) to both prevent progression of dysplasia to EAC and treat early esophageal cancer. Endoscopic therapy for early stage, particularly T1a (mucosally confined), EAC has been shown to lead to excellent long-term survival in several cohort studies with results comparable those obtained after esophagectomy.[4,23–26] Several studies have been published suggesting that the survival of cancers detected under surveillance is improved compared with those detected either in patients not under surveillance or in patients presenting after the onset of symptoms such as dysphagia. However, this is not universal, with some studies suggesting that the outcomes may not be improved in cancers detected by surveillance.[27–31] However, given that these studies are retrospective in nature, they are subject to both lead time bias (systematic error of apparent increased survival from detecting disease in an early stage) and length time bias (systematic error from screening detecting slower progressing disease with a longer preclinical period and better prognosis). These developments have spurred renewed interest in BE screening, leading to the development and ongoing assessment of minimally invasive (unsedated transnasal endoscopy, capsule sponge) and noninvasive tools (electronic nose) to detect BE, which can ultimately replace endoscopic screening.[32,33] In addition, the overall approach of BE screening followed by endoscopic surveillance for the detection of dysplasia or EAC has been found to be cost-effective by several modeling studies.[33–35]

However, several issues continue to exist that make widespread BE screening challenging. Indeed, more than 90% of EAC continue to be diagnosed in the absence of a prior BE diagnosis, depriving these patients of the potential benefit of surveillance.[36] Despite the increasing use of endoscopic evaluation of patients with gastroesophageal reflux disease (GERD), data suggest that this is often directed at patients who are likely at low risk for BE or EAC.[37] Elements desirable for a successful screening program for EAC are (1) A screening tool that is minimally or noninvasive, cost-effective, widely applicable, safe and accurate in the diagnosis of BE (and potentially BE related dysplasia); (2) A validated BE/EAC risk assessment tool, which allows screening to be targeted at those who are at substantial risk for developing BE/EAC; (3) A risk stratification tool that allows prediction of the risk of progression to high-grade dysplasia or EAC in those diagnosed with BE. Dysplasia, which is currently the only parameter used for risk stratification, is limited by sampling error and lack of interobserver agreement among pathologists, particularly for LGD. Hence, follow-up recommendations cannot be personalized on any other parameter than dysplasia; (4) Imaging techniques that offer the ability to detect dysplasia or neoplasia in BE mucosa; (5) Cost-effective tools for the treatment of dysplasia (to prevent development of EAC), or early carcinoma, once detected in screening or surveillance. Although excellent progress has been made on issues 4 and 5, issues 1, 2, and 3 remain to be definitively addressed.[38] Despite substantial data on the tolerability and accuracy of unsedated transnasal endoscopy, it has not been widely accepted as a tool for BE screening in the United States due to lack of acceptance from both physicians and, potentially, patients.[39–41] Encouraging data from the United Kingdom on the capsule sponge need to be validated in the United States.[42] Issue 3 is perhaps the most challenging at this time. Although several biomarkers to predict the risk of progression have been proposed, none is currently validated for use clinically. The low risk of progression in BE (overall) makes conduct of large prospective studies challenging. Screening recommendations from major gastroenterology societies are described in **Table 1**.

Current society recommendations suggest screening for BE in the presence of multiple risk factors, with most drawing an arbitrary line at 3 or more risk factors (see **Table 1**). Although there are substantial data on the association of individual risk factors with BE, there are very limited data on the additive or synergistic effect of multiple risk factors on BE prevalence. In a recent study, this question was

Table 1
Current Gastroenterology and Endoscopy Society guidelines for Barrett's esophagus screening

Society	Year	Targeted Population for Screening	Strength of Recommendation/ Level of Evidence
American College of Gastroenterology[8]	2016	Male patients with either more than 5 y of GERD or with more than weekly GERD symptoms AND at least 2 other risk factors: Age >50 y, central obesity (waist circumference >102 cm or WHR >0.9), Caucasian race, active/history of smoking, first-degree relative with BE or EAC	Strong recommendation and moderate level of evidence
British Society of Gastroenterology[9]	2014	Patients with GERD and at least 3 risk factors (age >50 y, Caucasian race, male sex, and obesity); threshold to be lowered in case of family history	Not Available and low-quality evidence
American Society for Gastrointestinal Endoscopy[7]	2012	Patients with multiple risk factors including male sex, white race, age older than 50 y, family history of BE, increased duration of reflux symptoms, smoking, and obesity	Not Available and very low-quality evidence
American Gastroenterological Association[6]	2011	Patients with multiple risk factors (age older than 50 y, white race, male sex, chronic GERD, hiatal hernia, obesity)	Not Available and low-quality evidence

investigated, and a strong correlation between the number of risk factors and the prevalence of BE was reported, with the risk of BE or erosive esophagitis increasing substantially (3.7-fold) in those with at least 3 or 4 risk factors and increasing to 5.7-fold in those with 5 or more risk factors, compared with those with 2 or fewer risk factors.[43]

RISK FACTORS FOR BARRETT'S ESOPHAGUS

The strongest risk factor for developing BE and subsequent EAC is GERD. Patients with GERD are 6 to 8 times more likely to have BE compared with those without GERD, and 5% to 15% of patients with GERD are diagnosed with BE at the time of endoscopy.[44–50] However, GERD is not a sensitive or specific predictor of BE. Several studies have shown comparable prevalence of BE in those with and without reflux symptoms.[51–53] The comparable prevalence may reflect the known lack of reflux symptoms in those with BE, due to mucosal hyposensitivity and the contribution of other risk factors.[54,55]

Obesity, as measured by both body mass index (BMI) and visceral adiposity, has more recently been described as an independent risk factor for BE. The incidence of obesity has increased in parallel with BE and EAC with more than 36% of the US population being obese in 2015.[56] A BMI of ≥30 was found to be associated with an increased risk (odds ratio [OR] 1.49, 95% confidence interval [CI] 1.24–1.8) of developing BE when compared with those with a BMI of less than 30 in a large meta-analysis in 2009.[57–61] BMI however does not take into account adipose tissue distribution. Visceral fat (which surrounds intra-abdominal organs) is more hormonally active than subcutaneous adipose tissue. It can be easily measured in the clinic by the waist-hip ratio (WHR), with values of ≥0.9 for men and ≥0.85 for women being associated with the highest risk of metabolic complications.[62] More recently in a systematic review and meta-analysis, visceral adiposity alone even after adjusting for reflux was associated with increased BE risk (adjusted OR 1.98, 95% CI 1.52–2.57).[63] Interestingly, this may hold true only for Caucasians, as a US case control study showed that the relationship between an increased WHR and BE was only significant for this group (OR 2.5, 95% CI 1.2–5.4) and not for those of African descent or Hispanics.[64] A similar strong and consistent relationship was also demonstrated between visceral adiposity and both esophagitis and EAC.

Another risk factor for BE is increasing age. Three studies have looked specifically at age and its relation to BE.[45,54,65] Male gender is also a risk factor for BE.[65] An association between smoking and BE, particularly when combined with GERD, has been reported.[66] However, not all studies have shown this association, even after stratifying by pack-year exposure, length of time smoking, or number of cigarettes per day.[67] Obstructive sleep apnea (OSA) is also a reflux and obesity–independent risk factor for BE.[68] Caucasian ethnicity is an independent risk factor for developing BE.[69] In a large cross-sectional study from the United Kingdom, Caucasians had a 2.9% prevalence of long-segment BE when compared with Asians (0.31%) and Afro-Caribbeans (0.2%).[70] This racial disparity was confirmed in a study from the United States that reported that Caucasians had a higher prevalence of BE when compared with Hispanics and those of African descent (6.1% vs 1.7% vs 1.6%, respectively).[71] Finally, family history of BE and EAC was also found to be associated with an increased risk of developing BE (OR 12.23, 95% CI, 3.34–44.76) in a case-control study by Chak and colleagues.[72] A summary of risk factors for developing BE is provided in **Table 2**.

Table 2
Summary of risk factors for developing Barrett's esophagus

Clinical Variable	Reference	Study Design	Sample Size	Results	Comments
Age	Eloubeidi & Provenzale,[54] 2001	Case control	211	Age ≥40 y independent predictor (P = .008)	Prospective study
	Johansson et al,[45] 2007	Case control	764	Prevalence increased by 5% by age (95% CI, 1–9)	Prospective study
	Edelstein et al,[65] 2009	Case control	615	OR per decade for BE 1.3 (95% CI, 1.1–1.5)	Adjusted OR for gender, WHR, and tobacco use
Male gender	Gerson et al,[74] 2001	Cohort	517	Logistic regression analysis (P = .05)	
	Cook et al,[82] 2005	Meta-analysis	N/A	Pooled male/female ratio, 1.96:1(95% CI, 1.77–2.17:1)	32 studies
	Edelstein et al,[65] 2009	Case control	615	OR, 1.5 (95% CI, 1.1–2.2)	
Ethnicity	Balasubramaniam et al,[69] 2012	Cohort	1058	Caucasian OR, 2.40 (95% CI, 1.42–4.03)	Prospective study
	Abrams et al,[71] 2008	Cross-Sectional	2100	Prevalence of BE in Caucasians 6.1% vs 1.7% and 1.6% for Hispanics and those of African descent, respectively	
	Ford et al,[70] 2005	Case-Control	20,310	Prevalence of BE in Caucasians 2.8% vs 0.31% and 0.2% for Asians and Afro-Caribbeans, respectively	
GERD symptoms	Conio et al,[44] 2002	Case control	451	OR 5.8 (95% CI, 4–8.4)	
	Johansson et al,[45] 2007	Case control	764	OR 2 (95% CI, 0.8–5)	Prospective study
	Anderson et al,[46] 2007	Case control	711	OR range 3.16–4.41 (95% CI, 1.08–14.6) depending on frequency, nocturnal symptoms, duration of GER (y)	

Obesity	Edelstein et al,[65] 2009	Case control	615	OR 1.7 (95% CI, 1.1–2.7) for BMI ≥30	Adjusted OR for age, gender, and smoking
	Singh et al,[63] 2013	Meta-analysis	N/A	OR 1.98 (95% CI, 1.52–2.57) with increased central adiposity	15 studies
	Kramer et al,[64] 2013	Case-Control	1258	OR 0.95–1.32 (95% CI, 0.47–2.4) for BMI ≥30, but OR 1.93–2.81 (95% CI, 0.79–7.99) for increased WHR	Adjusted for age, sex, race, *H pylori* infection, alcohol drinking, smoking, physical activity, and recruitment source
	Kamat et al,[57] 2009	Meta-analysis	N/A	OR 1.49 (95% CI, 1.24–1.8) for BMI ≥30	11 studies; unadjusted OR
Tobacco use	Cook et al,[66] 2012	Meta-analysis	N/A	OR 2.09 (95% CI, 1.54–2.83) for ever having smoked	5 studies
	Anderson et al,[46] 2007	Case Control	711	OR 1.41 (95% CI, 0.77–2.58) for current smoking	
	Thrift et al,[67] 2014	Case Control	1598	OR 1.09 (95% CI, 0.68–1.74) for current smoking	Prospective study
Family history	Chak et al,[72] 2002	Case Control	164	OR of 1.8 (95% CI, 1.1–3.2)	Adjusted for age, sex, and the presence of obesity
OSA	Leggett et al,[68] 2014	Case Control	262	OR 1.8 (95% CI, 1.1–3.2) for OSA	

RISK SCORES

With the establishment of ORs for different risk factors for developing BE, several easily computable clinical scoring tools have been devised to estimate a person's risk for having BE[73–77] (**Table 3**). Most of these rely on information that can be easily ascertained during the history and physical (age, gender, WHR, and smoking history), but one model devised by Thrift and colleagues[77] combined this information with serum biomarkers to increase the risk prediction to an area under the receiver operator curve (AUROC) of 0.85. Although this was improved compared with a model that is only used the frequency and duration of GER symptoms (AUROC of 0.74), the addition of serum markers may decrease the widespread applicability of such a model by increasing cost. The Michigan tool (M-BERET) has an available online probability calculator (http://mberet.umms.med.umich.edu/), but it has not been validated outside of its development cohort, of which 89% were Caucasian men from a Veterans Administration cohort.[76] The Brisbane model highlights the need to validate these types of tools in multiple cohorts. In their development cohort in Australia, the AUROC was 0.7, and when applied to an independent cohort in Washington State (United States), the AUROC dropped to 0.61.[73] The change in AUROC could partially be explained by the overmatching in the development cohort, where they used those with histology findings of reflux and not symptoms alone to define GERD. A recent model derived from a randomized trial in Olmsted County that compared the clinical effectiveness of different endoscopic modalities for BE screening reported a comparable AUROC (0.71) to other models.[43] Interestingly in this model, GERD was not an independent predictor of BE, with central obesity and male gender being the only significant predictors of BE. None of these models is currently used in the clinical arena because the risk threshold to screen for BE is yet undetermined.

Table 3
Barrett's esophagus risk assessment tools

Model	Variables	AUROC
Brisbane model[73]	Sex, age, tobacco use, BMI, highest level of education, & frequency of acid suppressant use	0.61 (validation cohort) 0.7 (development cohort)
Palo Alto model[74]	Sex, age, race, & severity of 7 symptoms	0.72
Mayo Clinic Rochester model[75]	Sex, age, 5-page questionnaire regarding GER symptoms, acid suppressant use, and 1-page questionnaire on somatization symptoms	0.76
Michigan prediction tool[76] http://mberet.umms.med.umich.edu/	Age, WHR, weekly GER symptoms, and pack-year smoking history	0.72
Houston model[77]	Age, duration of GER symptoms, sex, WHR, *H pylori* status, and multiple serum biomarkers (IL 12p70, IL6, IL8, IL10, and Leptin)	0.85
Olmsted County model[43]	Sex, age, GERD symptoms, central obesity, Caucasian ethnicity, smoking history, excess alcohol use (men: >2 alcoholic drinks per day; women: 1 alcoholic drink per day), and family history of BE or EAC	0.7118

As is evident from the AUROCs of models outlined in **Table 3**, their accuracy likely needs to be improved substantially before clinical application can be advocated. Notably, the model with the highest AUROC used additional biologically relevant variables such as circulating proinflammatory cytokines and adipokines, which are products of visceral adipose tissue, in addition to clinical variables. Other variables such as *Helicobacter pylori* status (inversely correlated with BE risk in several risk factors) and psychosomatic symptom scores (which may help adjust for symptoms not representative of true underlying GERD) may need to be considered to increase AUROC values to greater than 0.90, which may reflect a minimal threshold for widespread application.[78] Additional innovative markers, such as volatile organic compounds (circulating and exhaled), have been recently described, which may also help in predicting BE and may form part of a future BE risk score.[79] Attention is also more recently being directed at the oral and esophageal microbiome, which may have roles determining both the risk of and the pathogenesis of esophageal IM. Studies have found that a gram-negative predominant esophageal flora and some *Campylobacter* species are associated with BE.[80,81]

In the absence of clinically applicable risk scores to quantitatively assess BE risk, clinical practitioners continue to face the dilemma on how to identify those at substantial risk of BE and refer for definitive endoscopic evaluation. At least 2 recent Gastroenterology Society guidelines provide some granularity in terms of the number and nature of risk factors that can be used to determine potential eligibility for screening.[8,9] Both suggest limiting screening to those with chronic reflux symptoms (weekly or more for 5 years or more) and 2 or 3 additional risk factors (age, male gender, central obesity, smoking, and family history). These recommendations of course needs to be viewed in the overall perspective of patient performance status, life expectancy, and understanding of implications of a positive screen for BE. There is also an emerging consensus on the low yield of screening in women.

SUMMARY

Despite the exponential increase in the incidence of EAC and tremendous advances in the endoscopic treatment of BE-related dysplasia and early stage EAC, screening for the precursor lesion of EAC (BE) remains in evolution. There is mounting evidence that BE and EAC are associated with modifiable risk factors, primarily central obesity and gastroesophageal reflux. These risks, when combined with nonmodifiable risks such as age, Caucasian ethnicity, family history, and male gender, can be used as risk assessment tools. Although several risk assessment tools have been described, there is currently no validated and clinically applicable tool with reasonable accuracy to select the patients at most risk who could potentially benefit from screening. The risk threshold at which screening would be reasonable also needs to be defined. These risk assessment tools combined with a widely applicable minimally or noninvasive tool could form the basis of an EAC prevention strategy.

REFERENCES

1. Barrett NR. Chronic peptic ulcer of the oesophagus and 'oesophagitis'. Br J Surg 1950;38(150):175–82.
2. Hur C, Miller M, Kong CY, et al. Trends in esophageal adenocarcinoma incidence and mortality. Cancer 2013;119(6):1149–58.
3. Pohl H, Sirovich B, Welch HG. Esophageal adenocarcinoma incidence: are we reaching the peak? Cancer Epidemiol Biomarkers Prev 2010;19(6):1468–70.

4. Prasad GA, Wu TT, Wigle DA, et al. Endoscopic and surgical treatment of mucosal (T1a) esophageal adenocarcinoma in Barrett's esophagus. Gastroenterology 2009;137(3):815–23.
5. Sharma P, Katzka DA, Gupta N, et al. Quality indicators for the management of Barrett's esophagus, dysplasia, and esophageal adenocarcinoma: international consensus recommendations from the American Gastroenterological Association Symposium. Gastroenterology 2015;149(6):1599–606.
6. American Gastroenterological Association, Spechler SJ, Sharma P, et al. American Gastroenterological Association medical position statement on the management of Barrett's esophagus. Gastroenterology 2011;140(3):1084–91.
7. ASGE Standards of Practice Committee, Evans JA, Early DS, Fukami N, et al. The role of endoscopy in Barrett's esophagus and other premalignant conditions of the esophagus. Gastrointest Endosc 2012;76(6):1087–94.
8. Shaheen NJ, Falk GW, Iyer PG, et al, American College of Gastroenterology. ACG clinical guideline: diagnosis and management of Barrett's esophagus. Am J Gastroenterol 2016;111(1):30–50 [quiz: 51].
9. Fitzgerald RC, di Pietro M, Ragunath K, et al. British Society of Gastroenterology guidelines on the diagnosis and management of Barrett's oesophagus. Gut 2014;63(1):7–42.
10. Jung KW, Talley NJ, Romero Y, et al. Epidemiology and natural history of intestinal metaplasia of the gastroesophageal junction and Barrett's esophagus: a population-based study. Am J Gastroenterol 2011;106(8):1447–55 [quiz: 1456].
11. Thota PN, Vennalaganti P, Vennelaganti S, et al. Low risk of high-grade dysplasia or esophageal adenocarcinoma among patients with Barrett's esophagus less than 1 cm (irregular Z line) within 5 years of index endoscopy. Gastroenterology 2016. [Epub ahead of print].
12. Sharma P, Dent J, Armstrong D, et al. The development and validation of an endoscopic grading system for Barrett's esophagus: the Prague C & M criteria. Gastroenterology 2006;131(5):1392–9.
13. Spechler SJ, Fitzgerald RC, Prasad GA, et al. History, molecular mechanisms, and endoscopic treatment of Barrett's esophagus. Gastroenterology 2010;138(3):854–69.
14. Kelty CJ, Gough MD, Van Wyk Q, et al. Barrett's oesophagus: intestinal metaplasia is not essential for cancer risk. Scand J Gastroenterol 2007;42(11):1271–4.
15. Liu W, Hahn H, Odze RD, et al. Metaplastic esophageal columnar epithelium without goblet cells shows DNA content abnormalities similar to goblet cell-containing epithelium. Am J Gastroenterol 2009;104(4):816–24.
16. Chaves P, Crespo M, Ribeiro C, et al. Chromosomal analysis of Barrett's cells: demonstration of instability and detection of the metaplastic lineage involved. Mod Pathol 2007;20(7):788–96.
17. DeMeester SR, Wickramasinghe KS, Lord RV, et al. Cytokeratin and DAS-1 immunostaining reveal similarities among cardiac mucosa, CIM, and Barrett's esophagus. Am J Gastroenterol 2002;97(10):2514–23.
18. Bandla S, Peters JH, Ruff D, et al. Comparison of cancer-associated genetic abnormalities in columnar-lined esophagus tissues with and without goblet cells. Ann Surg 2014;260(1):72–80.
19. Bhat S, Coleman HG, Yousef F, et al. Risk of malignant progression in Barrett's esophagus patients: results from a large population-based study. J Natl Cancer Inst 2011;103(13):1049–57.

20. Khandwalla HE, Graham DY, Kramer JR, et al. Barrett's esophagus suspected at endoscopy but no specialized intestinal metaplasia on biopsy, what's next? Am J Gastroenterol 2014;109(2):178–82.
21. Kerkhof M, van Dekken H, Steyerberg EW, et al. Grading of dysplasia in Barrett's oesophagus: substantial interobserver variation between general and gastrointestinal pathologists. Histopathology 2007;50(7):920–7.
22. Curvers WL, ten Kate FJ, Krishnadath KK, et al. Low-grade dysplasia in Barrett's esophagus: overdiagnosed and underestimated. Am J Gastroenterol 2010; 105(7):1523–30.
23. Shaheen NJ, Sharma P, Overholt BF, et al. Radiofrequency ablation in Barrett's esophagus with dysplasia. N Engl J Med 2009;360(22):2277–88.
24. Phoa KN, van Vilsteren FG, Weusten BL, et al. Radiofrequency ablation vs endoscopic surveillance for patients with Barrett esophagus and low-grade dysplasia: a randomized clinical trial. JAMA 2014;311(12):1209–17.
25. Wani S, Drahos J, Cook MB, et al. Comparison of endoscopic therapies and surgical resection in patients with early esophageal cancer: a population-based study. Gastrointest Endosc 2014;79(2):224–32.e1.
26. Das A, Singh V, Fleischer DE, et al. A comparison of endoscopic treatment and surgery in early esophageal cancer: an analysis of surveillance epidemiology and end results data. Am J Gastroenterol 2008;103(6):1340–5.
27. Corley DA, Levin TR, Habel LA, et al. Surveillance and survival in Barrett's adenocarcinomas: a population-based study. Gastroenterology 2002;122(3):633–40.
28. Incarbone R, Bonavina L, Saino G, et al. Outcome of esophageal adenocarcinoma detected during endoscopic biopsy surveillance for Barrett's esophagus. Surg Endosc 2002;16(2):263–6.
29. Verbeek RE, Leenders M, Ten Kate FJ, et al. Surveillance of Barrett's esophagus and mortality from esophageal adenocarcinoma: a population-based cohort study. Am J Gastroenterol 2014;109(8):1215–22.
30. Ferguson MK, Durkin A. Long-term survival after esophagectomy for Barrett's adenocarcinoma in endoscopically surveyed and nonsurveyed patients. J Gastrointest Surg 2002;6(1):29–35 [discussion: 36].
31. van Sandick JW, van Lanschot JJ, Kuiken BW, et al. Impact of endoscopic biopsy surveillance of Barrett's oesophagus on pathological stage and clinical outcome of Barrett's carcinoma. Gut 1998;43(2):216–22.
32. Corley DA, Mehtani K, Quesenberry C, et al. Impact of endoscopic surveillance on mortality from Barrett's esophagus-associated esophageal adenocarcinomas. Gastroenterology 2013;145(2):312–9.e1.
33. Rubenstein JH, Sonnenberg A, Davis J, et al. Effect of a prior endoscopy on outcomes of esophageal adenocarcinoma among United States veterans. Gastrointest Endosc 2008;68(5):849–55.
34. Barbiere JM, Lyratzopoulos G. Cost-effectiveness of endoscopic screening followed by surveillance for Barrett's esophagus: a review. Gastroenterology 2009;137(6):1869–76.
35. Gerson LB, Groeneveld PW, Triadafilopoulos G. Cost-effectiveness model of endoscopic screening and surveillance in patients with gastroesophageal reflux disease. Clin Gastroenterol Hepatol 2004;2(10):868–79.
36. Dulai GS, Guha S, Kahn KL, et al. Preoperative prevalence of Barrett's esophagus in esophageal adenocarcinoma: a systematic review. Gastroenterology 2002; 122(1):26–33.

37. Kramer JR, Shakhatreh MH, Naik AD, et al. Use and yield of endoscopy in patients with uncomplicated gastroesophageal reflux disorder. JAMA Intern Med 2014;174(3):462–5.
38. Qumseya BJ, Wang H, Badie N, et al. Advanced imaging technologies increase detection of dysplasia and neoplasia in patients with Barrett's esophagus: a meta-analysis and systematic review. Clin Gastroenterol Hepatol 2013;11(12): 1562–70.e1-2.
39. Sami SS, Ragunath K, Iyer PG. Screening for Barrett's esophagus and esophageal adenocarcinoma: rationale, recent progress, challenges, and future directions. Clin Gastroenterol Hepatol 2015;13(4):623–34.
40. Sami SS, Subramanian V, Ortiz-Fernandez-Sordo J, et al. Performance characteristics of unsedated ultrathin video endoscopy in the assessment of the upper GI tract: systematic review and meta-analysis. Gastrointest Endosc 2015;82(5): 782–92.
41. Iyer PG, Chak A. Can endosheath technology open primary care doors to Barrett's esophagus screening by transnasal endoscopy? Endoscopy 2016;48(2): 105–6.
42. Lao-Sirieix P, Boussioutas A, Kadri SR, et al. Non-endoscopic screening biomarkers for Barrett's oesophagus: from microarray analysis to the clinic. Gut 2009;58(11):1451–9.
43. Crews NR, Johnson ML, Schleck CD, et al. Prevalence and predictors of gastroesophageal reflux complications in community subjects. Dig Dis Sci 2016;61(11): 3221–8.
44. Conio M, Filiberti R, Blanchi S, et al. Risk factors for Barrett's esophagus: a case-control study. Int J Cancer 2002;97(2):225–9.
45. Johansson J, Hakansson HO, Mellblom L, et al. Risk factors for Barrett's oesophagus: a population-based approach. Scand J Gastroenterol 2007;42(2):148–56.
46. Anderson LA, Watson RG, Murphy SJ, et al. Risk factors for Barrett's oesophagus and oesophageal adenocarcinoma: results from the FINBAR study. World J Gastroenterol 2007;13(10):1585–94.
47. Dent J, El-Serag HB, Wallander MA, et al. Epidemiology of gastro-oesophageal reflux disease: a systematic review. Gut 2005;54(5):710–7.
48. Shaheen NJ, Richter JE. Barrett's oesophagus. Lancet 2009;373(9666):850–61.
49. El-Serag HB, Sweet S, Winchester CC, et al. Update on the epidemiology of gastro-oesophageal reflux disease: a systematic review. Gut 2014;63(6):871–80.
50. Taylor JB, Rubenstein JH. Meta-analyses of the effect of symptoms of gastroesophageal reflux on the risk of Barrett's esophagus. Am J Gastroenterol 2010; 105(8):1729, 1730–7. [quiz: 1738].
51. Gerson LB, Shetler K, Triadafilopoulos G. Prevalence of Barrett's esophagus in asymptomatic individuals. Gastroenterology 2002;123(2):461–7.
52. Ward EM, Wolfsen HC, Achem SR, et al. Barrett's esophagus is common in older men and women undergoing screening colonoscopy regardless of reflux symptoms. Am J Gastroenterol 2006;101(1):12–7.
53. Zagari RM, Fuccio L, Wallander MA, et al. Gastro-oesophageal reflux symptoms, oesophagitis and Barrett's oesophagus in the general population: the Loiano-Monghidoro study. Gut 2008;57(10):1354–9.
54. Eloubeidi MA, Provenzale D. Clinical and demographic predictors of Barrett's esophagus among patients with gastroesophageal reflux disease: a multivariable analysis in veterans. J Clin Gastroenterol 2001;33(4):306–9.

55. Katzka DA, Castell DO. Successful elimination of reflux symptoms does not insure adequate control of acid reflux in patients with Barrett's esophagus. Am J Gastroenterol 1994;89(7):989–91.
56. Ogden CL, Carroll MD, Fryar CD, et al. Prevalence of obesity among adults and youth: United States, 2011-2014. NCHS Data Brief 2015;(219):1–8.
57. Kamat P, Wen S, Morris J, et al. Exploring the association between elevated body mass index and Barrett's esophagus: a systematic review and meta-analysis. Ann Thorac Surg 2009;87(2):655–62.
58. Shuster A, Patlas M, Pinthus JH, et al. The clinical importance of visceral adiposity: a critical review of methods for visceral adipose tissue analysis. Br J Radiol 2012;85(1009):1–10.
59. Oh TH, Byeon JS, Myung SJ, et al. Visceral obesity as a risk factor for colorectal neoplasm. J Gastroenterol Hepatol 2008;23(3):411–7.
60. Schapira DV, Clark RA, Wolff PA, et al. Visceral obesity and breast cancer risk. Cancer 1994;74(2):632–9.
61. von Hafe P, Pina F, Perez A, et al. Visceral fat accumulation as a risk factor for prostate cancer. Obes Res 2004;12(12):1930–5.
62. World Health Organization. Waist Circumference and Waist–Hip Ratio: report of a WHO expert consultation. Geneva, 2008, Accessed at: http://whqlibdoc.who.int/publications/2011/9789241501491_eng.pdf. Accessed on November 1, 2016.
63. Singh S, Sharma AN, Murad MH, et al. Central adiposity is associated with increased risk of esophageal inflammation, metaplasia, and adenocarcinoma: a systematic review and meta-analysis. Clin Gastroenterol Hepatol 2013;11(11):1399–412.e1.
64. Kramer JR, Fischbach LA, Richardson P, et al. Waist-to-hip ratio, but not body mass index, is associated with an increased risk of Barrett's esophagus in white men. Clin Gastroenterol Hepatol 2013;11(4):373–81.e1.
65. Edelstein ZR, Bronner MP, Rosen SN, et al. Risk factors for Barrett's esophagus among patients with gastroesophageal reflux disease: a community clinic-based case-control study. Am J Gastroenterol 2009;104(4):834–42.
66. Cook MB, Shaheen NJ, Anderson LA, et al. Cigarette smoking increases risk of Barrett's esophagus: an analysis of the Barrett's and Esophageal Adenocarcinoma Consortium. Gastroenterology 2012;142(4):744–53.
67. Thrift AP, Kramer JR, Richardson PA, et al. No significant effects of smoking or alcohol consumption on risk of Barrett's esophagus. Dig Dis Sci 2014;59(1):108–16.
68. Leggett CL, Gorospe EC, Calvin AD, et al. Obstructive sleep apnea is a risk factor for Barrett's esophagus. Clin Gastroenterol Hepatol 2014;12(4):583–8.e1.
69. Balasubramanian G, Singh M, Gupta N, et al. Prevalence and predictors of columnar lined esophagus in gastroesophageal reflux disease (GERD) patients undergoing upper endoscopy. Am J Gastroenterol 2012;107(11):1655–61.
70. Ford AC, Forman D, Reynolds PD, et al. Ethnicity, gender, and socioeconomic status as risk factors for esophagitis and Barrett's esophagus. Am J Epidemiol 2005;162(5):454–60.
71. Abrams JA, Fields S, Lightdale CJ, et al. Racial and ethnic disparities in the prevalence of Barrett's esophagus among patients who undergo upper endoscopy. Clin Gastroenterol Hepatol 2008;6(1):30–4.
72. Chak A, Lee T, Kinnard MF, et al. Familial aggregation of Barrett's oesophagus, oesophageal adenocarcinoma, and oesophagogastric junctional adenocarcinoma in Caucasian adults. Gut 2002;51(3):323–8.

73. Thrift AP, Kendall BJ, Pandeya N, et al. A clinical risk prediction model for Barrett esophagus. Cancer Prev Res (Phila) 2012;5(9):1115–23.
74. Gerson LB, Edson R, Lavori PW, et al. Use of a simple symptom questionnaire to predict Barrett's esophagus in patients with symptoms of gastroesophageal reflux. Am J Gastroenterol 2001;96(7):2005–12.
75. Locke GR, Zinsmeister AR, Talley NJ. Can symptoms predict endoscopic findings in GERD? Gastrointest Endosc 2003;58(5):661–70.
76. Rubenstein JH, Morgenstern H, Appelman H, et al. Prediction of Barrett's esophagus among men. Am J Gastroenterol 2013;108(3):353–62.
77. Thrift AP, Garcia JM, El-Serag HB. A multibiomarker risk score helps predict risk for Barrett's esophagus. Clin Gastroenterol Hepatol 2014;12(8):1267–71.
78. Wang C, Yuan Y, Hunt RH. Helicobacter pylori infection and Barrett's esophagus: a systematic review and meta-analysis. Am J Gastroenterol 2009;104(2):492–500 [quiz: 491, 501].
79. Chan DK, Zakko L, Visrodia KH, et al. Breath testing for Barrett's esophagus using exhaled volatile organic compound profiling with an electronic nose device. Gastroenterology 2017;152(1):24–6.
80. Yang L, Lu X, Nossa CW, et al. Inflammation and intestinal metaplasia of the distal esophagus are associated with alterations in the microbiome. Gastroenterology 2009;137(2):588–97.
81. Macfarlane S, Furrie E, Macfarlane GT, et al. Microbial colonization of the upper gastrointestinal tract in patients with Barrett's esophagus. Clin Infect Dis 2007;45(1):29–38.
82. Cook MB, Wild CP, Forman D. A systematic review and meta-analysis of the sex ratio for Barrett's esophagus, erosive reflux disease, and nonerosive reflux disease. Am J Epidemiol 2005;162(11):1050–61.

Alternatives to Traditional Per-Oral Endoscopy for Screening

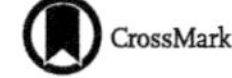

Judith Offman, PhD[a,*], Rebecca C. Fitzgerald, MD[b]

KEYWORDS

• Barrett's esophagus • Esophageal adenocarcinoma • Screening • Endoscopy
• Cell collection • Biomarkers • Transnasal endoscopy • Video capsule endoscopy

KEY POINTS

- Currently, diagnosis of Barrett's esophagus (BE) is dependent on endoscopy; however, this is not suitable for large-scale screening due to the invasive and expensive nature of the test.
- Less invasive tools such as transnasal and video capsule endoscopy are promising alternatives, but high costs are prohibitive for large-scale screening at the moment.
- Nonendoscopic screening methods are less invasive than endoscopic methods and can be more readily carried out in primary care, resulting in higher acceptability for patients.
- Large, randomized trials in the primary care setting are required to determine whether screening for BE is feasible and effective.

INTRODUCTION

The incidence of gastroesophageal reflux disease (GERD) has increased worldwide in the last 40 years.[1] One of the complications of GERD is Barrett's esophagus (BE), where esophageal squamous epithelium is replaced with columnar epithelium (metaplasia),[2] a process that can be viewed as a teleologic adaptation to reflux. BE predisposes patients to esophageal adenocarcinoma (EAC), a cancer with a very poor prognosis, carrying an overall 5-year survival of less than 15%.[3,4] Furthermore, the incidence of EACs has increased dramatically in high-income countries in the last 30 years.[5–7] Because GERD and obesity, which are the main risk factors linked to

Disclosure Statement: The authors disclose the following: R.C. Fitzgerald holds patents on the Cytosponge technology, which has been licensed by MRC Technology to Covidien GI Solutions (now Medtronic). R.C. Fitzgerald has no direct financial arrangement with Metronic. J. Offman has no conflict of interest to declare.

[a] Centre for Cancer Prevention, Wolfson Institute of Preventive Medicine, Barts and The London School of Medicine and Dentistry, Queen Mary University of London, Charterhouse Square, London EC1M 6BQ, UK; [b] MRC Cancer Unit, Hutchinson/MRC Research Centre, University of Cambridge, Box 197, Cambridge Biomedical Campus, Cambridge CB2 0XZ, UK
* Corresponding author.
E-mail address: j.m.offman@qmul.ac.uk

Gastrointest Endoscopy Clin N Am 27 (2017) 379–396
http://dx.doi.org/10.1016/j.giec.2017.02.002

BE and EAC,[8–10] are still increasing, EAC rates have been projected to also further increase.[6]

More than 50% of EAC cases are diagnosed in patients with GERD, who are presenting with alarm symptoms when the cancer is typically advanced.[11,12] Furthermore, it is estimated that only 20% to 25% of patients with the premalignant condition BE are diagnosed. Hence, there is little chance of altering the population mortality from EAC through BE surveillance and endoscopic treatment regimens.[12,13] For those patients who are diagnosed with BE, the impact of surveillance programs is controversial.[11,14–16] However, when performed well, surveillance of BE patients can significantly improve EAC outcomes, including cancer-related mortality, especially more recently using outpatient-based endoscopic therapies for early disease, which obviate the requirement for surgical intervention.[17] The question therefore arises whether screening could reduce mortality from esophageal cancer. Screening should be aimed at detecting early stage cancer, when it is easier to treat, or precancerous stages, when development of cancer can be prevented by removing the precancerous lesion. Screening programs have already been implemented for several cancers, for example, cervical or breast cancer.

RATIONALE FOR SCREENING

To prevent esophageal cancer, screening would be aiming to detect BE. The evidence would suggest that such a program would be in line with the Wilson and Jungner[18] criteria for the selection of conditions suitable for screening:

- The condition should be an important health problem.
  - The incidence of EAC is increasing in the western world.[5–7]
  - The survival is less than 15% at 5 years.[3,4]
- There should a recognizable latent stage.
  - BE is a precancerous stage with a long natural history that can be recognized by endoscopy and biopsy.
- There should be suitable treatments available.
  - Endoscopic intervention, using endoscopic resection and ablation techniques, can prevent progression from dysplasia to carcinoma.[19,20]
- Early detection should lead to a more favorable prognosis.
  - Patients with EAC diagnosed at an early stage (1 and 2) have a far better survival than patients diagnosed at stage 3 or 4.[3,21]
  - Evidence is currently not conclusive whether individuals diagnosed through surveillance programs experience improved survival.[12]

The magnitude of the problem is likely to be large because between 3% and 6% of individuals with GERD are estimated to have BE.[22] Therefore, in order to identify this number of cases, an affordable screening strategy, which is acceptable to the relevant population, is required. Currently, diagnosis of BE has been dependent on per-oral upper gastrointestinal endoscopy (EGD); **Fig. 1**A, for example, shows a diagnostic image. However, this is not suitable for population screening because of the invasive and expensive nature of the test. EGD not only costs on average £650 or $866 per patient[23] but also incurs indirect costs due to patients having to take time off work and require being accompanied.[24]

CURRENT GUIDELINES FOR DIAGNOSIS OF BARRETT'S ESOPHAGUS

The latest guidelines for the diagnosis of BE by the American College of Gastroenterology (ACG), British Society of Gastroenterology (BSG), Danish Society for

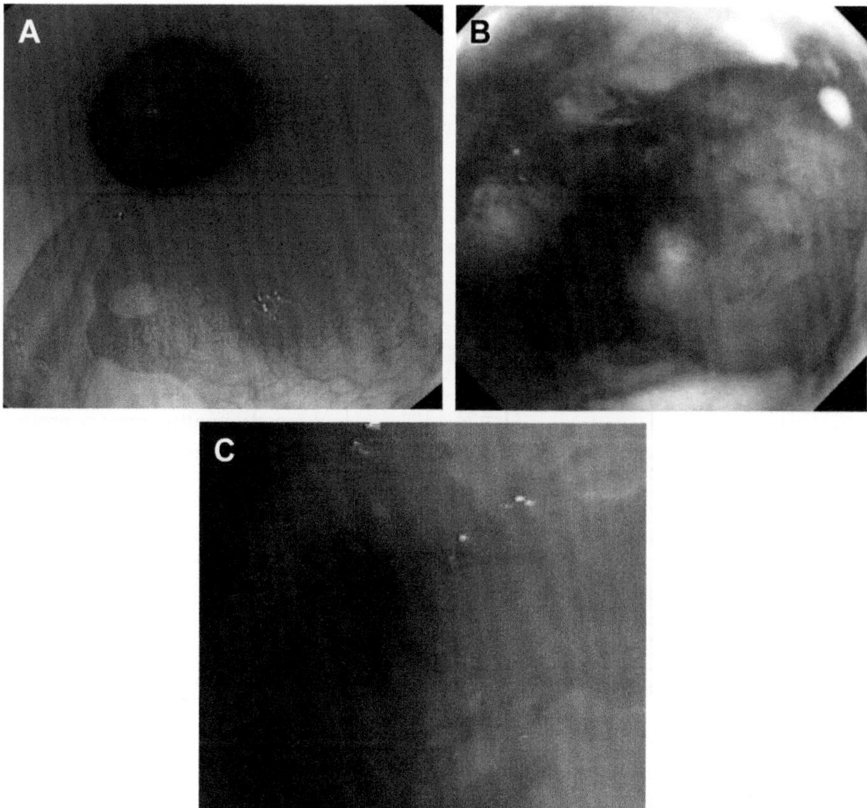

Fig. 1. Endoscopic diagnosis of Barrett's esophagus with conventional per-oral and office-based TNE. (*A*) High-resolution white light endoscopy (GIF-FQ260Z scope, Olympus, Japan). Barrett's esophagus appears as salmon red–colored mucosa and normal esophagus is pale pink. (*B*) Transnasal E.G. SCAN II (Medivators Inc., Minnearpolis, MN< USA) endoscopic view of a short segment of Barrett's esophagus. (*C*) Endosheath (EG530N; Fujinon, Fujifilm, Valhalla, NY) endoscopic diagnosis of Barrett's esophagus. This technology also allows biopsies for histologic confirmation.

Gastroenterology and Hepatology, French Society of Digestive Endoscopy, and Cancer Council Australia recommend the following[25–29]:

- EGD is considered the gold standard.
- Diagnosis should be based on visual evidence of columnar-lined epithelium.
- The length of the BE segment should be recorded using Prague criteria.
- Histologic confirmation with biopsies using the Seattle protocol should be performed.

However, their recommendations for screening for BE differ and are summarized in **Table 1**. None of the national guidelines recommend a population screening program, and, where discussed, it relies on endoscopy and is only recommended for patients with chronic GERD and several risk factors for BE and EAC. Despite general discussions of alternative screening methods, only the ACG guidelines suggest the use of an alternative screening method, which is unsedated transnasal endoscopy (TNE).[25]

Table 1
Recommendations for Barrett's esophagus screening

	American College of Gastroenterology[25]	British Society of Gastroenterology[26]	Danish Society for Gastroenterology and Hepatology[29]	French Society of Digestive Endoscopy[28]	Cancer Council Australia[27]
To be considered for	Men only with chronic and/or frequent GERD and 2 or more risk factors	Patients with chronic GERD and multiple risk factors	Patients with chronic, longstanding GERD at increased risk	N/C	N/C
Patients with family history	N/C	Threshold of risk factors can be lowered in presence of family history	N/C	N/C	N/C
Population screening	Not recommended	Not recommended	Not recommended	N/C	Not recommended
Alternative screening methods	TNE can be considered an alternative	N/C	N/C	N/C	N/C

Abbreviation: N/C, no comment.

EVALUATING NOVEL SCREENING TEST

A diagnostic screening test for BE should be accurate and cost-effective when applied on a population level. Furthermore, it should be simple to administer and acceptable to patients, so would ideally be performed in a nonhospital setting, for example, in a general practice.

When evaluating the performance of a novel clinical test, the most commonly used measures are sensitivity, specificity, predictive value, likelihood ratio, and under the receiver operating characteristic curve. An ideal screening test would be both highly sensitive, meaning with few false negative results, that is, few actual cases are missed, and highly specific, meaning producing few false positive results, that is, resulting in few subjects without the disease having to undergo follow-up procedures.[30] Suitable sensitivity and specificity should be individually assessed for each test and health care setting. For example, a screening test with low specificity would result in many individuals without BE having to undergo endoscopy, which would not be suitable in a health care setting with overstretched endoscopy clinics.

It is a common misconception that sensitivity and specificity of a test do not vary with disease prevalence, enabling comparison between different study populations. However, several studies have shown that test sensitivity and specificity are not as stable as assumed[31,32] and do vary with the prevalence and distribution of the disease in the sample population due to an effect called spectrum bias or spectrum effect.[33] For example, variation in disease prevalence between different study populations may result in differences of symptoms and disease severity, in turn resulting in variations of test sensitivity and specificity. In the case of BE, patients undergoing regular surveillance might, on average, have longer Barrett's fragments than undiagnosed patients in a screening population, which could impact test sensitivity and specificity. As the prevalence of BE is low in the screening population of interest, namely patients with chronic GERD, large studies would be required to accurately calculate measures of test accuracy like sensitivity and specificity. As this is often not possible, new tests are commonly validated in populations comprising a large proportion of BE patients undergoing surveillance, as can be seen in the studies cited in later discussion. Care must therefore be taken when comparing the performance of tests evaluated in different populations and interpreting test performances.

NOVEL SCREENING METHODS

Several alternative methods to EGD are currently being investigated, which are summarized in the following discussion and in **Table 2**.

Endoscopic Screening

Transnasal endoscopy

TNE is a less invasive alternative for visualizing the esophagus (**Fig.** 2B). This procedure uses a thinner-caliber scope, less than 6 mm in diameter.[34] It can be performed using only topical anesthetic, thus avoiding sedation, as gagging is prevented by avoiding contact with the root of the tongue, as would occur during oral intubation. Furthermore, the more compact design of TNE equipment and the use of disposable transnasal endosheath endoscopy (TEE) (**Fig.** 2C) obviating sterilization would allow office or mobile unit–based screening.[35,36]

Three randomized, crossover studies in GERD populations enriched with up to about 50% of BE surveillance patients compared the efficacy of TNE with EGD to detect BE. Jobe and colleagues[37] compared unsedated office-based TNE

Table 2
Characteristics on studies assessing alternative methods of diagnosing Barrett's esophagus

Type of Study	Study	Setting	Patient Group (n)	Method	BE Diagnosis	Se/Sp Compared to EGD (%)	No. of Side Effects	Acceptability Measures	Preferred Future Procedure
TNE (imaging and cell sampling for pathology)									
Jobe et al,[37] 2006	Randomized crossover	Tertiary care; USA	GERD (89) + BE (32)	Unsedated small-caliber endoscopy	Based on biopsy for ZAP grades I-III	Se: 84	3 complications	Endoscopic tolerability questionnaire	71% TNE vs 29% EGD
Shariff et al,[38] 2012	Randomized crossover	Tertiary care; UK	BE (49) + controls (46)	Unsedated TNE	Visible BE + IM on biopsy	98/100	No AEs	STAI + 10 point VAS	59% TNE vs 33% EGD
Shariff et al,[39] 2016	Randomized, crossover	Tertiary care; UK	BE + controls (21 total)	Transnasal disposable endosheath	Visible BE + biopsies according to 2005 BSG guidelines	100/100 for endoscopic diagnosis; 67/100 for histologic diagnosis	N/R	10-point VAS	60% TEE vs 25% EGD
Esophageal capsule endoscopy (imaging only)									
Koslowsky et al,[68] 2006	Prospective single screen	Tertiary care, Israel	GERD (42) + BE (8)	Untethered capsule	Visible BE + confirmation on biopsy	75/100 (4 fps); 100/100 (14 fps)	No AEs	N/I	N/I
Lin et al,[69] 2007	Prospective single screen	Tertiary care, USA	GERD (66) + BE (24)	Untethered capsule	Visible BE + IM on biopsy	67/84	2AEs	N/I	N/I
Galmiche et al,[44] 2008	Prospective single screen	Tertiary care, USA	GERD (77)	Untethered capsule	Visible BE + IM or GM on biopsy	71/99	No complications	N/I	N/I
Ramirez et al,[43] 2008	Prospective single screen	Tertiary care, USA	GERD (100)	Tethered capsule	Visible BE + IM on biopsy	78/82 (visual lesions); 93/78 (biopsy)	No complications	3 point VAS	81% ECE
Sharma et al,[70] 2008	Prospective single screen	Tertiary care, USA	GERD (41) + BE (53)	Untethered capsule	Visible BE + IM on biopsy	GERD patients: 67/87; BE patients: 79/78	No SAEs; AEs N/R	N/I	N/I
Gralnek et al,[71] 2008	Prospective single screen	Tertiary care, Israel	Esophageal disease, including BE (28)	Untethered capsule	Visible BE (ZAP classification)	100/74	No SAEs; AEs N/R	N/I	N/I

Delvaux et al,[72] 2008	Prospective single screen	Tertiary care, Germany/ Fance	GERD (32); BE (5), other esophageal conditions (61)	Untethered capsule	Visible BE ≥ 2 cm length	45/85	No complication	N/I	N/I
Bhardwaj, et al,[42] 2009	Meta-analysis	N/A	GERD (618, range 20–106)	Tethered and untethered	N/A	Pooled Se: 77 Pooled Sp: 86	N/A	N/A	N/A
Chavalitdhamrong et al,[45] 2011	Retrospective review of single screens	Tertiary care; USA	GERD (502)	Untethered capsule (Pillcam ESO)	Visible BE + confirmed columnar lining/IM on biopsy	Se: 83 (visual); 50 (IM)	N/A	N/I	N/I
Optical coherence tomography (imaging only)									
Evans et al,[47] 2007	Blinded, prospective trial (single screen)	Tertiary care; USA	Patients undergoing routine upper endoscopy including with IM (<1 cm) (113)	OCT with diagnostic algorithm (SCJ only)	IM on biopsy	Se for IM at SCJ: 81; Sp 66 or 57 depending on reader	N/R	N/I	N/I
Volumetric laser endomicroscopy (imaging only)									
Gora et al,[46] 2013	Single-screen pilot study	N/R; USA	Healthy (7) and EE (6)	Tethered capsule endomicroscopy	N/R	Se/Sp N/R; high-quality endomicroscopic images	No complications	N/I	92% VLE
Wolfsen et al,[48] 2015	Prospective, multicentre safety and feasibility study	Tertiary care, USA	Known or suspected EE (100)	Nvision VLE system	N/R	Se/Sp N/R; visualization of mucosa and submucosa in 87	2 AEs	N/I	N/I
Trindade et al,[49] 2016	Retrospective review of stored VLE images	Tertiary care; USA	Slide set of cardia, esophagus, EE (120)	Nvision VLE system	N/R	88/92 (nonneoplastic)	N/A	N/I	N/I

(*continued on next page*)

Table 2
(continued)

Type of Study	Study	Setting	Patient Group (n)	Method	BE Diagnosis	Se/Sp Compared to EGD (%)	No. of Side Effects	Acceptability Measures	Preferred Future Procedure
Nonendoscopic cell sampling devices combined with pathology									
Fennerty el al[50] 1995	Single-screen pilot study	Tertiary care; USA	BE (10)	Balloon cytology	Presence of IM	No goblet cells or definitive columnar cell dysplasia collected	N/R	N/I	N/I
Rader et al,[51] 2001	Single-screen pilot study	Tertiary care; USA	BE (11)	Flexible mesh catheter	Visible BE + IM on biopsy	Se 87	No complications	N/I	N/I
Nonendoscopic cell sampling devices combined with biomarkers									
Kadri et al,[56] 2010	Prospective cohort study	Primary care; UK	GERD (504)	Cytosponge-TFF3 test	Visible BE (≥C1) + IM on biopsy	73/94 (C ≥1); 90/94 (C ≥ 2)	No SAEs; AEs N/R	STAI, impact of events scale, 10-point VAS	N/I
Ross-Innes et al,[57] 2015	Case-control study	Tertiary care; UK	GERD (463) and BE (647)	Cytosponge-TFF3 test	Visible BE (≥C1 or ≥M3) + IM on biopsy	80/92 (C ≥ 1); 87/92 (C ≥ 3)	3 SAEs; AEs N/R	10-point VAS	N/I
Lao-Sirieix et al, (abstract)[54] 2015	Prospective single screen	Tertiary care; UK	BE (73)	Updated Cytosponge + TFF3 test	Visible BE (≥C1 or ≥M3) + IM on biopsy	Se: 92	no complications	10-point VAS	N/I
Blood biomarkers									
Bus et al,[65] 2016	Pilot study	Tertiary care; Netherlands	Controls (15), BE (41), EAC (59)	Circulating miRNAs	Visible BE + IM on biopsy	78/86 in validation cohort	N/R	N/I	N/I

Where sensitivity and specificity were not calculated as part of the study, the authors estimated these measures based on the information available.

Abbreviations: AE, adverse event; GM, gastric metaplasia; N/I, not investigated; N/R, not reported; SAE, serious adverse event; SCJ, squamocolumnar junction; Se, sensitivity; Sp, specificity; STAI, Spielberger State-Trait Anxiety Inventory; VAS, visual analogue scale; VLE, volumetric laser endomicroscopy.

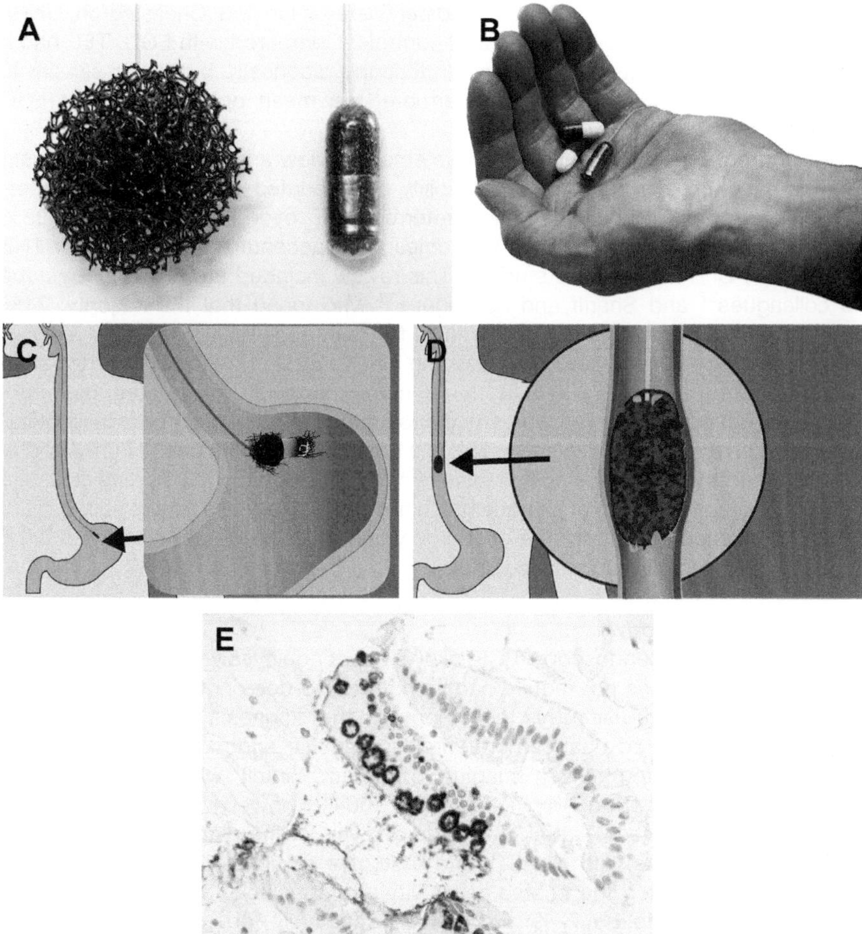

Fig. 2. Use of the Cytosponge test. (*A*) Expanded Cytosponge (*left*) and Cytosponge embedded in gelatin capsule (*right*). (*B*) The Cytosponge compared with paracetamol capsules in the palm of a hand. (*C*) The Cytosponge is swallowed, and the gelatin capsule dissolves in the stomach within 5 minutes. (*D*) The Cytosponge is retrieved by a nurse, collecting cells as it is pulled up. *The arrows* indicate the enlarged area containing the Cytosponge. (*E*) Immunohistochemical images (original magnification ×20), illustrating TFF3-positive staining in cells collected with the Cytosponge (Immunostaining for TFF3 with proprietary monoclonal antibody; BDDiagnostics, Durham, North Carolina, US).

(Olympus, Melville, NY, small caliber, diameter, 5.1 mm) with EGD in a study of 121 individuals and estimated the sensitivity for diagnosis of BE to be 84%. The agreement between the 2 approaches, however, was only moderate (kappa = 0.591). Patients undergoing EGD experienced significantly more anxiety, pain, gagging, and choking. Using an ultrathin endoscope (EG530N; Fujinon, Fujifilm, Valhalla, NY, diameter, 5.9 mm), Shariff and colleagues[38] found in a study of 95 individuals that TNE was an accurate and well-tolerated method for diagnosing BE with a sensitivity and specificity of 98% and 100%, respectively. Furthermore, they observed high correlation between the 2 modalities (R^2 = 0.97; P<.001). Shariff and colleagues[39] also investigated TEE (TNE–5000, DP Medical Systems Limited, Chessington, UK) in a small pilot study in 25 BE patients and controls. Compared with EGD, TEE had a sensitivity and specificity of 100% for endoscopy diagnosis, but lower sensitivity (66.7%) for histologic diagnosis. Furthermore, the mean optical quality of EGD was significantly better (**Fig. 1**).

Sami and colleagues[40] carried out a systematic review and meta-analysis to estimate the patient preference and acceptability of unsedated TNE. The pooled difference in proportion of patients who preferred TNE over EGD was 63% (95% confidence interval [CI], 49.0–76.0, 10 studies), and acceptability was high for TNE (85.2%; 95% CI, 79.1–89.9; 16 studies). This review included the 2 studies by Jobe and colleagues[37] and Shariff and colleagues[38] who found that the majority, 71% and 59% of patients, expressed a preference for TNE. Patients also reported a significantly better experience with TEE, preferring TEE to EGD.[38,39] However, a prospective randomized controlled trial in a community population of more than 400 patients did not observe increased participation rates for TEE when comparing invitations to EGD, TEE in a mobile van, or TEE in a hospital outpatient unit.[35] Furthermore, the cost of ultrathin devices is comparable to standard endoscopes, limiting its use to population screening of high-risk patients. In addition, to fully assess the suitability of TEE for population screening, the accuracy would have to be assessed in a large screening cohort in a community setting.

Video capsule endoscopy

Esophageal capsules endoscopy (ECE) allows direct noninvasive visualization of the esophagus, which does not require sedation, but also does not allow for taking of biopsies. Most studies using this technology for the diagnosis of BE were carried out using an untethered dual-camera wireless capsule endoscope (PillCam ESO, Given diagnostic system: Given Imaging, Yoqneam, Israel), which was approved by the US Food and Drug Administration in 2004[41]; however, tethered cameras have also been used (see **Table 2**). A meta-analysis of the diagnostic accuracy of ECE for BE in patients with GERD found 9 studies comprising a total of 618 patients.[42] They estimated the pooled sensitivity and specificity of ECE for the diagnosis of BE overall to be 77% and 86%, respectively (no CIs were provided). There was some variation in specificity observed when they either included studies using EGD (90%) or histologically confirmed intestinal metaplasia (IM) (73%) as the reference standard; however, the sensitivity remained the same (78%). Most study populations consisted of a combination of screening and BE surveillance populations; however, 2 of the studies included screening patients only. These 2 studies of 77 and 100 GERD patients reported sensitivities of 60% and 78% and specificities of 100% and 89%, respectively.[43,44] Chavalitdhamrong and colleagues[45] carried out a retrospective review of 502 ECE Pillcam ESO (Given diagnostic system: Given Imaging, Yoqneam, Israel) video files for patients with GERD to assess ECE video imaging. They identified 12 BE patients, which the authors used to estimate the sensitivity for BE diagnosis as 83% and 50% compared with visual inspection by EGD and histologic confirmation with IM, respectively. ECE was found to be safe in all studies; however, patient preference was only investigated in one study, where 81% of patients preferred ECE to EGD.[43]

When the cost-effectiveness of ECE compared with EGD was investigated though, the costs were found to be very similar, and the ability to perform the procedure without sedation is negated by the cost of ECE capsule and equipment.[24] Despite its attractiveness for screening because it is safe and does not require sedation, its costs currently seem prohibitive. Furthermore, this tool would have to be tested in an appropriate screening population to accurately estimate its accuracy.

Volumetric laser endomicroscopy

Volume laser endomicroscopy (VLE) is a new generation optical coherence tomography (OCT) that produces high-resolution cross-sectional images of the esophagus. Gora and colleagues have developed a tethered capsule microendoscopy, which involves swallowing an optomechanically engineered capsule that uses optical frequency domain imaging (OFDI) technology to provide 3-dimensional microscopic images of the digestive organs.[46] OFDI has previously been shown to have capability for the diagnosis of BE.[47] As the capsule travels through the digestive tract, it captures cross-sectional microscopic images at 30 μm (lateral) × 7 μm (axial), which can be used to reconstruct a 3-dimensional microscopic representation of the entire organ. In a small, proof-of-principle study in 7 healthy and 6 BE patients, this technology produced endomicroscopic images of the esophageal mucosa, which could distinguish between patients with and without BE.[46] Furthermore, 12 of the subjects reported a preference for tethered capsule endomicroscopy over EGD. Once the capsule is withdrawn, it can be disinfected for reuse, making it potentially inexpensive and feasible to be used for population screening.

A commercially available OFDI-based imaging system (Nivision VLE System, NinePoint Medical, Cambridge, Mass) was evaluated in a safety and feasibility study of 100 patients with BE, where the procedure was shown to be safe. VLE was successfully performed in 87 cases, enabling visualization of the mucosa and submucosa.[48] One hundred twenty stored Nivision VLE images of BE patients with and without dysplasia were evaluated retrospectively blinded to endoscopic and clinical findings.[49] As OCT and VLE are limited in differentiating between low-grade dysplasia and nondysplastic BE, they were combined in one group (nondysplastic BE). The overall agreement between users was excellent (kappa = 0.81; 95% CI, 0.79–0.83) when combining nonneoplastic BE and neoplastic BE; however, it was lower for nondysplastic BE with kappa = 0.66 (95% CI, 0.63–0.69). Compared with EGD, the sensitivity and specificity for nonneoplastic BE (nondysplastic and low-grade dysplasia) were 88% (95% CI, 83%-91%) and 92% (95% CI, 90%-94%), respectively. Even though this is a very promising new technology, the resolution of these images is still poor, and the technology requires further development. It also needs to be tested in several prospective controlled trials, both in BE and in screening populations, to assess suitability for BE screening in a GERD population. For the entirety of imaging modalities, one question that remains is whether an optical diagnosis can suffice without a tissue sample. With the current state-of-the-art, it is likely that a tissue biopsy will still be required to confirm the findings from these technologies.

Nonendoscopic Screening

The nonendoscopic screening methods described in the following discussion are less invasive than endoscopic methods and can be more readily carried out in primary care, resulting in higher acceptability for patients. In addition, by removing the requirement for a skilled operator, there is also the potential to reduce the cost.

Cell collection devices

Several relatively simple and low-cost nonendoscopic devices, including inflatable balloons and sponges, have been developed for collection of esophageal samples. An early study evaluated the use of a cytology balloon (Wilson Cook Medical, Inc.,

Winston-Salem, NC) for specimen collection from 10 BE patients; however, this device did not collect columnar cells from any of the patients, so was not suitable for BE screening.[50] Another pilot study investigated the use of a prototype flexible mesh catheter (Microvasive- Boston Scientific Corporation, Natick, Massachusetts, USA) for the diagnosis of BE in patients undergoing surveillance.[51] Of the 11 BE patients in the study, adequate specimens, defined as the presence of at least one glandular cell group, were obtained from 8 patients (73%), and the sensitivity among adequate samples was 87.5%. However, even though balloon cytology had a high sensitivity for EAC or BE with high-grade dysplasia (80%), the sensitivity was significantly lower for BE with low-grade dysplasia or without dysplasia (56%) when tested in a surveillance population.[52]

The combination of a modified cell collection device with a biomarker has proven more successful. The Cytosponge is a cell collection device developed at Cambridge University in the United Kingdom (Medical Research Council, London, UK). It is composed of a reticulated foam sphere approximately 30 mm in diameter compressed within a gelatin capsule and attached to a string (**Fig. 2**A, B). The patient swallows the capsule while holding onto the string. The gelatin capsule dissolves after 5 minutes, allowing the sponge to expand, and the sponge is pulled up from the stomach to the esophagus and mouth (see **Fig. 2**C, D). The cells it collects from the gastroesophageal junction and the entire length of the esophagus are processed and assessed for the presence of Trefoil Factor 3 (TFF3), a biomarker for BE (using a proprietary monoclonal antibody; BDDiagnostics, Durham, North Carolina, US) (**Fig. 2**E). TFF3 was identified in a gene expression study as a marker specifically for intestinal cells of BE, but not columnar cells derived from the normal gastric cardia or upper airways.[53]

The Cytosponge device combined with the TFF3 test has been tested in 4 clinical studies so far.[54–57] In an initial cohort study of more than 500 GERD patients selected from patients taking acid suppressants in primary care, the procedure was safe, and the vast majority of participants (99%) successfully swallowed the device.[56] Compared with EGD, the sensitivity and specificity of the test were 73.3% (95% CI, 44.9%–92.2%) and 93.8% (95% CI, 91.3%–95.8%), respectively, for circumferential length of BE of 1 cm or more (≥C1) and 90.0% (95% CI, 55.5%–99.6%) and 93.3% (95% CI, 90.9%–95.5%) for segments of 2 cm or more (≥C2). With 3% (15/501) of the study participants having an endoscopic diagnosis of BE, the sample size was not powered adequately to obtain accurate estimates of the sensitivity and specificity. A large case control study of more than 1000 patients (463 controls with dyspepsia and 647 BE cases) allowed more accurate evaluation of the safety, accuracy, and acceptability of this test.[57] The overall sensitivity of the Cytosponge-TFF3 test in this population was 79.9% (95% CI, 76.4%–83.0%) for ≥C1, which increased to 87.2% (95% CI, 83.0%–90.6%) for ≥C3. The specificity was 92.4% (95% CI, 89.5%–94.7%). The sensitivity increased to 89.7% (95% CI, 82.3%–94.8%) for patients having a repeat procedure. A commercial version of the Cytosponge device (Medtronic, Dublin, Ireland) in combination with the TFF3 test was found to have a higher overall sensitivity of 91.5% in a smaller prospective study (73 patients).[54]

The acceptability of the Cytosponge-TFF3 test was high with 82% of participants reporting low levels of anxiety before the test. Furthermore, the Cytosponge was rated favorably compared with endoscopy ($P<.001$). In a qualitative study investigating the acceptability of the Cytosponge using interviews and focus groups, the acceptability was found to be high, and participants perceived the test to be more comfortable and practical than endoscopy.[58]

It is noteworthy that the BEST1 and 2 trials have evaluated the accuracy and acceptability of the Cytosponge-TFF3 test in large, prospective trials; namely, a large GERD patient screening population (504 participants) to test feasibility and acceptability in primary care and a large BE enriched population in tertiary care (1110 participants) to obtain more accurate estimates of the test accuracy. Furthermore, a microsimulation of costs was carried out to compare the health benefits and cost-effectiveness of screening for BE by either Cytosponge or EGD versus no screening, which suggested that the Cytosponge test could be cost-effective when combined with endoscopic therapy.[59] This test therefore has the characteristics for a clinically acceptable screening tool: suitability for primary care, high acceptability and tolerability, low cost, and high accuracy. To further assess the suitability of the Cytosponge-TFF3 test, the BEST3 trial (Trial ID ISRCTN68382401) aiming to assess whether invitation to a Cytosponge-TFF3 test for patients with reflux symptoms will be effective in increasing the detection of BE in primary care and to evaluate its cost-effectiveness is due to start in 2017. Patient acceptability will also be evaluated in the BEST3 trial.

Circulating molecular markers

A blood-based screening test would be an appealing alternative, because these tests are less invasive, pose minimal risk to patients, and can be carried out in a primary care setting, all of which would increase patient acceptability and appeal. One example is detection of circulating microRNAs (miRNAs) as a method for diagnosing BE. miRNAs are approximately 21 to 25 nucleotides in length, are stable, and can be detected in circulating plasma.[60] They regulate numerous cellular processes, and dysregulation of their function has been associated with the pathogenesis of many diseases, including cancer.[61,62] Eleven studies, 7 of which specifically compared normal epithelium and nondysplastic BE, investigated miRNAs with high biomarker potential for screening and disease monitoring in the esophageal epithelium.[63] Overall, 5 biomarkers were identified as promising tissues markers for diagnosing BE. Cabibi and colleagues confirmed that circulating miRNA levels of 2 of these markers, miR-145 and miR-215, were significantly increased in BE compared with esophagitis controls[64]; however, these were not further validated in a larger population. In another pilot study, a different combination of 2 miRNAs, miR-194-5p and miR-451a, were significantly increased, and one, miR136, was significantly decreased in BE compared with controls.[65] These 3 miRNAs combined with an additional 3 miRNAs were further investigated in a larger validation study, and a combination of 4 of these miRNAs was found to be the most informative panel in distinguishing controls (15 patients) from BE (41 patients) with sensitivity and specificity of 78.4% (95% CI, 61.8%–90.2%) and 85.7% (95% CI, 57.2%–98.2%), respectively. A limitation of this study, however, was the fact that control patients did not have reflux symptoms, so the changes of miRNAs levels identified could simply be due to GERD. It seems feasible to detect BE using these blood-based miRNA markers; however, validation studies in larger cohorts are required.

Several different circulating autoantibodies, both alone and in combination, have also been investigated for early detection of esophageal cancer.[66] However, even though studies reported positive associations, the test sensitivities were too low and variability between studies was high.

Breath markers also represent an attractive method for cancer screening because it is noninvasive, provides results quickly, and is relatively cheap; however, studies are currently limited. One study identified a panel of breath volatile organic compounds (VOCs) that could be used to distinguish esophageal cancer from BE and benign conditions of the upper gastrointestinal tract, but these VOCs have not been investigated for diagnosis of BE yet.[67]

SUMMARY

BE is a condition that fulfills the criteria for a screening test in order to reduce population mortality from EAC. Endoscopy is the gold standard diagnostic tool; however, less invasive and more cost-effective alternatives are required. Several technologies have been studied, some of which are promising; however, most studies were carried out in high-prevalence populations, mostly in secondary care. As discussed, it is not appropriate to extrapolate the sensitivity and specificity of these new diagnostic tests developed and validated in high-prevalence secondary care populations to a screening scenario in a population with low prevalence because this could result in a decrease in sensitivity and increase in specificity.[31] Instead, well-powered studies carried out in the relevant populations are needed, and hence, careful consideration should be given to whether the test should be given to an enriched population according to their level of risk. In addition, studies should include evaluation of the acceptability and health economics before decisions can be made about implementing a new test in standard clinical care.

ACKNOWLEDGMENTS

We would like to thank UCL Health Creatives (London) for providing us with images for **Fig. 2**A–D. Furthermore, we would like to thank Drs Massimiliano Di Pietro for the images of **Fig. 1** and Shona MacRae for the image of **Fig. 2**E.

REFERENCES

1. Boeckxstaens G, El-Serag HB, Smout AJPM, et al. Symptomatic reflux disease: the present, the past and the future. Gut 2014;63(7):1185–93.
2. McDonald SA, Lavery D, Wright NA, et al. Barrett oesophagus: lessons on its origins from the lesion itself. Nat Rev Gastroenterol Hepatol 2015;12(1):50–60.
3. Eloubeidi MA, Mason AC, Desmond RA, et al. Temporal trends (1973-1997) in survival of patients with esophageal adenocarcinoma in the United States: a glimmer of hope? Am J Gastroenterol 2003;98(7):1627–33.
4. Cancer Research UK. Oesophageal cancer statistics. 2015. Available at: http://www.cancerresearchuk.org/health-professional/cancer-statistics/statistics-by-cancer-type/oesophageal-cancer. Accessed November 25, 2015.
5. Edgren G, Adami H-O, Weiderpass E, et al. A global assessment of the oesophageal adenocarcinoma epidemic. Gut 2013;62(10):1406–14.
6. Kong CY, Kroep S, Curtius K, et al. Exploring the recent trend in esophageal adenocarcinoma incidence and mortality using comparative simulation modeling. Cancer Epidemiol Biomarkers Prev 2014;23(6):997–1006.
7. Otterstatter MC, Brierley JD, De P, et al. Esophageal cancer in Canada: trends according to morphology and anatomical location. Can J Gastroenterol 2012; 26(10):723–7.
8. Ness-Jensen E, Gottlieb-Vedi E, Wahlin K, et al. All-cause and cancer-specific mortality in GORD in a population-based cohort study (the HUNT study). Gut 2016. [Epub ahead of print].
9. Kubo A, Corley DA. Body mass index and adenocarcinomas of the esophagus or gastric cardia: a systematic review and meta-analysis. Cancer Epidemiol Biomarkers Prev 2006;15(5):872–8.

10. Zhang Y. Epidemiology of esophageal cancer. World J Gastroenterol 2013; 19(34):5598–606.
11. Bhat SK, McManus DT, Coleman HG, et al. Oesophageal adenocarcinoma and prior diagnosis of Barrett's oesophagus: a population-based study. Gut 2015; 64(1):20–5.
12. Vaughan TL, Fitzgerald RC. Precision prevention of oesophageal adenocarcinoma. Nat Rev Gastroenterol Hepatol 2015;12(4):243–8.
13. Spechler SJ. Barrett esophagus and risk of esophageal cancer: a clinical review. JAMA 2013;310(6):627–36.
14. Corley DA, Mehtani K, Quesenberry C, et al. Impact of endoscopic surveillance on mortality from Barrett's esophagus-associated esophageal adenocarcinomas. Gastroenterology 2013;145(2):312–9.e1.
15. Verbeek RE, Leenders M, Ten Kate FJ, et al. Surveillance of Barrett's esophagus and mortality from esophageal adenocarcinoma: a population-based cohort study. Am J Gastroenterol 2014;109(8):1215–22.
16. Whiteman DC. Does a prior diagnosis of Barrett's oesophagus influence risk of dying from oesophageal adenocarcinoma? Gut 2015;64(1):5–6.
17. El-Serag HB, Naik AD, Duan Z, et al. Surveillance endoscopy is associated with improved outcomes of oesophageal adenocarcinoma detected in patients with Barrett's oesophagus. Gut 2016;65(8):1252–60.
18. Wilson JMG, Jungner G. Principles and practice of screening for disease. Geneva (Switzerland): WHO; 1968.
19. Shaheen NJ, Sharma P, Overholt BF, et al. Radiofrequency ablation in Barrett's esophagus with dysplasia. N Engl J Med 2009;360(22):2277–88.
20. Phoa K, van Vilsteren FI, Weusten BM, et al. Radiofrequency ablation vs endoscopic surveillance for patients with Barrett esophagus and low-grade dysplasia: a randomized clinical trial. JAMA 2014;311(12):1209–17.
21. Hur C, Miller M, Kong CY, et al. Trends in esophageal adenocarcinoma incidence and mortality. Cancer 2013;119(6):1149–58.
22. Cameron AJ, Zinsmeister AR, Ballard DJ, et al. Prevalence of columnar-lined (Barrett's) esophagus. Comparison of population-based clinical and autopsy findings. Gastroenterology 1990;99(4):918–22.
23. Inadomi JM, Somsouk M, Madanick RD, et al. A cost-utility analysis of ablative therapy for Barrett's esophagus. Gastroenterology 2009;136(7):2101–14.e1-6.
24. Rubenstein JH, Inadomi JM, Brill JV, et al. Cost utility of screening for Barrett's esophagus with esophageal capsule endoscopy versus conventional upper endoscopy. Clin Gastroenterol Hepatol 2007;5(3):312–8.
25. Shaheen NJ, Falk GW, Iyer PG, et al. ACG clinical guideline: diagnosis and management of Barrett's esophagus. Am J Gastroenterol 2016;111(1):30–50.
26. Fitzgerald RC, di Pietro M, Ragunath K, et al. British Society of Gastroenterology guidelines on the diagnosis and management of Barrett's oesophagus. Gut 2014; 63(1):7–42.
27. Whiteman DC, Appleyard M, Bahin FF, et al. Australian clinical practice guidelines for the diagnosis and management of Barrett's esophagus and early esophageal adenocarcinoma. J Gastroenterol Hepatol 2015;30(5):804–20.
28. Boyer J, Laugier R, Chemali M, et al. French Society of Digestive Endoscopy SFED guideline: monitoring of patients with Barrett's esophagus. Endoscopy 2007;39(09):840–2.
29. Hirota WK, Zuckerman MJ, Adler DG, et al. ASGE guideline: the role of endoscopy in the surveillance of premalignant conditions of the upper GI tract. Gastrointest Endosc 2006;63(4):570–80.

30. Maxim LD, Niebo R, Utell MJ. Screening tests: a review with examples. Inhal Toxicol 2014;26(13):811–28.
31. Usher-Smith JA, Sharp SJ, Griffin SJ. The spectrum effect in tests for risk prediction, screening, and diagnosis. BMJ 2016;353:i3139.
32. Leeflang MM, Rutjes AW, Reitsma JB, et al. Variation of a test's sensitivity and specificity with disease prevalence. CMAJ 2013;185(11):E537–44.
33. Ransohoff DF, Feinstein AR. Problems of spectrum and bias in evaluating the efficacy of diagnostic tests. N Engl J Med 1978;299(17):926–30.
34. Atar M, Kadayifci A. Transnasal endoscopy: technical considerations, advantages and limitations. World J Gastrointest Endosc 2014;6(2):41–8.
35. Sami SS, Dunagan KT, Johnson ML, et al. A randomized comparative effectiveness trial of novel endoscopic techniques and approaches for Barrett's esophagus screening in the community. Am J Gastroenterol 2015;110(1):148–58.
36. Peery AF, Hoppo T, Garman KS, et al. Feasibility, safety, acceptability and yield of office-based, screening transnasal esophagoscopy. Gastrointest Endosc 2012;75(5):945–53.e2.
37. Jobe BA, Hunter JG, Chang EY, et al. Office-based unsedated small-caliber endoscopy is equivalent to conventional sedated endoscopy in screening and surveillance for Barrett's esophagus: a randomized and blinded comparison. Am J Gastroenterol 2006;101(12):2693–703.
38. Shariff MK, Bird-Lieberman EL, O'Donovan M, et al. Randomized crossover study comparing efficacy of transnasal endoscopy with that of standard endoscopy to detect Barrett's esophagus. Gastrointest Endosc 2012;75(5):954–61.
39. Shariff MK, Varghese S, O'Donovan M, et al. Pilot randomized crossover study comparing the efficacy of transnasal disposable endosheath with standard endoscopy to detect Barrett's esophagus. Endoscopy 2016;48(02):110–6.
40. Sami SS, Subramanian V, Ortiz-Fernández-Sordo J, et al. Performance characteristics of unsedated ultrathin video endoscopy in the assessment of the upper GI tract: systematic review and meta-analysis. Gastrointest Endosc 2015;82(5):782–92.
41. Sharma VK, Eliakim R, Sharma P, et al. ICCE Consensus for esophageal capsule endoscopy. Endoscopy 2005;37(10):1060–4.
42. Bhardwaj A, Hollenbeak CS, Pooran N, et al. A meta-analysis of the diagnostic accuracy of esophageal capsule endoscopy for Barrett's esophagus in patients with gastroesophageal reflux disease. Am J Gastroenterol 2009;104(6):1533–9.
43. Ramirez FC, Akins R, Shaukat M. Screening of Barrett's esophagus with string-capsule endoscopy: a prospective blinded study of 100 consecutive patients using histology as the criterion standard. Gastrointest Endosc 2008;68(1):25–31.
44. Galmiche JP, Sacher-Huvelin S, Coron E, et al. Screening for esophagitis and Barrett's esophagus with wireless esophageal capsule endoscopy: a multicenter prospective trial in patients with reflux symptoms. Am J Gastroenterol 2008;103(3):538–45.
45. Chavalitdhamrong D, Chen GC, Roth BE, et al. Esophageal capsule endoscopy for evaluation of patients with chronic gastroesophageal reflux symptoms: findings and its image quality. Dis Esophagus 2011;24(5):295–8.
46. Gora MJ, Sauk JS, Carruth RW, et al. Tethered capsule endomicroscopy enables less invasive imaging of gastrointestinal tract microstructure. Nat Med 2013;19(2):238–40.
47. Evans JA, Bouma BE, Bressner J, et al. Identifying intestinal metaplasia at the squamocolumnar junction by using optical coherence tomography. Gastrointest Endosc 2007;65(1):50–6.

48. Wolfsen HC, Sharma P, Wallace MB, et al. Safety and feasibility of volumetric laser endomicroscopy in patients with Barrett's esophagus (with videos). Gastrointest Endosc 2015;82(4):631–40.
49. Trindade AJ, Inamdar S, Smith MS, et al. Volumetric laser endomicroscopy in Barrett's esophagus: interobserver agreement for interpretation of Barrett's esophagus and associated neoplasia among high-frequency users. Gastrointest Endosc 2016. [Epub ahead of print].
50. Fennerty MB, DiTomasso J, Morales TG, et al. Screening for Barrett's esophagus by balloon cytology. Am J Gastroenterol 1995;90(8):1230–2.
51. Rader AE, Faigel DO, Ditomasso J, et al. Cytological screening for Barrett's esophagus using a prototype flexible mesh catheter. Dig Dis Sci 2001;46(12): 2681–6.
52. Falk GW, Chittajallu R, Goldblum JR, et al. Surveillance of patients with Barrett's esophagus for dysplasia and cancer with balloon cytology. Gastroenterology 1997;112(6):1787–97.
53. Lao-Sirieix P, Boussioutas A, Kadri SR, et al. Non-endoscopic screening biomarkers for Barrett's oesophagus: from microarray analysis to the clinic. Gut 2009;58(11):1451–9.
54. Lao-Sirieix P, Debiram -Beecham I, Sarah K, et al. 54 evaluation of a minimally-invasive cytosponge esophageal cell collection system in patients with Barrett's esophagus. Gastroenterology 2015;148(4):S-16.
55. Lao-Sirieix P, Rous B, O'Donovan M, et al. Non-endoscopic immunocytological screening test for Barrett's oesophagus. Gut 2007;56(7):1033–4.
56. Kadri SR, Lao-Sirieix P, O'Donovan M, et al. Acceptability and accuracy of a non-endoscopic screening test for Barrett's oesophagus in primary care: cohort study. BMJ 2010;341:c4372.
57. Ross-Innes CS, Debiram-Beecham I, O'Donovan M, et al. Evaluation of a minimally invasive cell sampling device coupled with assessment of trefoil factor 3 expression for diagnosing Barrett's esophagus: a multi-center case-control study. PLoS Med 2015;12(1):e1001780.
58. Freeman M, Offman J, Walter FM, et al. Acceptability of the Cytosponge procedure for detecting Barrett's oesophagus: A qualitative study. BMJ 2017;7(3): e013901.
59. Benaglia T, Sharples LD, Fitzgerald RC, et al. Health benefits and cost effectiveness of endoscopic and nonendoscopic cytosponge screening for Barrett's esophagus. Gastroenterology 2013;144(1):62–73.e6.
60. Mitchell PS, Parkin RK, Kroh EM, et al. Circulating microRNAs as stable blood-based markers for cancer detection. Proc Natl Acad Sci U S A 2008;105(30): 10513–8.
61. Calin GA, Croce CM. MicroRNA signatures in human cancers. Nat Rev Cancer 2006;6(11):857–66.
62. Farazi TA, Hoell JI, Morozov P, et al. MicroRNAs in human cancer. In: Schmitz U, Wolkenhauer O, Vera J, editors. MicroRNA cancer regulation: advanced concepts, bioinformatics and systems biology tools. Dordrecht (The Netherlands): Springer Netherlands; 2013. p. 1–20.
63. Mallick R, Patnaik SK, Wani S, et al. A systematic review of esophageal microRNA markers for diagnosis and monitoring of Barrett's esophagus. Dig Dis Sci 2016; 61(4):1039–50.
64. Cabibi D, Caruso S, Bazan V, et al. Analysis of tissue and circulating microRNA expression during metaplastic transformation of the esophagus. Oncotarget 2016;7(30):47821–30.

65. Bus P, Kestens C, Ten Kate FJW, et al. Profiling of circulating microRNAs in patients with Barrett's esophagus and esophageal adenocarcinoma. J Gastroenterol 2016; 51(6):560–70.
66. Yazbeck R, Jaenisch SE, Watson DI. From blood to breath: new horizons for esophageal cancer biomarkers. World J Gastroenterol 2016;22(46):10077–83.
67. Kumar S, Huang J, Abbassi-Ghadi N, et al. Mass spectrometric analysis of exhaled breath for the identification of volatile organic compound biomarkers in esophageal and gastric adenocarcinoma. Ann Surg 2015;262(6):981–90.
68. Koslowsky B, Jacob H, Eliakim R, et al. PillCam ESO in esophageal studies: improved diagnostic yield of 14 frames per second (fps) compared with 4 fps. Endoscopy 2006;38(1):27–30.
69. Lin OS, Schembre DB, Mergener K, et al. Blinded comparison of esophageal capsule endoscopy versus conventional endoscopy for a diagnosis of Barrett's esophagus in patients with chronic gastroesophageal reflux. Gastrointest Endosc 2007;65(4):577–83.
70. Sharma P, Wani S, Rastogi A, et al. The diagnostic accuracy of esophageal capsule endoscopy in patients with gastroesophageal reflux disease and Barrett's esophagus: a blinded, prospective study. Am J Gastroenterol 2008; 103(3):525–32.
71. Gralnek IM, Adler SN, Yassin K, et al. Detecting esophageal disease with second-generation capsule endoscopy: initial evaluation of the PillCam ESO 2. Endoscopy 2008;40(04):275–9.
72. Delvaux M, Papanikolaou IS, Fassler I, et al. Esophageal capsule endoscopy in patients with suspected esophageal disease: double blinded comparison with esophagogastroduodenoscopy and assessment of interobserver variability. Endoscopy 2008;40(01):16–22.

Effectiveness and Cost-Effectiveness of Endoscopic Screening and Surveillance

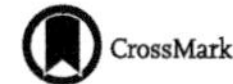

Nina Saxena, MD, John M. Inadomi, MD*

KEYWORDS

- Mass screening • Endoscopy • Surveillance • Cost-effectiveness
- Barrett's esophagus • Esophageal adenocarcinoma

KEY POINTS

- Although there are no prospective trials confirming the effectiveness of endoscopic screening and surveillance to reduce mortality from esophageal adenocarcinoma, retrospective data suggest that individuals at elevated risk may benefit from endoscopy.
- Studies published to date rely on data generated before widespread use of endoscopic radiofrequency ablation; therefore, the impact of endoscopic treatment in the context of screening and surveillance is unknown.
- Endoscopic eradication therapy in individuals with Barrett's esophagus and high-grade dysplasia is cost-effective compared with surveillance or no screening.
- Endoscopic eradication therapy in individuals with Barrett's esophagus without dysplasia is not a cost-effective intervention compared with surveillance.
- Endoscopic eradication therapy in individuals with Barrett's esophagus and low-grade dysplasia may be cost-effective compared with surveillance but this depends on the accuracy of the histopathologic diagnosis of dysplasia.

INTRODUCTION

Over the past several decades, the incidence of esophageal adenocarcinoma in the United States has been increasing and long-term survival remains poor.[1,2] Barrett's esophagus is a highly prevalent, premalignant condition that can progress in certain individuals to esophageal adenocarcinoma. Screening is the mechanism through which populations may be assessed to identify individuals who have a disease or preclinical condition that predisposes to disease. Surveillance is the program though which these at-risk individuals are periodically examined to identify disease at a stage

Division of Gastroenterology, Department of Medicine, University of Washington School of Medicine, 1959 Northeast Pacific Street, Box 356424, Seattle, WA 98195, USA
* Corresponding author.
E-mail address: jinadomi@medicine.washington.edu

Gastrointest Endoscopy Clin N Am 27 (2017) 397–421
http://dx.doi.org/10.1016/j.giec.2017.02.005
1052-5157/17/Published by Elsevier Inc.

amenable to cure. National guidelines suggest screening in selected populations with surveillance among individuals who have been diagnosed with Barrett's esophagus.[3,4]

The evidence to support screening and surveillance endoscopy, however, is variable and based on retrospective cohort and case-control studies. Moreover, the separation of effects between screening and surveillance are not possible to discern in these studies because of the limitations of the databases in which these studies were conducted. This article reviews the current evidence examining the effectiveness of prior endoscopy, for either screening or surveillance, to reduce mortality from esophageal adenocarcinoma. With the limitations of effectiveness studies in mind, this article also summarizes studies that have estimated the potential cost-effectiveness of screening and surveillance programs.

The ideal study to assess the effectiveness of endoscopic screening and surveillance would be a clinical trial of subjects who did not know whether they had Barrett's esophagus and randomizing them to undergo screening upper endoscopy to identify those with Barrett's esophagus compared with no endoscopic screening. Surveillance endoscopy would be performed in subjects with Barrett's esophagus at intervals based on whether dysplasia was present and endoscopic eradication therapy would be performed for subjects diagnosed with dysplasia or intramucosal cancer, reserving esophagectomy for subjects with more extensive malignancy. The primary outcome of this study would be comparison of cancer mortality with secondary endpoints of cancer incidence, stage, and overall mortality. This study would provide high-quality evidence to support the clinical practice of endoscopic screening with surveillance to reduce mortality from esophageal adenocarcinoma. Such a study, however, would require thousands of participants and decades of follow-up because cancer occurs only in 0.1% to 0.5% annually among patients with Barrett's esophagus.

THE EFFECTIVENESS OF ENDOSCOPIC SCREENING AND SURVEILLANCE TO REDUCE MORTALITY FROM ESOPHAGEAL ADENOCARCINOMA

The current state of knowledge of the effectiveness of endoscopic screening and surveillance to reduce cancer mortality is limited to retrospective studies such as case-control and cohort studies. Case-control studies compare subjects who died of esophageal adenocarcinoma with controls who either did not have esophageal adenocarcinoma or who had esophageal adenocarcinoma but did not die of cancer. Both study types look back in time to determine which subjects received endoscopy and calculate an odds ratio (OR), which represents the odds of having received endoscopy among cases compared with controls. The OR is often a difficult concept to grasp because it does not directly express the reduction in risk achieved with endoscopic surveillance. However, the prevalence of cancer is not known in a case-control study and is set by the investigators by assigning the proportion of cases to controls and, for this reason, the risk reduction cannot be calculated. It should be noted, however, that when the incidence of disease is low (eg, 1% or lower) the OR approximates the risk ratio and one can generally infer that the result is equivalent to the cancer reduction achieved with endoscopic screening and surveillance.

The other type of study design that has been used to estimate the effectiveness of endoscopic screening and surveillance is the retrospective cohort study. This design can identify a cohort of subjects who had Barrett's esophagus or were at risk for developing Barrett's esophagus and determine their cancer incidence and mortality over a period of time. Alternatively, one can identify a cohort of subjects with esophageal adenocarcinoma and compare those who died of cancer with those who did not die of cancer. Subjects who received endoscopy can be compared with those who did not receive endoscopy and a hazard ratio, or the chance of cancer mortality among subjects who had undergone endoscopy divided by the chance of cancer mortality among subjects who had not undergone endoscopy. The advantage of the cohort study compared with a case-control study is that the incidence of cancer is known so a risk ratio can be calculated. The disadvantage is that assembly of a cohort may be difficult because not all information may be available, follow-up may be incomplete, and there may be a large proportion of subjects who drop out.

In all retrospective studies there is a considerable risk of bias, which usually falsely increases the apparent benefit of an intervention. There is almost certainly a presence of selection bias of individuals who receive endoscopy. They are generally healthier and, therefore, more likely to survive than individuals who do not receive endoscopy. There is lead-time bias, which is the detection of asymptomatic, preclinical cancer by endoscopy, which may only increase the detection time of individuals with cancer without truly increasing life-years. Finally, length-time bias occurs when slowly growing cancers are more likely detected during endoscopy than rapidly growing cancers, which artificially creates the appearance that endoscopic screening and surveillance prolongs survival.

Investigators can mitigate the impact of bias but they do not eliminate the possibility that conclusions may be based on confounded analyses due to problems such as lead-time or length-time bias. There are statistical techniques that can be used to adjust for these problems, including propensity scores and instrumental variable analysis. When a randomized clinical trial is not performed, a propensity score may be developed in the attempt to determine the likelihood that an individual would receive endoscopy, which can be used to identify and adjust for selection bias. Similarly, an instrumental variable analysis estimates the likelihood that an individual receives endoscopy and may identify and adjust for unmeasured confounders that influence the observed effect of endoscopy. Dose-effects can be examined to see whether increased exposure to endoscopy increases its effectiveness, which raises the confidence that endoscopy is the cause of improved outcomes.

STUDIES OF THE EFFECTIVENESS OF ENDOSCOPIC SCREENING OR SURVEILLANCE

The authors conducted a systematic review of English-language publications in PubMed from August 2001 through August 2016 with the following Medical Subject Headings (MeSH) search terms to retrieve studies of the effectiveness of endoscopy to reduce mortality from esophageal adenocarcinoma: Barrett's esophagus, esophageal cancer, screening, surveillance, and endoscopy. Literature was limited to human research, clinical studies and English language (US and English spelling of terms were examined). This search retrieved 8405 article titles, of which 51 reported either the incidence or mortality from esophageal adenocarcinoma. Thirty-seven were excluded because they lacked a comparison group of individuals not undergoing endoscopic surveillance or did not report the difference in mortality from esophageal adenocarcinoma. Fourteen studies examined whether prior endoscopy reduced mortality from esophageal adenocarcinoma and are summarized in **Table 1**. Note that most studies included adenocarcinoma of the gastric cardia or esophagogastric junction because these were difficult to separate from esophageal adenocarcinoma. Importantly, all studies were retrospective and most used administrative or billing data that could not differentiate between a screening and surveillance endoscopy; for this reason the term surveillance will be used in the remainder of this article to designate the performance of an upper endoscopy before the diagnosis of cancer.

Table 1
Effectiveness of endoscopic screening and surveillance to reduce mortality from esophageal adenocarcinoma

Author, Year	Design	Population	Surveillance Definition	Outcome	Cancer Mortality (95% CI)
Kastelein et al,[15] 2016	Cohort	EAC only[a]	EGD for surveillance	HR	0.8 (0.3–1.8) stage 0 EAC; HR 0.7 (0.4–1.2) stage 1 EAC; neither significant
Royston et al,[75] 2016	Cohort	BE (with or without intestinal metaplasia)	EGD for surveillance	HR	0.64 (0.30–1.48) not significant
Bhat et al,[14] 2015	Cohort	EAC only	BE diagnosis >6 mo before cancer	HR	0.39 (0.27–0.58)
Verbeek et al,[13] 2014	Cohort	EAC only	EGD for surveillance	HR	0.79 (0.64–0.92)
Corley et al,[16] 2013	Case-Control	Cases: EAC or EGJ cancer death; controls: BE	EGD for surveillance $\leq$3 y before cancer	OR	0.99 (0.36–2.75) no improved survival
Cooper et al,[12] 2009	Cohort	EAC only	EGD or BE diagnosis 6 mo–3 y before cancer	HR	EGD 0.66 (0.47–0.93); BE 0.0.45 (0.25–0.80)
Rubenstein et al,[17] 2008	Cohort	EAC or gastric cardia adenocarcinoma	EGD 1–5 y before cancer	HR	0.93 (0.58–1.50) no improved survival
Kearney et al,[11] 2003	Case-control	Cases: EAC or gastric cardia cancer death; controls: GERD	EGD $\geq$1 y before cancer	OR	0.66 (0.45–0.96)
Cooper et al,[9] 2002	Cohort	EAC or gastric cardia adenocarcinoma (separate)	EGD $\geq$1 y before cancer	HR	EAC 0.73 (0.57–0.93); cardia not significant
Corley et al,[10] 2002	Cohort	EAC or gastric cardia adenocarcinoma	EGD for surveillance	HR	0.2 (0.1–0.7)
Incarbone et al,[7] 2002	Cohort	EAC only	EGD for surveillance	Median survival	48 mo vs 24 mo (P<.01)
Ferguson & Durkin,[8] 2002	Cohort	EAC only	EGD	Median survival	107 mo vs 12 mo (P<.001)
van Sandick et al,[6] 1998	Cohort	EAC or EGJ adenocarcinoma	BE diagnosis $\geq$6 mo before cancer	Cancer mortality	85.9% vs 43.3% log rank P = .0029 (significantly better)
Peters et al,[5] 1994	Cohort	EAC cardia not specified	EGD	Cancer mortality	chi2 5.8 (significantly better)

Abbreviations: BE, Barrett's esophagus; EAC, esophageal adenocarcinoma; EGD, esophagogastroduodenoscopy; EGJ, esophagogastric junction; GERD, gastroesophageal reflux disease; HR, hazards ratio; OR, odds ratio.

[a] Comparison between observed and expected survival.

Two studies conducted in the 1990s exemplified the retrospective cohort analysis that has been the predominant form of study design used to examine the benefit of endoscopic surveillance.[5,6] Both concluded that endoscopic surveillance successfully reduced mortality from esophageal adenocarcinoma. Studies published in 2002 also used a retrospective cohort study design to demonstrate that subjects with esophageal adenocarcinoma who had received prior endoscopy had significantly better median survival than subjects with esophageal adenocarcinoma not receiving prior endoscopy.[7,8]

More recent studies of this topic have reported either hazards ratios (HRs) (for cohort studies) or ORs (for case-control studies) when comparing surveillance effects on esophageal adenocarcinoma mortality. Cooper and colleagues[9] reported that in a cohort of subjects diagnosed with esophageal adenocarcinoma, those who had undergone surveillance, defined as receipt of an upper endoscopy 1 year or more before the diagnosis of cancer, had a 27% reduction in mortality compared with subjects with esophageal adenocarcinoma who had not undergone surveillance (HR 0.73, 95% CI 0.57–0.93). Corley and colleagues[10] reported an impressive 80% reduction in cancer mortality (HR 0.2, 95% CI 0.1–0.7) among subjects with esophageal adenocarcinoma who had undergone endoscopic surveillance compared with subjects with esophageal adenocarcinoma who had not received surveillance. Kearney and colleagues[11] conducted a case-control study of subjects with gastroesophageal reflux comparing cases who had died of esophageal adenocarcinoma with controls who did not die of esophageal adenocarcinoma and reported a 34% reduction in cancer mortality (adjusted OR 0.66, 95% CI 0.45, 0.96) among individuals who had received an upper endoscopy greater than 1 year before the esophageal adenocarcinoma diagnosis.

Cooper and colleagues[12] conducted a second cohort study of subjects with esophageal adenocarcinoma but defined surveillance by an administrative code that identified a diagnosis of Barrett's esophagus 6 months to 3 years before esophageal adenocarcinoma instead of receipt of endoscopy. This could potentially reduce the bias of endoscopy performed for symptoms of cancer or for persistent symptoms and limit the surveillance group to a more select population who were recognized as being at higher risk for development of esophageal adenocarcinoma. The hazard of death was reduced by 55% compared with subjects who developed esophageal adenocarcinoma without a prior diagnosis of Barrett's esophagus.

Subsequent studies have largely demonstrated an improvement in survival among subjects with cancer who received endoscopic surveillance. Verbeek and colleagues[13] demonstrated a 21% cancer mortality reduction in a cohort of Dutch esophageal adenocarcinoma subjects who were diagnosed with Barrett's esophagus and underwent adequate surveillance compared with those who did not receive surveillance. Bhat and colleagues[14] reported a diagnosis of Barrett's esophagus before the diagnosis of cancer to be protective against cancer death (HR 0.39, 95% CI 0.27–0.58).

In contrast to most studies that report a survival advantage among subjects who undergo surveillance endoscopy, there are a few studies that failed to demonstrate a benefit. Kastelein and colleagues[15] reported a 20% reduction in cancer mortality among a cohort of subjects with Barrett's esophagus followed for a median of 7 years compared with national statistics of cancer survival; however, this was not statistically significant. Corley and colleagues[16] performed a case-control study using the same (Kaiser) database as their previous cohort study to compare subjects with Barrett's esophagus who died of esophageal adenocarcinoma with controls with Barrett's esophagus who did not die of esophageal adenocarcinoma. In contrast to the positive results of their cohort study, they reported that receipt of surveillance endoscopy performed within 3 years before the diagnosis of esophageal adenocarcinoma was not associated with improved cancer survival (OR 0.99, 95% CI 0.36–2.75). Cases were less likely to have received surveillance endoscopy and cancer stage was earlier but these findings were not statistically significant. However, despite the large dataset, the actual sample of subjects on which the analyses were based was small, which produced a large confidence interval. In addition, the study data were generated before the widespread use of endoscopic radiofrequency ablation (RFA) to treat dysplasia in Barrett's esophagus.

Rubenstein and colleagues[17] conducted a retrospective controlled cohort study of gastroesophageal reflux disease subjects with esophageal adenocarcinoma and identified those who received endoscopy 1 to 5 years before the diagnosis of cancer (excluding endoscopy within the year before cancer diagnosis that may have been performed for cancer symptoms). They had among of the longest follow-up periods and, perhaps because of this, their findings (HR 0.93, 95% CI 0.58–1.50) failed to demonstrate an improvement in survival with endoscopic surveillance. Importantly, they were able to demonstrate that use of a shorter follow-up period (5 years) was associated with significant mortality reduction with endoscopic surveillance, possibly revealing lead-time bias in other studies with shorter follow-up. The take-home message from that study could be that longer follow-up may reduce or eliminate the observed benefit from endoscopic surveillance that may be a result of lead-time bias.

There are several limitations of the published literature examining the effectiveness of endoscopic screening and surveillance on cancer mortality that may explain the discrepancies between published studies. The main limitation regarding the lack of randomized clinical trials has already been highlighted. Another important limitation is that the data used in all published analyses were collected before the widespread use of RFA to treat subjects with dysplasia and Barrett's esophagus.[18–20] Photodynamic therapy (PDT) may have been available but limited mainly to academic or large referral centers.[21,22] Before endoscopic eradication therapy, the role of surveillance was mainly to identify subjects with cancer in whom esophagectomy could be performed in the hopes of curing cancer. It is hoped that future cohort and case-control studies will be able to detect significant reduction in cancer incidence and improvements in cancer survival when endoscopic screening and surveillance is coupled with endoscopic eradication therapy using mucosal resection and RFA.

COST-EFFECTIVENESS OF SCREENING AND SURVEILLANCE

Medical decision analysis is a process that allows 2 or more competing medical management theories to be quantitatively compared using probability theory. A cost-effectiveness analysis (CEA) includes the costs of these strategies to identify the most beneficial strategy in a resource-limited environment. Previous guidelines for the conduct of CEA have been published.[23–25] The purpose of this article is to present the cost-effectiveness analyses involving the screening, surveillance, and management of Barrett's esophagus.

COST-EFFECTIVENESS ANALYSIS: DEFINITIONS

Costs

Costs in a CEA represent the resources forgone by society to provide medical care, and differ from charges, which often vary from costs based on profit structures, the bargaining power of payers and providers, and accounting inaccuracies. Costs can be direct or indirect. Direct costs include both the direct health and non–health care costs associated with an intervention.[24,26] In the case of Barrett's esophagus, for example, direct medical costs may include the costs of an endoscopy, pathologic evaluation, medications, and the use of medical facilities. Direct non–health care costs may include the cost of transportation to an appointment or the cost of childcare. In addition, some studies may also report indirect costs, which are costs incurred from lost productivity, such as the lost wages incurred from a day of work that was missed for an endoscopy, or lost productivity from death.[26,27] Most of the included studies focus on direct health care costs, based on data regarding reimbursements from the Center for Medicare and Medicaid Services.

Incremental Cost-Effectiveness Ratio

The purpose of cost-effectiveness analyses is to compare the outcomes and costs of competing medical management strategies. As such, they must use metrics that can be easily quantified and compared. Both the absolute costs and the outcomes, reported frequently in total life-years or quality-adjusted life-years (QALYs), should be reported in a CEA. If a strategy is both less costly and has improved outcomes over another, then this is defined as a dominant strategy. More often, however, a strategy with an improved outcome will also incur a greater cost. These strategies can be compared by using the incremental cost-effectiveness ratio, which is the difference in cost divided by the difference in outcomes.[27]

Previous studies have suggested that society is willing to pay between $50,000 and $100,000 per QALY in the United States. This threshold is called the willingness-to-pay (WTP) threshold, and is based largely on historical norm because this was described as the cost per life year gained from performing hemodialysis on patients with renal failure.[24]

Discounting

Discounting reflects a preference toward possessing money, goods, and services in the present rather than in the future. This concept allows the model to account for the opportunity cost lost by spending money in the present to derive future benefit and generally reflects the amount of money that would have been gained had the funds spent on a medical intervention been invested instead. Discounting also applies to the time preferences patients have for health benefits; although delaying care may be cost-effective, patients will prefer to have excellent health earlier rather than postponing this to a future date. In most studies, the discount rate was between 3% and 5% (see later discussion).[26]

Utilities

Utilities allow for patient preferences of certain health states to be quantified and thereby incorporated into a CEA. Most models define perfect health as a 1, and death as a 0. The morbidity associated with different health states can be translated into a numeric value to thereby weight the outcomes. For example, symptomatic esophageal adenocarcinoma is often given a utility of 0.5.[24–26]

Sensitivity Analysis

Economic models require assumptions regarding the input values of various variables used in the model (parameter assumptions) and the manner in which variables are associated (structural assumptions). Uncertainty inherently exists within these assumptions and can affect the results of a CEA. Sensitivity analyses can examine the degree of uncertainty by varying the input models within reasonable clinical bounds to assess for significant changes in outcome. A 1-way sensitivity outcome alters a single variable at a time. In the example of Barrett's esophagus, this may involve decreasing the prevalence of Barrett's esophagus in a population with gastroesophageal reflux disease to assess whether screening remains cost-effective. A multivariable sensitivity analysis alters many variables simultaneously, the most common of which is the Monte Carlo simulation in which each variable is represented by a probability distribution. The simulation is run multiple times, for which different values are selected from these distributions at random. A model with a low degree of uncertainty will have the same outcome despite these changes in inputs.[26]

STUDIES OF THE COST-EFFECTIVENESS OF SCREENING AND SURVEILLANCE TO REDUCE MORTALITY FROM ESOPHAGEAL ADENOCARCINOMA

The authors conducted a systematic review of English-language publications from August 2001 through August 2016, using a PubMed MeSH search with the following terms: Barrett's esophagus, esophageal neoplasms diagnosis, health care economics, and organizations. Journal articles were included if they quantified both the costs and the effectiveness of a surveillance strategy, with effectiveness measured in either life-years or QALYs gained.

ENDOSCOPIC SCREENING BEFORE THE AVAILABILITY OF ENDOSCOPIC RADIOFREQUENCY ABLATION

As shown in **Table 2**, 9 studies have been published assessing the cost-effectiveness of screening the population for Barrett's esophagus.[28–36] Of the 9 screening studies, 6 were published before the advent of endoscopic ablation.[31–36] All were Markov simulations and in 5 the screening population consisted of 50-year-old men with gastroesophageal reflux, as recommended by the American College of Gastroenterology guidelines.[3] One study analyzed a subject population of 50-year-old subjects of either sex with chronic gastroesophageal reflux disease.[35]

All studies found endoscopic screening and surveillance of subjects with gastroesophageal reflux disease to be cost-effective if the WTP threshold was less than $100,000, meaning that society would be willing to pay up to $100,000 for each QALY gained.[31–36] Of these, 2 simulated esophagectomy for high-grade dysplasia (HGD),[31,35] 3 simulated surveillance for HGD,[33,34,36] and 1 compared both strategies.[32] Five of these studies showed a cost-effectiveness that was generally between $4000 and $15,000 per QALY gained, whereas Nietert and colleagues[35] calculated a higher cost-effectiveness of $87,000 per QALY, although it is worth noting that they used a lower Barrett's esophagus prevalence and a lower esophageal adenocarcinoma incidence than other studies. When these factors were adjusted to values used in other studies in their sensitivity analyses, the cost-effectiveness decreased below $50,000 per QALY gained.

ENDOSCOPIC SURVEILLANCE BEFORE THE AVAILABILITY OF ENDOSCOPIC RADIOFREQUENCY ABLATION

Two studies discussed not only screening but also the cost-effectiveness of various surveillance schedules. Inadomi and colleagues[33] examined the cost-effectiveness of endoscopically screening 50-year-old white men with gastroesophageal reflux disease symptoms with surveillance in those diagnosed with Barrett's esophagus. Within this model, subjects found to have HGD were managed with intense surveillance every 3 months, with an esophagectomy if cancer was discovered. Screening in this population was found to be cost-effective; however, the incremental cost of surveillance for subjects with Barrett's esophagus without dysplasia at 5-year intervals was almost

Table 2
Cost-effectiveness of screening to reduce mortality from esophageal adenocarcinoma

Author, Year	Population	Strategies	HGD Treatment	Health-Adjusted Life Expectancy	Cost	Cost-effectiveness	Most Cost-Effective if WTP <$100K
Benaglia et al,[30] 2013	50-y-o men with GERD	No screening	—	67.964	$132	Base case	Cytosponge with RFA/EMR for HGD
		Cytosponge	RFA/EMR	67.979	$373	$15,724	
		Endoscopy	RFA/EMR	67.977	$431	$22,167	
		UTE if 50% endoscopy cost	RFA/EMR	69.973	$319	$19,134	
		if 75% cost	RFA/EMR	69.973	$364	$23,767	
		if 100% cost	RFA/EMR	69.973	$409	$28,401	
		Cytosponge	Esophagectomy	67.973	$380	$26,004	
		Endoscopy	Esophagectomy	67.972	$437	$36,462	
Gupta et al,[28] 2011	50-y-o subjects undergoing screening colonoscopy	No screening	—	68.0789	$480	Base case	No screening
		Screening only	RFA/EMR	68.0828	$933.00	$115,664	
		Screening and surveillance	RFA/EMR	68.0849	$957.00	$79,882	
Gerson et al,[31] 2007[a]	50-y-o men with GERD	No screening	—	68.3	$901	Base case	Screening with EGD
		Screening with ECE	Esophagectomy	68.36	$2392	$24,850	
		Screening with EGD	Esophagectomy	68.54	$1988	$4530	
Rubenstein et al,[34] 2007	50-y-o white men with GERD	No screening	—	66.47	$102	Base case	Screening with EGD
		Screening with EGD	Surveillance	66.66	$2304	$11,245	
		Screening ECE	Surveillance	66.64	$2348	$13,208	
Rubenstein & Inadomi,[36] 2006	50-y-o white men with GERD	No screening	—	66.466	$104	Base case	Screening and surveillance
		Screening and surveillance	Surveillance	66.637	$2443	$13,721	
Rubenstein et al,[29] 2005	50-y-o white men with GERD	No screening	—	66.466	$104	Base case	Biomarker-guided esophagectomy
		Dysplasia-guided surveillance	Surveillance	66.637	$2444	$14,211	
		Biomarker-guided surveillance	Surveillance	66.691	$2536	$10,809	
		Biomarker-guided esophagectomy	—	66.707	$2291	$9055	

(*continued on next page*)

Table 2
(continued)

Author, Year	Population	Strategies	HGD Treatment	Health-Adjusted Life Expectancy	Cost	Cost-effectiveness	Most Cost-Effective if WTP <$100K
Gerson et al,[32] 2004[a]	50-y-o men with GERD	No screening, esophagectomy and endoscopic therapy for cancer	—	68.16	$655	Base case	Surveillance of dysplastic and nondysplastic BE, with esophagectomy and endoscopic therapy for HGD
		Surveillance of nondysplastic and dysplastic BE	Surveillance	68.25	$1890	$13,722	
		Surveillance of nondysplastic and dysplastic BE	Esophagectomy	68.21	$1883	$24,560	
		Surveillance of nondysplastic and dysplastic BE	Esophagectomy and endoscopic therapy	68.27	$1920	$11,500	
		Surveillance of dysplastic BE only	Surveillance	68.21	$1614	$19,180	
		Surveillance of dysplastic BE only	Esophagectomy and Endoscopic therapy	68.21	$1623	$19,360	
Nietert et al,[35] 2003	50-y-o subjects with GERD	No screening	—	69.3266	$11,785	—	UTE
		UTE	Esophagectomy	69.3326	$12,119	$55,764	
		Standard endoscopy	Esophagectomy	69.3329	$12,332	$86,883	
Inadomi et al,[33] 2003	50-y-o white men with GERD	No screening	—	66.466	$104	—	Screening with surveillance of dysplasia only
		Surveillance of dysplastic BE only	Surveillance	66.624	$1748	$10,440	
		Surveillance of dysplastic BE and ND BE at various intervals	—	—	—	—	
		q5 y	Surveillance	66.624	$2053	$12,336	
		q4 y	Surveillance	66.624	$2153	$12,946	
		q3 y	Surveillance	66.625	$2309	$13,894	
		q2 y	Surveillance	66.626	$2587	$15,579	

Health-adjusted life expectancy: discounted health-adjusted life expectancies from the starting age of each cohort.

Cost-effectiveness: incremental cost as compared with base cost, obtained from each study or calculated based on information given.

All costs are given as they were presented in the study and have not been adjusted based on inflation.

Abbreviations: ECE, esophageal capsule endoscopy; EMR, endoscopic mucosal resection; HGD, high-grade dysplasia; UTE, ultrathin endoscopy.

[a] Outcomes in life-years instead of QALYs.

$600,000 per QALY gained compared with limiting surveillance to those subjects with dysplasia. Small changes to the assumptions within the model, such the cancer incidence, the rates of progression from HGD to cancer, the prevalence of Barrett's esophagus in gastroesophageal reflux disease, and the utility state associated with esophagectomy could increase the incremental cost per QALY, although these almost always stayed below the $50,000 per QALY benchmark. The investigators concluded that screening high-risk individuals to detect Barrett's esophagus with neoplasia could be cost-effective but, because the development of esophageal adenocarcinoma is fairly rare in patients with nondysplastic Barrett's esophagus, the costs of surveillance endoscopies are likely of limited additional value in that population.

In contrast, Gerson and colleagues[32] concluded that surveillance of patients with Barrett's esophagus even in the absence of dysplasia was cost-effective. Several differences between the 2 models can help explain these differences. Gerson and colleagues[32] assumed higher rates of progression from nondysplastic Barrett's esophagus and low-grade dysplasia (LGD) to cancer. They defined outcomes based on life-years and did not incorporate subject preferences for health states or utilities that could otherwise address the decrease in quality of life experiences after an esophagectomy.[33]

Two other studies evaluated surveillance of subjects diagnosed with Barrett's esophagus before the availability of endoscopic ablation (**Table 3**). Sonnenberg and colleagues[37] compared no surveillance with a schedule of endoscopy every 2 years for all subjects with Barrett's esophagus with esophagectomy for HGD and found that surveillance was cost-effective. In contrast to these findings, Garside and colleagues[38] evaluated the cost-effectiveness of surveillance in the United Kingdom and reported that surveillance of nondysplastic Barrett's esophagus every 3 years, LGD every year, and HGD every 3 months was both more costly and less effective than a strategy of no surveillance. It is worth noting that the study differed from others in that they assigned a significant decrease in quality of life for subjects with Barrett's esophagus, assuming that these subjects also suffered from severe gastroesophageal reflux disease. It is also relevant that the study was conducted in the United Kingdom with costs in 2004 pounds, which may be difficult to extrapolate to a US model of care delivery.

OTHER SCREENING MODALITIES

Ultrathin Endoscopy

As previously described, the direct costs of endoscopic examinations in a screening and surveillance program can be fairly high. However, these examinations also require sedation, which can result in indirect costs from lost wages of both the patient and the driver and discourage patients from seeking the necessary care. Therefore, several alternative modalities of screening have been explored in an effort to reduce the costs of care. Nietert and colleagues[35] analyzed the cost-effectiveness of ultrathin endoscopy (UTE), which uses an ultrathin, 3.1 mm diameter scope that can be passed into the esophagus without sedation, although with some loss of optical quality and the inability to obtain biopsies. A strategy of no screening was compared with screening with standard endoscopy or with UTE. Those in the UTE arm who were identified as having a columnar-lined esophagus would then undergo standard endoscopy to confirm the presence of Barrett's esophagus. They concluded that UTE was more cost-effective than standard endoscopy within a plausible range of costs of UTE.

These results contrast with a study by Benaglia and colleagues[30] who reported that unless UTE was 50% or less than the cost of standard endoscopy it was unlikely to be

Table 3
Cost-effectiveness of endoscopic surveillance without endoscopic therapy

Author, Year	Population	Strategies	HGD Treatment	Health-Adjusted Life Expectancy	Cost	Cost-effectiveness	Most Cost-Effective at WTP <$100K
Garside et al,[38] 2006[a]	55-y-o men with BE	No surveillance	None	67.03	£2.951	Dominant	No surveillance
		Surveillance	None	66.98	£3.869	—	
Sonnenberg et al,[37] 2002[b]	60-y-o subjects with BE	No surveillance	None	0.263	$7829	—	Surveillance q2 y
		Surveillance q2 y	Esophagectomy	0.511	$12,257	$16,965/life-years saved	

Health-adjusted life expectancy: discounted health-adjusted life expectancies from the starting age of each cohort.
Cost-effectiveness: incremental cost as compared with base cost, obtained from each study or calculated based on information given.
All costs are given as they were presented in the study and have not been adjusted based on inflation.
[a] UK health technology assessment.
[b] Outcomes in life-years saved through prevention of death from EAC.

cost-effective. This study accounted for lost wages associated with anesthesia, which should have biased the model toward UTE over standard endoscopy. Countering this effect, however, Nietert and colleagues[35] used a lower incidence of Barrett's esophagus and cancer than other studies that would have led to fewer standard endoscopies following UTE.

Esophageal Capsule Endoscopy

Esophageal capsule endoscopy (ECE), which uses a wireless pill-sized capsule, has also been evaluated as a potential means of screening. Unlike standard endoscopy, ECE can be conducted in less than 30 minutes in an office setting. Those patients with the visual appearance of columnar mucosa by ECE can then undergo standard endoscopy with biopsy. Both Rubenstein and colleagues[34] and Gerson and Lin[31] evaluated the cost-effectiveness of ECE compared with strategies of no surveillance and standard endoscopy, accounting for both direct costs and for lost wages that would be incurred from esophagogastroduodenoscopy (EGD) with sedation. In each study, given the decreased sensitivity of ECE compared with standard endoscopy and the fairly high cost of ECE, standard endoscopy was found to have both improved outcomes and lower cost compared with ECE, making EGD the dominant strategy.

Markers of Cancer

The difficulty in developing a cost-effective strategy for esophageal adenocarcinoma screening is that only a very small minority of patients with Barrett's esophagus will ever develop esophageal adenocarcinoma, with estimations of annual incidence ranging between 0.12% and 0.63%.[39–42] Most patients with Barrett's esophagus ultimately die of causes other than esophageal adenocarcinoma,[42] calling into question the cost-effectiveness of ongoing surveillance endoscopy. Current methods of screening and surveillance rely on the presence of dysplasia as a marker of higher risk; however, the interobserver variability for interpreting dysplasia is high, and dysplasia itself frequently regresses back to a nondysplastic state.[43–45]

Therefore, the effectiveness and cost-effectiveness of screening could be greatly improved with the use of a more sensitive and specific biomarker than dysplasia that could accurately recognize those patients who are likely to develop esophageal adenocarcinoma, ideally even in the absence of gastroesophageal reflux disease symptoms.[46] Rubenstein and colleagues[29] evaluated the cost-effectiveness of biomarker-based surveillance and biomarker-guided esophagectomy and found that if a biomarker had greater than 95% specificity, biomarker-guided esophagectomy was the most cost-effective strategy. For biomarker-guided surveillance to be cost-effective, the test would need to be 80% sensitive and specific with a cost of $100.

Multiple studies have reported particular genetic biomarkers with associations between the development of esophageal adenocarcinoma, including p16,[47] DNA methylation,[48–50] tumor suppressor gene p53,[51] and aneuploidy or abnormal tetraploidy.[52,53] A study by Galipeau and colleagues[54] found that using a combination of 17p loss of heterozygosity, 9p loss of heterozygosity, and DNA content tetraploidy and aneuploidy could allow for better prediction of esophageal adenocarcinoma development than the use of any single marker. Subsequently, Gordon and colleagues[55] compared strategies of no surveillance, endoscopic surveillance, and a hypothetical biomarker-based surveillance with biomarker-positivity defined as the presence 3 of these abnormalities. This panel was assumed to predict the progression from Barrett's esophagus to esophageal adenocarcinoma with 40.7% sensitivity and

98.0% specificity. The investigators concluded that biomarker-based surveillance could be more cost-effective than standard endoscopic surveillance alone.

There has also been growing interest in the cytosponge, an ingestible gelatin capsule comprised of compressed mesh attached to a string. The capsule is swallowed and retrieved, allowing for cytologic sampling of the esophagus. Using analysis for trefoil factor 3, an immunohistochemical marker for Barrett's esophagus, the test has a sensitivity of 73.35% and specificity of 93.8% for Barrett's esophagus.[56] A microsimulation study performed by Benaglia and colleagues[30] showed that cytosponge screening followed by endoscopic mucosal resection (EMR) and RFA for HGD was the most cost-effective strategy, with a cost of $15,000 per QALY gained compared with no screening, which was less than the $22,000 per QALY gained by screening with standard endoscopy.

ENDOSCOPIC ABLATION FOR HIGH-GRADE DYSPLASIA

Photodynamic Therapy

Four studies have assessed the cost-effectiveness of PDT for the management of HGD compared with surveillance strategies or esophagectomy (**Table 4**).[57–60] In all studies, PDT was cost-effective, with cost-effective ratios of between $12,000 and $47,000 per QALY. Discrepancies between studies largely correlated with whether or not the model accounted for the possibility of recurrent dysplasia and malignancy in subject who have successfully undergone PDT. The models were sensitive to assumptions regarding the effectiveness of PDT; however, even when the parameters were altered to allow for lower rates of success with PDT, it remained a cost-effective alternative to surveillance and esophagectomy.

Radiofrequency Ablation

Over the past several years, RFA, with or without EMR for nodular dysplasia, has become the preferred method of management for HGD. RFA is less morbid than esophagectomy, has a high rate of metaplastic eradication, has low rates of dysplasia recurrence, and is now the recommended first-line therapy for HGD in national guidelines.[3,4] Six studies have examined the cost-effectiveness of RFA for HGD, comparing it to surveillance and/or esophagectomy (**Table 5**).[61–66] In all of these studies, the use of RFA with or without EMR dominated esophagectomy, in that it provided more QALYs gained at a lower cost.

Inadomi and colleagues[64] more specifically compared various ablation modalities, including RFA, PDT, and argon plasma coagulation, with strategies of surveillance or immediate esophagectomy. They found that RFA was cost-effective for subjects with Barrett's esophagus and HGD, with a cost of $5800 per QALY gained. PDT ablation allowed for slightly improved outcomes but was not cost-effective. Sensitivity analysis showed that this outcome depends on the rates of eradication of metaplasia and dysplasia with RFA, the cost of RFA, and RFA-associated complications.

MANAGEMENT OF NONDYSPLASTIC BARRETT'S ESOPHAGUS AND LOW-GRADE DYSPLASIA

Surveillance

Although the management of HGD with endoscopic eradication therapy has become accepted practice, the most cost-effective management of Barrett's esophagus with LGD is controversial (**Table 6**). Current guidelines vary in their primary recommendations for patients with LGD and surveillance every 6 to 12 months or endoscopic therapy may be considered.[3,4] However, it remains unclear as to whether these are

Table 4
Cost-effectiveness of surveillance with photodynamic therapy

Author, Year	Population	Strategies	Health-Adjusted Life Expectancy	Cost	Cost-effectiveness	Most Cost-Effective at WTP <$100K
Comay et al,[57] 2007[a]	50-y-o male with HGD	Surveillance	61.85	$17,817	Base	PDT
		PDT	67.04	$22,381	$879	
		Esophagectomy	65.85	$24,963	$1787	
Vij et al,[60] 2004	55-y-o white men with HGD	Esophagectomy	66.817	$24,045	Base	PDT followed by surveillance
		Surveillance	66.819	$28,850	$2,402,500	
		PDT followed by esophagectomy for recurrent HGD	67.243	$45,525	$50,423	
		PDT followed by surveillance for recurrent HGD	67.307	$47,300	$47,410	
Shaheen et al,[59] 2004	50-y-o white men with HGD	No surveillance	63.9	$748	Base	PDT
		Esophagectomy	64.89	$34,857	$34,454	
		Surveillance	64.96	$34,724	$32,053	
		PDT	65.51	$41,998	$25,621	
Hur et al,[58] 2003	55-y-o male with HGD	Surveillance	64.96	$27,800	Base	PDT
		Esophagectomy	64.44	$41,000	Dominated by surveillance	
		PDT	66.61	$48,000	$12,400	

Health-adjusted life expectancy: discounted health-adjusted life expectancies from the starting age of each cohort.
Cost-effectiveness: incremental cost compared with base cost obtained from each study or calculated based on information given.
All costs are given as they were presented in the study and have not been adjusted based on inflation.
[a] Costs in 2003 Canadian dollars (US $1 = CDN $1.34).

Table 5
Cost-effectiveness of surveillance with radiofrequency ablation of high-grade dysplasia

Author, Year	Population	Strategies	Health-Adjusted Life Expectancy	Cost	Cost-effectiveness	Most Cost-Effective at WTP <$100K
Hu et al,[62] 2016	65-y-o subjects with HGD	Surveillance	75.21	$66,800	Base	RFA
		Esophagectomy	76.44	$74,300	$6098	—
		RFA	76.47	$52,000	Dominant	—
Kastelein et al,[65] 2015	55-y-o male with ND BE, surveillance q5 y	None	67.62	€5.695	Base	RFA
		RFA	67.87	€7.019	€5.283	—
		Esophagectomy	67.64	€13.965	€413.500	—
	55-y-o male with LGD, surveillance q5 y	None	65.95	€21.806	Base	RFA
		RFA	66.91	€24.562	€4.922	—
		Esophagectomy	66.33	€50.909	€76.587	—
Hur et al,[63] 2012	50-y-o subjects with HD	Surveillance	66.036	$71,288	Base	RFA
		RFA	66.74	$45,679	Dominant	—
Boger et al,[61] 2010	64-y-o male with HD	Esophagectomy	77.8	£8555	Base	RFA
		RFA	78.2	£6653	Dominant	—
Pohl et al,[66] 2009	65-y-o male with early Barrett's esophageal cancer	RFA	69.88	$17,408	Dominant	RFA
		Esophagectomy	69.59	$27,830	—	—
Inadomi et al,[64] 2009	50-y-o subjects with HGD	None	62.43	$1859	Base	RFA
		RFA with surveillance	65.67	$20,776	$5839.00	—
		APC with surveillance	65.62	$22,117	$6350.47	—
		PDT with surveillance	65.67	$34,580	$10,099.07	—
		Surveillance	64.82	$48,354	$19,453.97	—
		Esophagectomy	65.02	$58,973	$22,051.74	—

Health-adjusted life expectancy: discounted health-adjusted life expectancies from the starting age of each cohort.
Cost-effectiveness: incremental cost compared with base cost, obtained from each study or calculated based on information given.
All costs are given as they were presented in the study and have not been adjusted based on inflation.
Abbreviations: APC, argon plasma coagulation; ND, nondysplastic.

Table 6
Cost-effectiveness of surveillance for nondysplastic Barrett's esophagus and low-grade dysplasia

Author, Year	Population	Strategies	HGD Treatment	Health-Adjusted Life Expectancy	Cost	Cost-effectiveness	Most Cost-Effective for WTP <$100K
Kastelein et al,[65] 2015	55-y-o men with ND BE	No surveillance	None	67.62	€5.695	Base case	ND BE: surveillance q5 y with RFA for HGD
		Surveillance:					
		q5 y	RFA	67.87	€7.019	€5.283	
		q5 y	Esophagectomy	67.64	€13.965	€413.500	
		q4 y	RFA	67.89	€7.821	€7.874	
		q3 y	RFA	67.9	€9.005	€11.821	
	55-y-o men with LGD	No surveillance	None	65.95	€21.806	Base case	If WTP €35K, then q3 y; If €80K, then q year with RFA for HGD
		Surveillance:					
		q5 y	RFA	66.91	€24.562	€4.922	
		q5 y	Esophagectomy	66.33	€50.909	€76.587	
		q4 y	RFA	66.99	€28.964	€6.883	
		q3 y	RFA	67.09	€32.071	€9.004	
		q2 y	RFA	67.19	€36.242	€11.642	
		q1 y	RFA	67.27	€42.086	€15.364	
Gordon et al,[55] 2014	50-y-o subjects with BE	No surveillance	None	62.04	$5226	Base case	No surveillance
		Surveillance q2 y for ND BE and q6 mo for BE with LGD	RFA	62.19	$14,659	$60,858	
Hur et al,[63] 2012	50-y-o subjects with LGD	Surveillance	Surveillance	66.709	$33,963	Base case	Initial RFA
		Surveillance	RFA	66.879	$26,517	Dominated surveillance	
		Initial RFA for LGD	N/A	66.987	$28,486	$18,231 as compared with surveillance with RFA for HGD	
	50-y-o subjects with ND BE	Surveillance	Surveillance	66.873	$19,315	Base case	Surveillance with RFA for HGD
		Surveillance	RFA	66.932	$16,435	Dominated surveillance	
		Initial RFA	—	66.996	$24,422	$41,520	

(*continued on next page*)

Table 6
(continued)

Author, Year	Population	Strategies	HGD Treatment	Health-Adjusted Life Expectancy	Cost	Cost-effectiveness	Most Cost-Effective for WTP <$100K
Das et al,[76] 2009	50-y-o men with ND BE	No surveillance	—	67.959	$2894	Base case	No surveillance
		Surveillance ND BE q3 y, LGD qyear, HGD q3 mo	Surveillance, esophagectomy if high-risk	68.076	$13,016	$86,434	
		Initial RFA	N/A	68.259	$21,919	$63,416	
Inadomi et al,[64] 2009	50-y-o subjects with LGD	No surveillance	None	64.71	$687	Base case	Ablation without surveillance
		Ablation without surveillance	None	65.78	$12,540	$11,078	
		APC ablation with surveillance	Surveillance	65.73	$13,881	$12,935	
		RFA ablation with surveillance	Surveillance	65.78	$14,409	$12,824	
		Surveillance	Surveillance	65.38	$16,210	$23,169	
		PDT ablation with surveillance	Surveillance	65.75	$28,017	$26,279	
	50-y-o subjects with ND BE	No surveillance	None	65.19	$471	Base case	Ablation without surveillance
		Ablation without surveillance	None	65.83	$10,876	$16,258	
		Surveillance with RFA for incident dysplasia	RFA	65.67	$10,933	$21,796	
		APC ablation with surveillance	Surveillance	65.77	$12,512	$20,760	
		MPEC ablation with surveillance	Surveillance	65.81	$12,691	$19,710	
		RFA with Surveillance	Surveillance	65.83	$13,268	$19,995	

Health-adjusted life expectancy: discounted health-adjusted life expectancies from the starting age of each cohort.
Cost-effectiveness: incremental cost compared with base cost obtained from each study or calculated based on information given.
All costs are given as they were presented in the study and have not been adjusted based on inflation.

cost-effective strategies. Earlier studies, before the advent of endoscopic therapy, showed mixed results regarding the ideal surveillance interval and the utility of surveillance of nondysplastic Barrett's esophagus.[32,33] A more recent study by Kastelein and colleagues[65] analyzed the change in cost-effectiveness associated with various different surveillance intervals for nondysplastic Barrett's esophagus and LGD, with subjects undergoing RFA ablation if HGD was diagnosed. Surveillance endoscopy of subjects with LGD every 3 years was cost-effective with €32,000 per QALY gained. At an interval of every year, the incremental increase in cost was €76,000 per QALY gained, which is within the WTP threshold in the Netherlands. Gordon and colleagues[55] similarly found that surveillance of nondysplastic Barrett's esophagus every 2 years and LGD every 6 months was not cost-effective if the WTP was $50,000 per QALY gained, although could become effective with intervals of every 3 years and every 1 year, respectively. The general consensus of these studies is that the ideal interval for surveillance is likely at around 1 year for LGD and between 3 and 5 years for nondysplastic Barrett's esophagus, as has been incorporated into the current guidelines.[3,4]

Endoscopic Ablation of Low-Grade Dysplasia

LGD is a particularly challenging entity because multiple epidemiologic studies have shown significant variation with regard to its risk of progression to esophageal adenocarcinoma.[67] Although some studies suggest that the rate of progression to cancer is similar to that of HGD,[68] others report that it behaves more similarly to nondysplastic Barrett's esophagus.[69,70] Even the diagnosis of LGD is challenging because multiple studies have shown significant interobserver and intraobserver variation of pathologic diagnosis. Barrett's esophagus frequently occurs in the setting of gastroesophageal reflux disease, which can lead to inflammatory changes in the esophagus that can be misinterpreted as dysplasia.[43,45] Furthermore, the distribution of LGD within the esophagus is highly variable because it can be spotty, diffuse, unifocal, or multifocal and, therefore, it lends itself to sampling error even when the proper Seattle protocol (4-quadrant jumbo biopsy forces every 1–2 cm along the visible Barrett's esophagus length) is used.[69] Even when LGD is correctly diagnosed, multiple studies have shown varying incidences of regression to nondysplastic Barrett's esophagus and, therefore, the value of performing ablation in patients who may regress without any intervention is unclear.

Hur and colleagues[63] found that initial RFA for LGD was cost-effective compared with a strategy of surveillance with RFA reserved for HGD, with a cost of $18,200 per QALY gained. Their analysis was sensitive to both the rates of progression from LGD to esophageal adenocarcinoma and the WTP threshold of society, although RFA for LGD remained the preferred strategy at a wide range of progression rates and in most trials in a multivariable sensitivity analysis. The cost of RFA ablation strategies is increased by the need for ongoing surveillance after intestinal metaplasia has been eradicated. Therefore, Inadomi and colleagues[64] explored a strategy in which, following ablation, surveillance was either continued for all subjects or reserved only for those with residual intestinal metaplasia. They calculated that ablation without surveillance for subjects in whom eradication had been achieved offered the greatest benefit at the lowest cost compared with other strategies.

Endoscopic Ablation of Nondysplastic Barrett's Esophagus

The use of RFA for the initial management of nondysplastic Barrett's esophagus appears to be not cost-effective. Hur and colleagues[63] found that initial RFA costs between $118,000 and $205,000 per QALY compared with a strategy of surveillance alone. Interestingly, Inadomi and colleagues[64] found that initial RFA ablation could be cost-effective but only if complete ablation was achieved in a high proportion of subjects and if discontinuation of surveillance after ablation were a clinically viable option. Given the fairly high recurrence rates of intestinal metaplasia in post-RFA patients, estimated to be around one-third by some reports,[71] ongoing endoscopy after RFA will likely be continued in clinical practice. Therefore, surveillance of nondysplastic Barrett's esophagus with ablation for dysplasia remains a more cost-effective solution.

CHEMOPREVENTION

One study reported that aspirin with endoscopic surveillance is more effective and less costly than surveillance alone.[72] A more recent study assessed the cost-effectiveness of both aspirin and statin use in combination with endoscopic surveillance and found that the use of aspirin with ongoing surveillance was more cost-effective than surveillance alone.[73] The combination of statin with surveillance, with or without aspirin, was found to further increase QALYs gained but at a cost of between $150,000 and $860,000 per QALY. Another study reported that nonsteroidal anti-inflammatory drugs (NSAIDs) in combination with surveillance were more effective than surveillance alone, with a cost of less than $30,000 per QALY gained.[74] Of note, none of these studies assessing the use of aspirin or nonaspirin NSAIDs incorporated the use of ablation for HGD and, therefore, a comprehensive analysis of the influence these medications have on both outcomes and cost remains unclear.

SUMMARY

Guidelines for the screening and surveillance of Barrett's esophagus continue to evolve as the incidence of esophageal adenocarcinoma increases, identification of individuals at highest risk for cancer improves, and management of dysplasia evolves. The studies reviewed in this article highlight that much remains unknown with regard to the actual effects of screening and surveillance to reduce mortality from esophageal adenocarcinoma. Economic analyses illustrate that endoscopic therapy for HGD is cost-effective and likely improves clinical outcomes without significant increases in cost. The management of LGD is less clear and is further complicated by difficulties in the diagnosis of LGD, with high interobserver and intraobserver variability, and the possibility of regression to nondysplastic Barrett's esophagus. Current management of nondysplastic Barrett's esophagus continues to focus on surveillance, although this may change if the cost and morbidity from endoscopic procedures decreases, or if treatment is successful to the point that surveillance can be discontinued after ablation.

The variability between the referenced studies highlights current gaps in knowledge. Assumptions about the transition rates from nondysplastic states or LGD to esophageal adenocarcinoma may not be accurate and small changes in these rates could shift effectiveness from 1 strategy to another. Heartburn is an imperfect symptom to identify individuals who should be screened and dysplasia is an imperfect marker to identify those at risk for development of cancer. Advances in diagnosis, such as genetic and epigenetic biomarkers or cytosponge offer promising strategies to help focus screening efforts on those individuals who are most likely to develop esophageal adenocarcinoma.

REFERENCES

1. El-Serag HB, Sweet S, Winchester CC, et al. Update on the epidemiology of gastro-oesophageal reflux disease: a systematic review. Gut 2014;63(6):871–80.

2. Hur C, Miller M, Kong CY, et al. Trends in esophageal adenocarcinoma incidence and mortality. Cancer 2013;119(6):1149–58.
3. Shaheen NJ, Falk GW, Iyer PG, et al. American College of G. ACG clinical guideline: diagnosis and management of Barrett's esophagus. Am J Gastroenterol 2016;111(1):30–50 [quiz: 51].
4. Spechler SJ, Sharma P, Souza RF, et al. American Gastroenterological Association medical position statement on the management of Barrett's esophagus. Gastroenterology 2011;140(3):1084–91.
5. Peters JH, Clark GW, Ireland AP, et al. Outcome of adenocarcinoma arising in Barrett's esophagus in endoscopically surveyed and nonsurveyed patients. J Thorac Cardiovasc Surg 1994;108(5):813–21 [discussion: 821–2].
6. van Sandick JW, van Lanschot JJ, Kuiken BW, et al. Impact of endoscopic biopsy surveillance of Barrett's oesophagus on pathological stage and clinical outcome of Barrett's carcinoma. Gut 1998;43(2):216–22.
7. Incarbone R, Bonavina L, Saino G, et al. Outcome of esophageal adenocarcinoma detected during endoscopic biopsy surveillance for Barrett's esophagus. Surg Endosc 2002;16(2):263–6.
8. Ferguson MK, Durkin A. Long-term survival after esophagectomy for Barrett's adenocarcinoma in endoscopically surveyed and nonsurveyed patients. J Gastrointest Surg 2002;6(1):29–35 [discussion: 36].
9. Cooper GS, Yuan Z, Chak A, et al. Association of prediagnosis endoscopy with stage and survival in adenocarcinoma of the esophagus and gastric cardia. Cancer 2002;95(1):32–8.
10. Corley DA, Levin TR, Habel LA, et al. Surveillance and survival in Barrett's adenocarcinomas: a population-based study. Gastroenterology 2002;122(3):633–40.
11. Kearney DJ, Crump C, Maynard C, et al. A case-control study of endoscopy and mortality from adenocarcinoma of the esophagus or gastric cardia in persons with GERD. Gastrointest Endosc 2003;57(7):823–9.
12. Cooper GS, Kou TD, Chak A. Receipt of previous diagnoses and endoscopy and outcome from esophageal adenocarcinoma: a population-based study with temporal trends. Am J Gastroenterol 2009;104(6):1356–62.
13. Verbeek RE, Leenders M, Ten Kate FJ, et al. Surveillance of Barrett's esophagus and mortality from esophageal adenocarcinoma: a population-based cohort study. Am J Gastroenterol 2014;109(8):1215–22.
14. Bhat SK, McManus DT, Coleman HG, et al. Oesophageal adenocarcinoma and prior diagnosis of Barrett's oesophagus: a population-based study. Gut 2015;64(1):20–5.
15. Kastelein F, van Olphen SH, Steyerberg EW, et al. Impact of surveillance for Barrett's oesophagus on tumour stage and survival of patients with neoplastic progression. Gut 2016;65(4):548–54.
16. Corley DA, Mehtani K, Quesenberry C, et al. Impact of endoscopic surveillance on mortality from Barrett's esophagus-associated esophageal adenocarcinomas. Gastroenterology 2013;145(2):312–9.e1.
17. Rubenstein JH, Sonnenberg A, Davis J, et al. Effect of a prior endoscopy on outcomes of esophageal adenocarcinoma among United States veterans. Gastrointest Endosc 2008;68(5):849–55.
18. Shaheen NJ, Sharma P, Overholt BF, et al. Radiofrequency ablation in Barrett's esophagus with dysplasia. N Engl J Med 2009;360(22):2277–88.
19. Fleischer DE, Overholt BF, Sharma VK, et al. Endoscopic radiofrequency ablation for Barrett's esophagus: 5-year outcomes from a prospective multicenter trial. Endoscopy 2010;42(10):781–9.

20. Shaheen NJ, Overholt BF, Sampliner RE, et al. Durability of radiofrequency ablation in Barrett's esophagus with dysplasia. Gastroenterology 2011;141(2):460–8.
21. Overholt BF, Panjehpour M, Halberg DL. Photodynamic therapy for Barrett's esophagus with dysplasia and/or early stage carcinoma: long-term results. Gastrointest Endosc 2003;58(2):183–8.
22. Overholt BF, Lightdale CJ, Wang KK, et al. Photodynamic therapy with porfimer sodium for ablation of high-grade dysplasia in Barrett's esophagus: international, partially blinded, randomized phase III trial. Gastrointest Endosc 2005;62(4): 488–98.
23. Russell LB, Gold MR, Siegel JE, et al. The role of cost-effectiveness analysis in health and medicine. Panel on Cost-Effectiveness in Health and Medicine. JAMA 1996;276(14):1172–7.
24. Weinstein MC, Siegel JE, Gold MR, et al. Recommendations of the panel on cost-effectiveness in health and medicine. JAMA 1996;276(15):1253–8.
25. Siegel JE, Weinstein MC, Russell LB, et al. Recommendations for reporting cost-effectiveness analyses. Panel on cost-effectiveness in health and medicine. JAMA 1996;276(16):1339–41.
26. Inadomi JM. Cost considerations in implementing a screening and surveillance strategy for Barrett's oesophagus. Best Pract Res Clin Gastroenterol 2015; 29(1):51–63.
27. Gold MR. Cost-effectiveness in health and medicine. New York: Oxford University Press; 1996.
28. Gupta N, Bansal A, Wani SB, et al. Endoscopy for upper GI cancer screening in the general population: a cost-utility analysis. Gastrointest Endosc 2011;74(3): 610–24.e2.
29. Rubenstein JH, Vakil N, Inadomi JM. The cost-effectiveness of biomarkers for predicting the development of oesophageal adenocarcinoma. Aliment Pharmacol Ther 2005;22(2):135–46.
30. Benaglia T, Sharples LD, Fitzgerald RC, et al. Health benefits and cost effectiveness of endoscopic and nonendoscopic cytosponge screening for Barrett's esophagus. Gastroenterology 2013;144(1):62–73.e6.
31. Gerson L, Lin OS. Cost-benefit analysis of capsule endoscopy compared with standard upper endoscopy for the detection of Barrett's esophagus. Clin Gastroenterol Hepatol 2007;5(3):319–25.
32. Gerson LB, Groeneveld PW, Triadafilopoulos G. Cost-effectiveness model of endoscopic screening and surveillance in patients with gastroesophageal reflux disease. Clin Gastroenterol Hepatol 2004;2(10):868–79.
33. Inadomi JM, Sampliner R, Lagergren J, et al. Screening and surveillance for Barrett esophagus in high-risk groups: a cost-utility analysis. Ann Intern Med 2003; 138(3):176–86.
34. Rubenstein JH, Inadomi JM, Brill JV, et al. Cost utility of screening for Barrett's esophagus with esophageal capsule endoscopy versus conventional upper endoscopy. Clin Gastroenterol Hepatol 2007;5(3):312–8.
35. Nietert PJ, Silverstein MD, Mokhashi MS, et al. Cost-effectiveness of screening a population with chronic gastroesophageal reflux. Gastrointest Endosc 2003; 57(3):311–8.
36. Rubenstein JH, Inadomi JM. Defining a clinically significant adverse impact of diagnosing Barrett's esophagus. J Clin Gastroenterol 2006;40(2):109–15.
37. Sonnenberg A, Soni A, Sampliner RE. Medical decision analysis of endoscopic surveillance of Barrett's oesophagus to prevent oesophageal adenocarcinoma. Aliment Pharmacol Ther 2002;16(1):41–50.

38. Garside R, Pitt M, Somerville M, et al. Surveillance of Barrett's oesophagus: exploring the uncertainty through systematic review, expert workshop and economic modelling. Health Technol Assess 2006;10(8):1–142, iii-iv.
39. Bhat S, Coleman HG, Yousef F, et al. Risk of malignant progression in Barrett's esophagus patients: results from a large population-based study. J Natl Cancer Inst 2011;103(13):1049–57.
40. de Jonge PJ, van Blankenstein M, Looman CW, et al. Risk of malignant progression in patients with Barrett's oesophagus: a Dutch nationwide cohort study. Gut 2010;59(8):1030–6.
41. Hvid-Jensen F, Pedersen L, Drewes AM, et al. Incidence of adenocarcinoma among patients with Barrett's esophagus. N Engl J Med 2011;365(15):1375–83.
42. Sikkema M, de Jonge PJ, Steyerberg EW, et al. Risk of esophageal adenocarcinoma and mortality in patients with Barrett's esophagus: a systematic review and meta-analysis. Clin Gastroenterol Hepatol 2010;8(3):235–44 [quiz: e232].
43. Alikhan M, Rex D, Khan A, et al. Variable pathologic interpretation of columnar lined esophagus by general pathologists in community practice. Gastrointest Endosc 1999;50(1):23–6.
44. Montgomery E, Bronner MP, Goldblum JR, et al. Reproducibility of the diagnosis of dysplasia in Barrett esophagus: a reaffirmation. Hum Pathol 2001;32(4):368–78.
45. Reid BJ, Haggitt RC, Rubin CE, et al. Observer variation in the diagnosis of dysplasia in Barrett's esophagus. Hum Pathol 1988;19(2):166–78.
46. di Pietro M, Alzoubaidi D, Fitzgerald RC. Barrett's Esophagus and cancer risk: how research advances can impact clinical practice. Gut Liver 2014;8(4):356–70.
47. Wong DJ, Paulson TG, Prevo LJ, et al. p16(INK4a) lesions are common, early abnormalities that undergo clonal expansion in Barrett's metaplastic epithelium. Cancer Res 2001;61(22):8284–9.
48. Alvi MA, Liu X, O'Donovan M, et al. DNA methylation as an adjunct to histopathology to detect prevalent, inconspicuous dysplasia and early-stage neoplasia in Barrett's esophagus. Clin Cancer Res 2013;19(4):878–88.
49. Jin Z, Cheng Y, Gu W, et al. A multicenter, double-blinded validation study of methylation biomarkers for progression prediction in Barrett's esophagus. Cancer Res 2009;69(10):4112–5.
50. Kaz AM, Wong CJ, Luo Y, et al. DNA methylation profiling in Barrett's esophagus and esophageal adenocarcinoma reveals unique methylation signatures and molecular subclasses. Epigenetics 2011;6(12):1403–12.
51. Dulak AM, Stojanov P, Peng S, et al. Exome and whole-genome sequencing of esophageal adenocarcinoma identifies recurrent driver events and mutational complexity. Nat Genet 2013;45(5):478–86.
52. Reid BJ, Prevo LJ, Galipeau PC, et al. Predictors of progression in Barrett's esophagus II: baseline 17p (p53) loss of heterozygosity identifies a patient subset at increased risk for neoplastic progression. Am J Gastroenterol 2001;96(10):2839–48.
53. Rabinovitch PS, Longton G, Blount PL, et al. Predictors of progression in Barrett's esophagus III: baseline flow cytometric variables. Am J Gastroenterol 2001; 96(11):3071–83.
54. Galipeau PC, Li X, Blount PL, et al. NSAIDs modulate CDKN2A, TP53, and DNA content risk for progression to esophageal adenocarcinoma. PLoS Med 2007; 4(2):e67.
55. Gordon LG, Mayne GC, Hirst NG, et al. Cost-effectiveness of endoscopic surveillance of non-dysplastic Barrett's esophagus. Gastrointest Endosc 2014;79(2):242–56.e6.

56. Kadri SR, Lao-Sirieix P, O'Donovan M, et al. Acceptability and accuracy of a non-endoscopic screening test for Barrett's oesophagus in primary care: cohort study. BMJ 2010;341:c4372.
57. Comay D, Blackhouse G, Goeree R, et al. Photodynamic therapy for Barrett's esophagus with high-grade dysplasia: a cost-effectiveness analysis. Can J Gastroenterol 2007;21(4):217–22.
58. Hur C, Nishioka NS, Gazelle GS. Cost-effectiveness of photodynamic therapy for treatment of Barrett's esophagus with high grade dysplasia. Dig Dis Sci 2003;48(7):1273–83.
59. Shaheen NJ, Inadomi JM, Overholt BF, et al. What is the best management strategy for high grade dysplasia in Barrett's oesophagus? A cost effectiveness analysis. Gut 2004;53(12):1736–44.
60. Vij R, Triadafilopoulos G, Owens DK, et al. Cost-effectiveness of photodynamic therapy for high-grade dysplasia in Barrett's esophagus. Gastrointest Endosc 2004;60(5):739–56.
61. Boger PC, Turner D, Roderick P, et al. A UK-based cost-utility analysis of radiofrequency ablation or oesophagectomy for the management of high-grade dysplasia in Barrett's oesophagus. Aliment Pharmacol Ther 2010;32(11–12):1332–42.
62. Hu Y, Puri V, Shami VM, et al. Comparative effectiveness of esophagectomy versus endoscopic treatment for esophageal high-grade dysplasia. Ann Surg 2016;263(4):719–26.
63. Hur C, Choi SE, Rubenstein JH, et al. The cost effectiveness of radiofrequency ablation for Barrett's esophagus. Gastroenterology 2012;143(3):567–75.
64. Inadomi JM, Somsouk M, Madanick RD, et al. A cost-utility analysis of ablative therapy for Barrett's esophagus. Gastroenterology 2009;136(7):2101–14.e1-6.
65. Kastelein F, van Olphen S, Steyerberg EW, et al. Surveillance in patients with long-segment Barrett's oesophagus: a cost-effectiveness analysis. Gut 2015;64(6):864–71.
66. Pohl H, Sonnenberg A, Strobel S, et al. Endoscopic versus surgical therapy for early cancer in Barrett's esophagus: a decision analysis. Gastrointest Endosc 2009;70(4):623–31.
67. Yousef F, Cardwell C, Cantwell MM, et al. The incidence of esophageal cancer and high-grade dysplasia in Barrett's esophagus: a systematic review and meta-analysis. Am J Epidemiol 2008;168(3):237–49.
68. von Rahden BH, Stein HJ, Weber A, et al. Critical reappraisal of current surveillance strategies for Barrett's esophagus: analysis of a large German Barrett's database. Dis Esophagus 2008;21(8):685–9.
69. Sharma P, Falk GW, Weston AP, et al. Dysplasia and cancer in a large multicenter cohort of patients with Barrett's esophagus. Clin Gastroenterol Hepatol 2006;4(5):566–72.
70. Wani S, Falk GW, Post J, et al. Risk factors for progression of low-grade dysplasia in patients with Barrett's esophagus. Gastroenterology 2011;141(4):1179–86.
71. Guarner-Argente C, Buoncristiano T, Furth EE, et al. Long-term outcomes of patients with Barrett's esophagus and high-grade dysplasia or early cancer treated with endoluminal therapies with intention to complete eradication. Gastrointest Endosc 2013;77(2):190–9.
72. Hur C, Nishioka NS, Gazelle GS. Cost-effectiveness of aspirin chemoprevention for Barrett's esophagus. J Natl Cancer Inst 2004;96(4):316–25.
73. Choi SE, Perzan KE, Tramontano AC, et al. Statins and aspirin for chemoprevention in Barrett's esophagus: results of a cost-effectiveness analysis. Cancer Prev Res (Phila) 2014;7(3):341–50.

74. Sonnenberg A, Fennerty MB. Medical decision analysis of chemoprevention against esophageal adenocarcinoma. Gastroenterology 2003;124(7):1758–66.
75. Royston C, Caygill C, Charlett A, et al. The evolution and outcome of surveillance of Barrett's oesophagus over four decades in a UK District General Hospital. Eur J Gastroenterol Hepatol 2016;28(12):1365–73.
76. Das A, Wells C, Kim HJ, et al. An economic analysis of endoscopic ablative therapy for management of nondysplastic Barrett's esophagus. Endoscopy 2009;41(5):400–8.

The Role of Adjunct Imaging in Endoscopic Detection of Dysplasia in Barrett's Esophagus

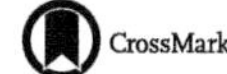

Pujan Kandel, MD, Michael B. Wallace, MD, MPH*

KEYWORDS

• Barrett's esophagus • Imaging • Optical chromoendoscopy

KEY POINTS

- Advances in imaging technologies have demonstrated promise in early detection of dysplasia and cancer in Barrett's esophagus (BE).
- Optical chromoendoscopy (eg, narrow-band imaging [NBI]), dye-based chromoendoscopy, and novel technologies such as confocal laser endomicroscopy have provided the opportunity to visualize the cellular and subcellular structures.
- Currently, only NBI and acetic acid chromoendoscopy have reached benchmarks for clinical use to guide biopsy.
- New-generation optical tomography (volumetric laser endomicroscopy) has demonstrated significant promise in dysplasia detection in BE given its quick and wide-field, cross-sectional, high-resolution imaging.

BACKGROUND

Barrett's esophagus (BE) is a condition in which the distal squamous epithelium of the esophagus is replaced with columnar epithelium and there is presence of histologically proven intestinal metaplasia (IM). Gastroesophageal reflux disease is a major risk factor for BE and development of esophageal adenocarcinoma (EAC). The evolution of EAC starts from the sequence of low-grade dysplasia (LGD); high-grade dysplasia (HGD); and, eventually, EAC.[1] The incidence of EAC is rising in United States.[2] For the diagnosis of BE, at least 8 random biopsies, as well as targeted sampling of visible

---

Conflicts of Interest: M.B. Wallace reports grant support from Boston Scientific, Medtronic, Cosmo pharmaceuticals, and equity interest in iLumen. None of these entities are discussed in this article.
Department of Gastroenterology and Hepatology, Mayo Clinic Florida, 4500 San Pablo Road, Jacksonville, FL 32224, USA
* Corresponding author.
E-mail address: wallace.michael@mayo.edu

http://dx.doi.org/10.1016/j.giec.2017.02.007

mucosal abnormalities, should be obtained to increase the yield of IM on histology in patients with suspected BE.[3] However, in patients with a short segment (1–2 cm) in which 8 biopsies in not obtainable, at least 4 biopsies per centimeter of circumferential BE should be obtained. IM (with goblet cells) is required for the diagnosis of BE because it is suspected to be the predominant type of esophageal columnar epithelium that predisposes to cancer. The missed rates of dysplastic or neoplastic lesions with standard protocol biopsies in patients with BE is as great as 57%.[4] The introduction of advanced imaging technologies has increased the detection of dysplasia and has reduced the number of biopsies in patients with BE.[5] Early detection of precursor lesions during surveillance endoscopy and subsequent classification into categories such as no dysplasia, LGD, and HGD increases the survival in patients with EAC.[3,6] New advanced imaging is rapid, easy to use and acquisitions of high-resolution (HR) images have made these modalities an important tool for surveillance endoscopy in BE. This article discusses the new technologies and adjunct imaging in BE. Various imaging technologies used to identify red flag lesions in BE are illustrated in **Table 1**.[7]

Table 1
Optical technologies for Barrett's esophagus

Technology	Advantages	Disadvantages
Standard white light endoscopy	Wide-field imaging, widely available, no contrast	Limited sensitivity and specificity
High-definition white light endoscopy	Wide-field imaging, improved image quality, no contrast	Cost of upgrading entire endoscopy system, utility evaluated in small studies
Dye-based chromoendoscopy	Wide-field imaging, mucosal enhancement	Time consuming, tedious, requires contrast, contrast may be harmful, contrast often does not equally distribute over the mucosa
Optical chromoendoscopy	Wide-field imaging, mucosal enhancement, no staining agent, user-friendly, can be used as targeted biopsy	Unclear if there is added benefit to HR-WLE alone
Autofluorescence imaging	Wide-field imaging, high-sensitivity, no exogenous contrast	High false-positive rate, utility evaluated in small pilot studies
Confocal laser endomicroscopy	In vivo histology, probe can be used in any endoscope	Near-field imaging, expensive, requires fluorescein, interpretation of imaging
Optical coherence tomography	In vivo assessment of tissue architecture, no contrast, ability for subsurface imaging	Near-field imaging, early in development
nVision volumetric laser endomicroscopy	Cross-sectional wide-field imaging, no use of dye, high sensitivity and accuracy	Restricted to tertiary referral centers, expensive, limited clinical data
Molecular imaging	Molecular targets with high sensitivity and specificity	Early stage, restricted to preclinical models, limited clinical data on humans

OPTICAL CHROMOENDOSCOPY: NARROW-BAND IMAGING

Optical chromoendoscopy is a well-established imaging technology for visualization of esophageal mucosal surface. Narrow-band imaging (NBI) improves the resolution of mucosal surface with the use of special light filters or optical enhancement software without the use of dye spraying. First described by Gono and colleagues[8] in 2004, NBI uses different frequencies of light wavelengths for imagining of mucosal surfaces. It filters white light into 2 specific wavelengths: shorter wavelength blue light (415 nm) and longer wavelength green light (540 nm), which are strongly absorbed by hemoglobin. Blue light highlights superficial capillary vessels, whereas green light highlights subepithelial vessels with identification of subtle mucosal changes. Having similar technology and principles to NBI, Flexible Intelligent Chromoendoscopy (FICE; Fujinon, Inc, Wayne, NJ, USA) and i-SCAN (Pentax Medical, Montvale, NJ, USA) are optical chromoendoscopies that optically enhance different components of lights, such as red, green and blue, which are useful for visualization of superficial and vascular structures. There are fewer studies describing the efficacy of FICE and i-SCAN for detection of BE neoplasia in combination with acetic acid.[9,10]

Several studies demonstrate NBI to have higher diagnostic accuracy in detecting IM and HGD when compared with standard definition white light imaging.[11–16] BE and HGD do have characteristic vascular and mucosal patterns that are identified on optical chromoendoscopy (**Fig. 1**).[11]

HGD has irregular blood vessels with disrupted mucosa, whereas IM has a flat, villous-appearing mucosal pattern with long branching vessels. There have been several systems proposed for characterization of BE surface patterns with NBI but none have been widely validated. Recently, investigators from Europe, United States, and Japan, known as the Barrett's International NBI Group (BING), have developed and validated the NBI classification system for identification of dysplasia and cancer in patients with BE. Vascular and mucosal patterns of each NBI images were classified as regular and irregular on consensus by the BING group (**Table 2**). Regular mucosal patterns were demonstrated by circular, ridged or villous, or tubular patterns, and

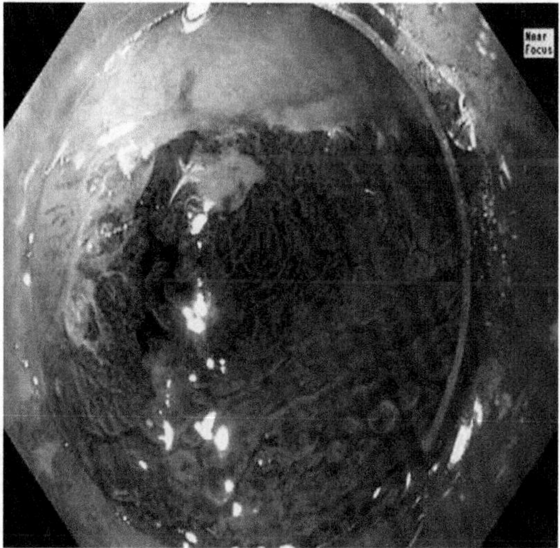

Fig. 1. BE with HGD dysplasia. Note the dilated and irregular vascular and mucosal pattern immediately adjacent to squamocolumnar junction.

Table 2
Narrow-band imaging classification of Barrett's epithelium according to the Barrett's International NBI Group criteria

Morphologic Characteristics	Classification
Mucosal pattern	
Circular, ridged or villous, or tubular pattern	Regular
Absent or irregular patterns	Irregular
Vascular pattern	
Blood vessels situated regularly along or between mucosal ridges and/or those showing normal, long branching patterns	Regular
Focally or diffusely distributed vessels not following normal architecture of the mucosa	Irregular

From Sharma P, Bergman JJ, Goda K, et al. Development and validation of a classification system to identify high-grade dysplasia and esophageal adenocarcinoma in Barrett's Esophagus using narrow-band imaging. Gastroenterology 2016;150(3):591–8.

irregular mucosa was demonstrated by absent or irregular surface patterns (**Figs. 2** and **3**). Regular vascular patterns were recognized by blood vessels located along or between mucosal ridges and/or those showing normal long branching patterns. Irregular vascular patterns were recognized by focally or diffusely distributed vessels

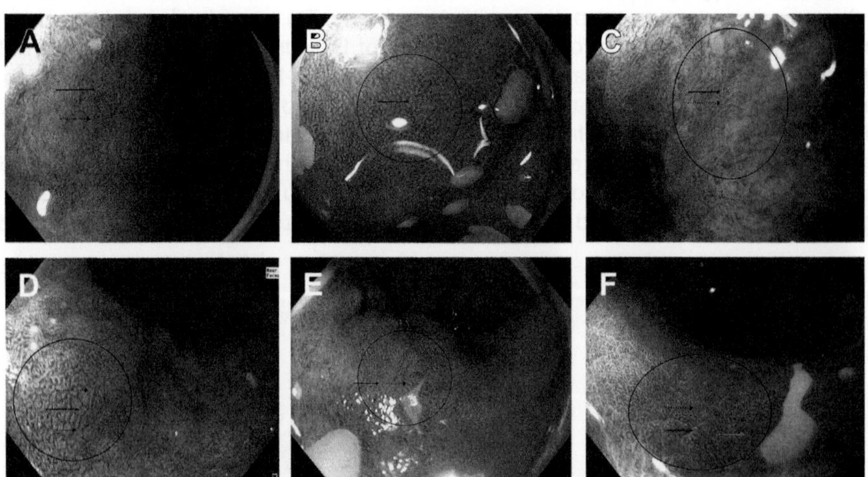

Fig. 2. (*A*) HR image of non dysplastic barrett's esophagus (NDBE) using NBI. Presence of circular mucosal patterns (*solid arrow*) that are orderly arranged blood vessels that clearly follow the mucosal architecture (*dashed arrows*). (*B*) Circular mucosal patterns are arranged in a regular fashion and blood vessels follow normal architecture of mucosa (*solid arrow*). (*C*) Circular mucosal patterns (*solid arrow*) are arranged in an orderly fashion and blood vessels follow the mucosal ridges (*dashed arrows*). (*D*) Ridge or villous mucosal patterns (*solid arrows*) are arranged in a regular fashion and blood vessels are arranged in a normal architecture between the ridges (*dashed arrows*). (*E*) Circular mucosal patterns (*solid arrow*) are arranged in an orderly fashion and blood vessels follow the normal mucosa (*dashed arrows*). (*F*) Circular (*solid black arrow*) and ridge or villous (*red arrow*) mucosal patterns arranged in a normal fashion and blood vessels follow the normal architecture of mucosal ridge (*dashed arrows*). (*Adapted from* Sharma P, Bergman JJ, Goda K, et al. Development and validation of a classification system to identify high-grade dysplasia and esophageal adenocarcinoma in Barrett's Esophagus using narrow-band imaging. Gastroenterology 2016;150(3):591–8; with permission.)

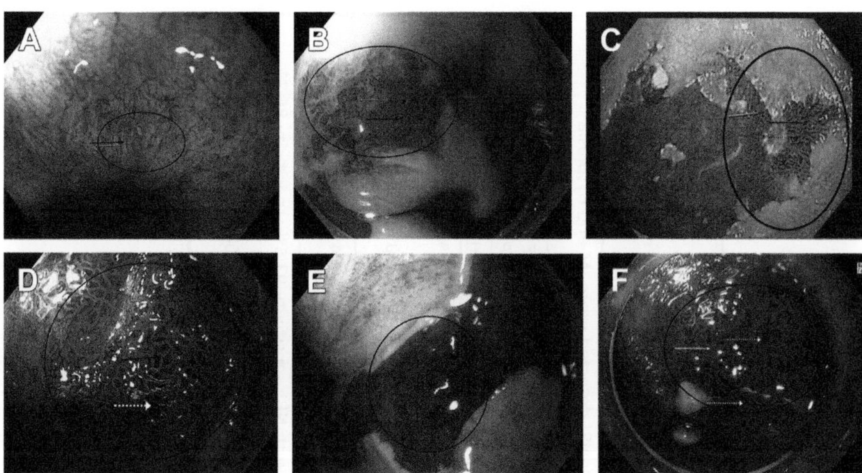

Fig. 3. (*A*) HR image of dysplastic BE using NBI. Irregular mucosal and vascular patterns in BE patient using NBI; irregular mucosal (*black arrow*) and vascular patterns (*red arrow*). (*B*) Irregular mucosal (*black arrow*) and vascular patterns (*red arrow*). Vessels do not follow the normal architecture of the mucosa. (*C*) Irregular mucosal (*solid black arrow*) and vascular patterns (*dashed arrows*). Red arrow shows area on the mucosa where vessels are arranged in a regular fashion that follows the normal architecture of the mucosa. (*D*) Irregular mucosal and vascular patterns (*dashed arrows*). Focally or diffusely distributed vessels do not follow the normal architecture of the mucosa (*black arrow*). (*E*) Irregular mucosal and vascular patterns (*solid arrow*) and the regularly arranged mucosal and vascular pattern (*dashed arrows*). (*F*) Irregular mucosal (*solid arrow*) and vascular patterns (*dashed arrows*). (*Adapted from* Sharma P, Bergman JJ, Goda K, et al. development and validation of a classification system to identify high-grade dysplasia and esophageal adenocarcinoma in Barrett's Esophagus using narrow-band imaging. Gastroenterology 2016;150(3):591–8; with permission.)

not following the normal architecture of the mucosa (see **Figs. 2** and **3**). The BING criteria identified patients with dysplasia with 85% overall accuracy, 80% sensitivity, 81% positive predictive value (PPV), and 85% negative predictive value (NPV). When dysplasia was assessed with high confidence, these values were 92%, 91%, 89%, and 95%, respectively. The interobserver agreement between experts was substantial (kappa value [κ] 0.68).[17] This was an internally validated system for identification of dysplasia and EAC in patients with BE based on NBI results.

Studies comparing NBI and white light endoscopy (WLE) in detecting dysplasia in BE are illustrated in **Table 3**. Results from prospective studies have shown that NBI was superior to WLE for the detection of dysplasia and IM[18] and was able to identify more patients with dysplasia and HGD.[19] In a recent meta-analysis of 14 studies with a total of 843 subjects, NBI increased the diagnostic yield for detection of dysplasia or cancer by 34% compared with WLE with random biopsies (risk difference [RD] = 0.34; 95% CI 0.14–0.56, *P*<.0001). In subgroup analysis, there was no difference in NBI and chromoendoscopy.[20] Results from the systematic review and meta-analysis performed by the American Society of Gastrointestinal Endoscopy (ASGE) have shown sensitivity, NPV, and specificity of NBI is 94%, 97%, and 94%. Thus, the ASGE technology committee has endorsed NBI to guide targeted biopsies for detection of dysplasia during surveillance of patients with nondysplastic BE and to replace the use of random biopsies for routine surveillance.[21] However, results from a few studies have demonstrated that there was no improvement in diagnostic yield of HGD or early

Table 3
Studies comparing efficacy of narrow-band imaging with white light endoscopy in Barrett's esophagus

Study	Study Design	Subjects, Number	Lesions, Number	Histologic Reference Standard	Results
Pascarenco et al,[18] 2016	Prospective cohort	84	256	Dysplasia, IM	Dysplasia and IM: NBI detected more IM and dysplasia than WLE (*P* = .01)
Sharma et al,[25] 2013	RCT	123	977	BE, dysplasia	Detection of BE with NBI is equal to WLE NBI detected more dysplasia than WLE (*P* = .1)
Wolfsen et al,[19] 2008	RCT (tandem)	65	—	BE, dysplasia	Detection of dysplasia with NBI is more than WLE (57% vs 43%)
Anagnostopoulos et al,[15] 2007	Cross-sectional	50	344	BE, HGD	Detection of BE with NBI: sensitivity 100%, specificity 78.8%, PPV 93.5%, NPV 100% Detection of HGD with NBI: sensitivity 90%, specificity 100%, PPV 99.2%, NPV 100%
Kara et al,[11] 2006	Descriptive study	63	161	BE, HGD	Detection of HGD with NBI: sensitivity 94%, specificity 76%, PPV 64%, NPV 98%
Sharma et al,[13] 2006	Prospective cohort	51	204	BE, HGD	Detection of BE with NBI: sensitivity 93.5%, specificity 86.7%, PPV 94.7% Detection of HGD with NBI: sensitivity 100%, specificity 98.7%, PPV 95.3%

Abbreviation: RCT, randomized controlled trial.

neoplasia when NBI was compared with HR-WLE alone.[22–24] In a multicenter, randomized, controlled crossover trial, Sharma and colleagues[25] found that there was no difference in detection rate of IM comparing NBI with targeted biopsies versus HR-WLE with standard protocol biopsies, although detecting higher proportion of dysplasia (30% vs 21%, P = .1) with fewer number of biopsies per subject (3.6 vs 7.6, P<.001) in the NBI group. NBI has been shown to be similar to dye-based chromoendoscopy in the assessment of Barrett's epithelium.[20] In a study comparing i-SCAN and acetic acid, there was no difference in diagnosing IM (57% vs 66%, P = .75). Similarly, a study comparing indigo carmine and NBI showed a similar detection rate of HGD and early neoplasia in BE (93% vs 86%, P = 1).

There are several advantages of NBI, including push-button ease of use, visualization of both mucosal and vascular patterns, and integration into standard endoscopy. Although there remains a lack of a well-defined standard for mucosal and vascular patterns classification, it remains an easy and effective endoscopic technology in targeting high-risk lesions arising in a background of BE.

OPTICAL COHERENCE TOMOGRAPHY

Optical coherence tomography (OCT) is an advanced noninvasive cross-sectional imaging modality for evaluation of BE. Its principle is similar to that of ultrasound imaging, except that it uses infrared light waves rather than sound waves. OCT devices provide subsurface imaging with longitudinal and spatial high resolution of the microstructure of tissues. The axial resolution is 10 times better than that of high-frequency endoscopic ultrasound but the depth of penetration is limited to 1 to 3 mm. OCT devices use a low-power infrared light with a wavelength ranging from 750 to 1300 nm with the scattering of light on tissue surface. Scattering occurs when the light interacts with dense structures (eg, nuclei) in the tissue surface and the image formation depends on the difference in optical backscattering properties of the tissue. OCT images are generated from measuring the echo time delay and the intensity of back-scattering of light.[26,27] The use of OCT in the gastrointestinal tract goes back more than a decade to when the technology was mainly based on time-domain OCT, which is limited to small fields of view and slower imaging processing.

Several studies have been published in imaging of Barrett's metaplasia with OCT, which can easily differentiate the gastric cardia and normal squamous mucosa.[28–31] Diagnostic accuracy of OCT in detecting BE and dysplasia in various studies are illustrated in **Table 4**. Results from a prospective study showed the sensitivity and specificity of OCT in detecting dysplasia was 68% and 82%, respectively.[32] Similarly, another study used OCT in detecting HGD/intramucosal cancer and showed a sensitivity of 83% and specificity of 75%.[33] Some studies have explored the benefit of OCT in detection of the buried Barrett's glands after radio frequency ablation (RFA). In an ex vivo study by Cobb and colleagues,[33] in which 2-dimensional OCT was used in 14 subjects who underwent surgery for HGD or cancer in BE. OCT corresponded to histology in buried Barrett's glands in ablation-naïve subjects. OCT demonstrated buried glands in 10 of 14 (71%) subjects that were missed by prior endoscopic biopsy.

VOLUMETRIC LASER ENDOMICROSCOPY

Volumetric laser endomicroscopy (VLE) is a second-generation OCT imaging technique that uses near-infrared light to produce real-time cross-sectional images. It is a wide-field detector of dysplasia and neoplasia in BE. It consists of a balloon-based OCT device containing a 3.7 mm probe, designed to fit through a therapeutic endoscope's channel. The distal end of the balloon should be positioned 1 cm distal

Table 4
Diagnostic accuracy and efficiency of optical coherence tomography in Barrett's esophagus and dysplasia in various studies

Study	Study Design	Subjects, Number	Lesions, Number	Histologic Reference Standard	Results
Poneros et al,[34] 2001	Retrospective and prospective cohort	121	288	IM	In retrospective analysis: 100% sensitive and 93% specific Prospective analysis: 97% sensitive and 92% specific
Isenberg et al,[32] 2005	Prospective cohort	33	314	Dysplasia	Detection of dysplasia, sensitivity 68%, specificity 82%, PPV 53%, and NPV 89% Accuracy 78%
Tao et al,[35] 2012	Retrospective cohort	9	—	BE, dysplasia	OCT shows distinct difference between subjects requiring subsequent RFA treatment after complete eradication of IM as a result of recurrent BE vs subjects who maintained treatment response on long-term endoscopic follow-up
Lee et al,[36] 2015	Retrospective cohort	13	—	NDBE, HGD	Enface OCT of NDBE showed uniformly distributed, oval or circular surface mucosa pattern Enface OCT of HGD showed nonuniform, irregular and distorted mucosal pattern with enlarged and elongated cysts

Abbreviation: NDBE, nondysplastic Barrett's esophagus.

to the gastroesophageal junction. The probe helically scans the esophageal surface from the distal to the proximal end of the balloon, obtaining a 360° evaluation with 7 μm resolution and 3 mm depth. A registration line is seen on the balloon and is matched with the registration line on the cross-sectional imaging to allow orientation and localization of suspicious lesions for further biopsy sampling.[37]

NvisionVLE (nVLE; NinePoint Medical Inc, Bedford, MA, USA) is now commercially available and approved by the Food and Drug Administration to help target neoplasia. VLE increases the detection of persistent or recurrent BE and dysplasia that could not be visualized in WLE.[38] VLE offers higher resolution compared with high-definition electronic chromoendoscopy and a much larger field of view compared with confocal laser endomicroscopy (CLE) at 6 cm times the full circumference versus 250 square microns for probe-based CLE (pCLE) and is substantially faster at 60 to 90 seconds for a full scan (**Fig. 4**).

The OCT scoring index (OCT-SI) was the first scoring system used for detection of dysplasia. Based on glandular architecture and signal intensity, normal mucosa was distinguished from metaplasia, dysplasia, and neoplasia. Normal squamous esophageal mucosa appears as layered horizontal architecture without glands in the epithelium, whereas IM is seen as loss of the layered architecture, without surface pits and crypts, and glands seen in the epithelium. Homogeneous scattering is suggestive of HGD or cancer.[39] An OCT-SI higher or equal to 2 was found to have a sensitivity of 83% and a specificity of 75% for detection of dysplasia (**Figs. 5**A and **6**).[39,40]

To create a new scoring system with better diagnostic yield, a new VLE diagnostic algorithm (VLE-DA) was proposed based on identified features associated with dysplasia: atypical gland counts and effacement of the VLE mucosal layer. Diagnostic accuracy of nVLE in detecting BE and dysplasia in various studies is illustrated in **Table 5**. In a cross-sectional study, 50 endoscopic mucosal resection specimens were evaluated by pCLE and VLE, and both VLE-DA and OCT-SI were applied. The

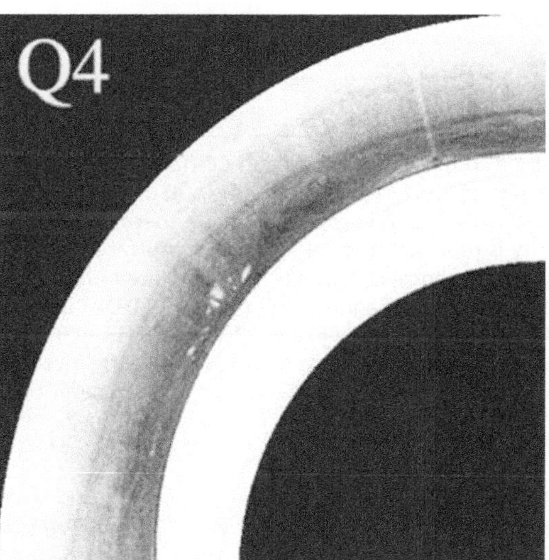

Fig. 4. VLE image (nVLE) showing irregular white structures (*arrow*) in the mucosa with a dark, overlying epithelium (*small arrow*), suggestive of HGD. The image represents one-quarter circumference taken from a full circumference 6 cm length scan.

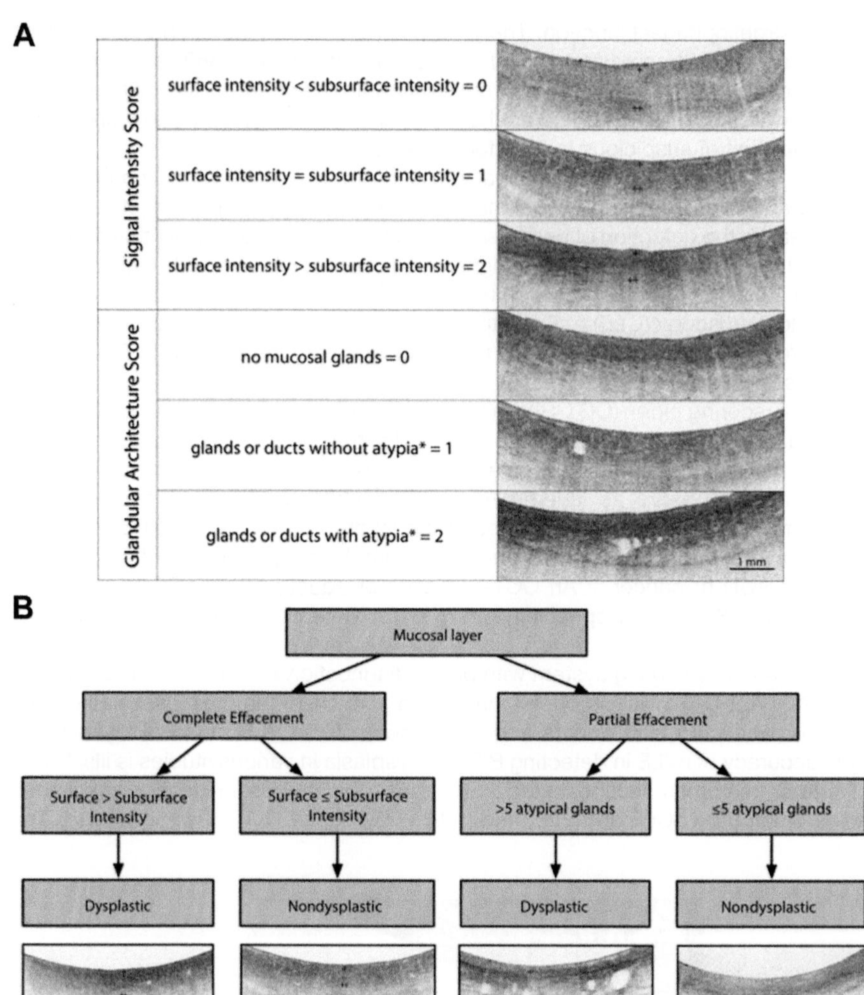

Fig. 5. (*A*) OCT-SI is used to diagnose dysplasia in BE. To calculate dysplasia score, 2 criteria were included (surface-to-subsurface signal intensity and glandular architecture). A score of 2 or more is associated with a sensitivity of 83% and a specificity of 75% for dysplasia. The surface signal intensity is represented by + and the subsurface intensity by ++. Glandular atypia is defined by the presence of irregular and/or dilated glands. *, measuring surface and subsurface intensity. (*B*) VLE diagnostic algorithm (VLE-DA) index. The sensitivity and specificity of VLE-DA is 86% (95% CI 69–96) and 88% (95% CI 66–99). (*Adapted from* Leggett CL, Gorospe EC, Chan DK, et al. Comparative diagnostic performance of volumetric laser endomicroscopy and confocal laser endomicroscopy in the detection of dysplasia associated with Barrett's esophagus. Gastrointest Endosc 2016;83(5):880–8.e2; with permission.)

diagnostic accuracy was 77% for pCLE, 67% for OCT-SI, and 87% for VLE-DA. The interobserver agreement of OCT-SI was fair (κ 0.39), of pCLE was moderate (κ 0.46), and of VLE-DA was substantial (κ 0.83) (**Fig. 5**B).[42] To date, this is the only study comparing the diagnostic yield of VLE and pCLE. Furthermore, these findings were confirmed by a multicenter cross-sectional study that showed that VLE has a high diagnostic accuracy for histology types based on VLE registry images.[42] VLE can

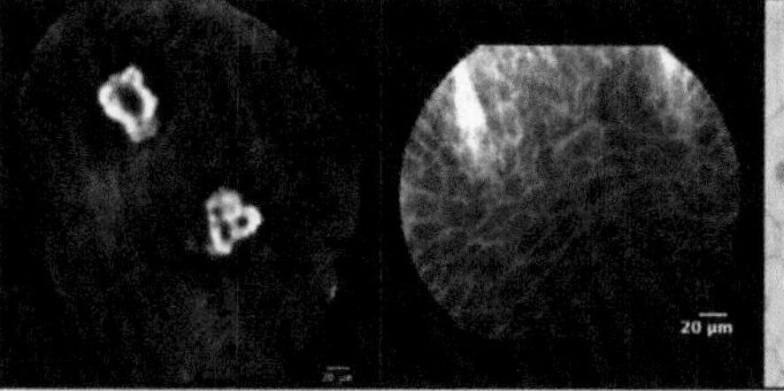
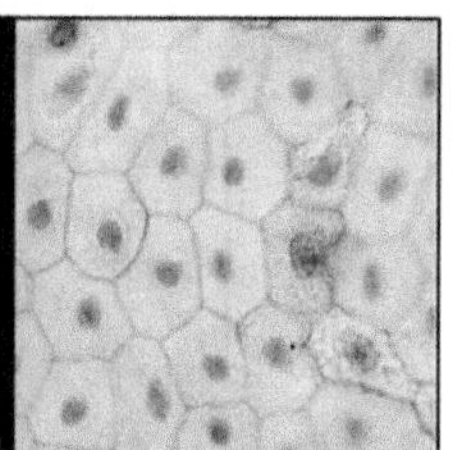

Normal Squamous Epithelium
• Flat cells without crypts or villi
• Bright vessels within papillae (intra papillary capillary loops)
20 μm

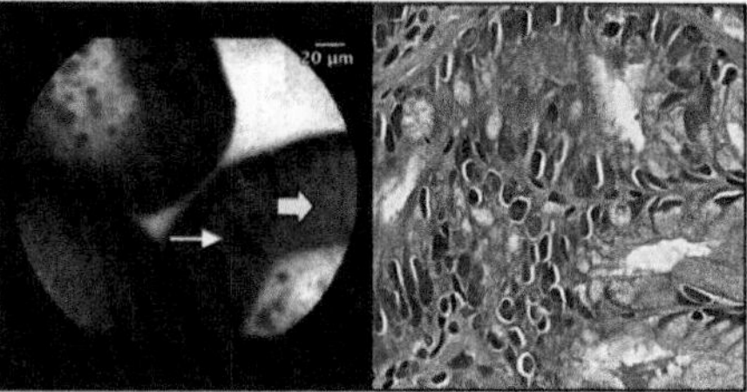

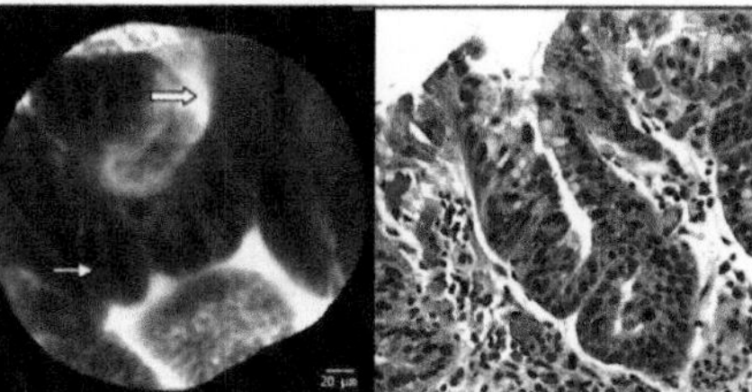

High-Grade Dysplasia
• Villiform structures
• Dark, irregularly thickened epithelial borders (arrow)
• Dilated irregular vessels (block arrow)

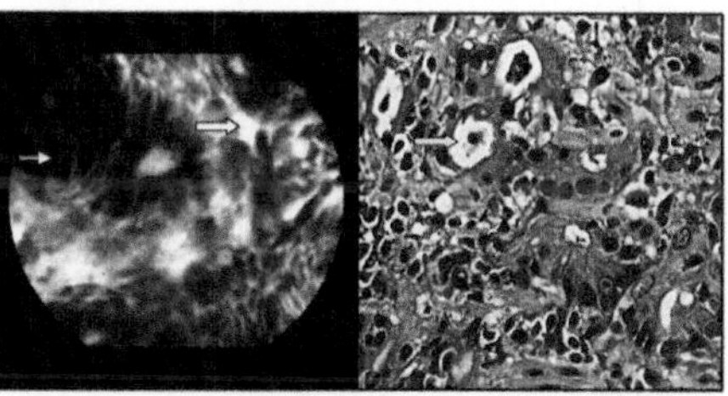

Adenocarcinoma
• Disorganized/loss of villiform structure and crypts
• Dark columnar cells (thin arrow)
• Dilated irregular vessels (block arrow)

Fig. 6. Miami classification of Barrett's neoplasia. (*From* Wallace M, Lauwers GY, Chen Y, et al. Miami classification for probe-based confocal laser endomicroscopy. Endoscopy 2011;43(10):882–91; with permission.)

potentially change the treatment of patients misdiagnosed with BE without dysplasia; however, data are just emerging. A case series reported 6 subjects with long-segment BE and IM on HR-WLE plus NBI and random biopsies, in which VLE was subsequently performed. On VLE, 3 cases had patterns consistent with HGD, 2 with LGD, and 1 with intramucosal cancer. These findings were confirmed with

Table 5
Volumetric laser endomicroscopy diagnostic accuracy

Study	Study Design	Subjects, Number	Histologic Reference Standard	Results
Leggett et al,[41] 2016	Prospective cohort	27	BE, dysplasia	VLE-DA: sensitivity 86%, specificity 88%, accuracy 87%, VLE-DA vs OCT-SI accuracy (87% vs 67%, $P = .01$), for pCLE 76%, 79%, and 77%, respectively
Trindale et al,[50] 2016	Prospective, multicenter study, Interobserver agreement	—	GC, NS, NDBE, DBE	Overall agreement among users (κ = 0.81, 95% CI 0.79–0.83); for esophageal squamous and gastric cardia (κ = 0.95 and 0.86, 95% CI 0.92–0.98 and 0.83–0.89, respectively); for NDBE and DBE (κ = 0.66 and 0.79, 95% CI 0.63–0.69 and 0.75–0.82, respectively) Accuracy for identifying NS, GC, NDBE, and DBE are 99% (95% CI 98–100), 97% (95% CI 95–99), 93% (95% CI 88–98), 95% (CI 91%–99%), respectively
Swager et al,[51] 2016	Retrospective cohort	—	NDBE, HGD/cancer	Sensitivity and specificity for overall diagnosis of (NDBE or neoplasia) 89% and 31%, respectively Sensitivity and specificity based on the highest VLE prediction score for worst histology 91% and 31%, respectively AUC 0.74 (95% CI 0.57–0.92)
Swager et al,[52] 2016	Retrospective cohort, develop and validate VLE prediction score for early BE neoplasia	—	NBE, HGD/cancer	ROC curve of prediction score: AUC of 0.83 (95% CI 0.69–0.96) in learning phase, AUC of 0.81 (95% CI 0.71–0.90) in validation phase Sensitivity and specificity of 85% and 68%, respectively, in learning; 83% and 71%, respectively, in validation phase at cut-off value of >8 points
Leggett et al,[53] 2015	Retrospective cohort	20	Non-neoplastic (SE, nondysplastic BE, LGD), neoplastic (HGD, intramucosal carcinoma)	VLE-DA: sensitivity 100% (95% CI 46–100), specificity 67% (95% CI 39–87), NPV 100% (95% CI 66–100), PPV 50% (95% CI 20–80)
Wolfsen et al,[54] 2015	Prospective, multicenter study	100	Adenocarcinoma, HGD, LGD, IM, normal squamous cells	VLE was completed in 87 of 100 cases (87%), well-tolerated, able to visualize mucosa and submucosa
Wallace et al 2014[55]	Prospective, cross-sectional, multicenter	67	BE, dysplasia	For ≥2 OCT dysplasia score, sensitivity 98%, specificity 23%; for ≥3 sensitivity 81%, specificity 48% in detecting of any grade of dysplasia Agreement for BE diagnosis (κ = 0.89) and for dysplasia (κ = 0.51) BE: sensitivity 100%, specificity 33%
Leggett et al,[56] 2014	Retrospective cohort	32	Dysplasia, nondysplasia	For ≥3 OCT dysplasia score, sensitivity 98%, specificity 68%, κ = 0.81

Abbreviations: AUC, area under the curve; DBE, dysplastic Barrett's esophagus; GC, gastric cardia; NS, normal squamous; ROC, receiver operating characteristic; SE, squa-

Table 6
Diagnostic accuracy of volumetric laser endomicroscopy with computer-aided image-interpretation of Barrett's epithelium

Study	Study Design	Subjects, Images (Number)	Histologic Reference Standard	Results
Diaz-Rodriguez & Singh,[48] 2015	Retrospective cohort	38, 60	NDBE, DBE, BED, GC, NS	Accuracy in distinguishing GC from NDBE 77% and BED 93% Accuracy in distinguishing NS from NDBE 83% and BED 83% Distinguishing NDBE from BED sensitivity 86% and specificity 93%
Swager et al,[49] 2016	Retrospective cohort	60 images	NDBE, HGD and early adenocarcinoma	Detection of BE neoplasia: sensitivity 93%, specificity 70%, and accuracy 82% AUC = 0.91

Abbreviation: BED, dysplastic barretts

histology and management was modified in all cases.[42] Furthermore, the role of VLE has expanded to evaluate submucosal structures. In a recent prospective tandem study, VLE revealed that most post-RFA submucosal glandular structures are normal histologic structures and do not represent buried Barrett's glands, which may lead to recurrence of Barrett's epithelium.[43] VLE may be a promising tool for surveillance to detect persistent or recurrent BE neoplasia following RFA or endoscopic mucosal resection.[44–47]

Interpretation of VLE is complex due to large number of images and complicated architecture, although software to highlight abnormalities is in late stages of development. Several feasibility studies have been conducted to see the diagnostic accuracy of computer-aided detection of dysplasia in BE with ex vivo VLE images analysis (**Table 6**). Results from these studies have demonstrated good diagnostic accuracy[48,49] in detecting BE dysplasia. Compared with traditional random biopsies, VLE can help better to identify potential lesions for targeted biopsies or resection. Computer-aided detection of dysplasia in BE with VLE images is a novel approach that could guide better surveillance programs in BE in the future. In addition, further studies are needed to validate these preliminary findings in in vivo VLE scans.

In conclusion, VLE is a promising, rapidly evolving, safe, and easy to use as a wide-field detector of neoplasia in BE with high interobserver agreement. However, in vivo correlation of images with histopathology, and its diagnostic yield when performed in community hospitals is needed.

CONFOCAL LASER ENDOMICROSCOPY

CLE is an important focal imaging technology that provides microscopic imaging of the mucosa of gastrointestinal tract in real time during the endoscopic procedure, similar to histology. The magnification is produced up to 1000 times, allowing the pinpoint visualization of cellular structures. CLE is an emerging technology that may help decrease or possibly avoid the need for biopsy. CLE is based on the principle of tissue excitation in which florescent dye is administered, most commonly fluorescein sodium, to create a contrast for visualization of mucosal surface with a low-power focused blue laser light of wavelength 488 nm. The laser light is passed through the pinhole and is focused at a selected depth in the tissue of interest with a huge spatial resolution. The reflected light is then focused onto the detection system by the lens.

CLE has traditionally been available in 2 systems. The pCLE (Mauna Kea Technologies, Paris, France) uses a small caliber flexible optical probe that is inserted though the accessory channel of a traditional endoscope. In the endoscope-integrated CLE (Pentax Medical, Montvale, NJ, USA), a confocal fluorescence microscope is integrated into the distal tip of a conventional endoscope, although this system is no longer clinically available. The integrated system allows the visualization of depth up to 250 μm, whereas the probe-based system allows fixed-depth tissue visualization between 70 to 130 μm for standard probes and 55 and 65 μm for the high-definition probes.[57] The main objective of pCLE is to differentiate neoplastic from non-neoplastic tissue in real time by performing a virtual optical biopsies. This will helps achieve 2 goals: decrease the number of traditional biopsies and allow immediate treatment decisions in real time during endoscopy, thereby decreasing the costs and increasing the efficiency of patient care. Classification has been standardized, termed the Miami classification, to diagnose and differentiate BE, HGD, and adenocarcinoma for the CLE user.[58]

Diagnostic accuracy of CLE in detecting BE and dysplasia in various studies is illustrated in **Table 7**. In a prospective study, the sensitivity and specificity of in vivo imaging to detect BE was 98.1% and 92.9%, and neoplasia was 94.1% and 98.4%, respectively.[59] Several studies have demonstrated that CLE-targeted biopsies are superior to traditional 4-quadrant random biopsies protocol (see **Table 3**). In a multicenter study, HR-WLE in combination with CLE increased the neoplasia detection in subjects with BE compared with HR-WLE alone.[60] Similarly, in a randomized controlled trial (RCT), subjects undergoing BE surveillance were randomized either to receive HR-WLE with conventional random biopsies or HR-WLE with CLE-targeted biopsies. CLE increased the neoplasia detection rate from 40% to 96% (P<.01) and improved the diagnostic yield (22% vs 6%, P = .02).

There are several limitations of CLE. Because the imaging is restricted to a small area of mucosa, there is always possibility of sampling error. In an RCT, 2 of 39 subjects with BE-associated HGD were missed by CLE but detected with WLE-guided traditional biopsies.[61] Precise matching of CLE image and subsequent targeted biopsy of mucosa is always challenging. Another limitation is that published research studies are mainly limited to expert academic settings. The value of CLE in community is still unestablished; therefore, use of this technology may prove to be impractical to the practicing gastroenterologist.

AUTOFLUORESCENCE IMAGING

Autofluorophores are biological substances capable of emitting fluorescence light when excited by short wavelength light (395–475 nm). This phenomenon is known as autofluorescence.[67] Normal and dysplastic tissues have different concentrations and distribution of fluorophores, therefore emitting distinct patterns of fluorescence light. Dysplasia and neoplasia appear blue or violet, whereas normal mucosa and

Table 7
Diagnostic accuracy of CLE in evaluation of BE, dysplasia or cancer

Study	Study Design	Subjects, Number	Histologic Reference Standard	Results
Kiesslich et al,[59] 2006	Prospective cohort	63	BE and Barrett's-associated neoplasia	For BE: sensitivity 98.1% and specificity 94.1% For cancer: sensitivity 92.9% and specificity 98.4%
Pohl et al,[62] 2008	Prospective, multicenter	38	HGD or carcinoma, BE with or without LGD	Sensitivity 75%, NPV 98.8%
Dunbar et al,[61] 2009	Crossover study	39	HGD or carcinoma	Diagnostic yield comparing CLE-TB vs WLE with random biopsies (33.7% vs 17.2%, $P = .01$)
Wallace et al,[63] 2010	Prospective cohort	—	HGD or adenocarcinoma	Detection of dysplasia: sensitivity 88%, specificity 96% Interobserver agreement, $\kappa = 0.72$
Bajbouj et al,[64] 2010	Prospective cohort	68	HGD, carcinoma	Real time: optical biopsies: sensitivity 12%, specificity 97% compared with conventional 4-quadrant biopsies
Sharma et al,[60] 2011	RCT (tandem)	164	HGD, carcinoma	pCLE with HD-WLE increased sensitivity and specificity for HGD and adenocarcinoma detection compared with HD-WLE alone ($P = .02$)
Di Pietro et al,[65] 2013	Prospective cohort	23	NDBE, BED, HGD, and cancer	Detection of HGD/cancer: sensitivity 100%, specificity 68% For any grade of dysplasia: sensitivity 63%, specificity 77%
Canto et al,[66] 2014	RCT	192	BE, dysplasia	Endoscope-integrated CLE-targeted biopsy increased the diagnostic yield for neoplasia 3 × compared with WLE with random biopsies (22% vs 6% = 0.02)
Leggett et al,[41] 2016	Prospective cohort	27	BE, dysplasia	Detection of dysplasia: sensitivity 76%, specificity 79%, PPV 89%, NPV 63%

metaplasia appear green[67,68] (**Fig. 7**). This technology has been used as a wide-field detector of neoplastic lesions in BE.

Studies evaluating efficacy of autofluorescence imaging (AFI) imaging in BE, dysplasia and cancer are illustrated in **Table 8**. Earlier uncontrolled studies suggested that video AFI potentially improved the detection of early neoplasia in subjects with BE, given its high sensitivity.[67] Further multicenter, randomized, crossover studies showed that AFI following HR endoscopy (HRE) for detection of HGD/EAC had false-positive rates as high as 71% to 81%.[69,70] To overcome this downside, AFI was added to trimodal endoscopes with HRE and NBI, giving place to the endoscopic trimodal imaging (ETMI).[71] Data regarding the role of ETMI are conflicting. Some prospective, multicenter studies showed that AFI followed by targeted inspection with NBI reduced the false-positive rate to 24% to 48%.[69,70,72] Although 2 randomized crossover trials showed that the targeted histologic yield of ETMI for detection of HGD/EAC was better than that of standard video endoscopy, both of these techniques showed persistently high false-positive rates (90% and 83%, respectively).[72] Furthermore, an analysis of pooled data from 3 uncontrolled prospective studies and 2 randomized crossover trials showed that the diagnostic and therapeutic value of AFI was limited to 2% compared with WLE. This study also showed a pooled false-positive rate of 78%, which was found to be higher in community hospitals.[73]

One prospective tandem study evaluating the role of AFI-targeted pCLE showed that the sensitivity and specificity for detecting any grade of dysplasia increased compared with AFI-targeted NBI (96.4% and 74.1% vs 57.1% and 74.1%).[74] Furthermore, adding tissue-based biomarkers (aneuploidy, cyclin A, p53) reduced the false-positive rate of pCLE by 50%. Although, these results were promising, they did not fulfill the diagnostic yield requirements to replace WLE with random biopsies.

In conclusion, AFI can identify dysplasia in lesions seen as inconspicuous and flat on endoscopy; however, these lesions rarely contain more advanced stages of neoplasia than those identified by adequate inspection with WLE.[73] For this reason, it cannot replace random biopsies and is not widely used clinically.

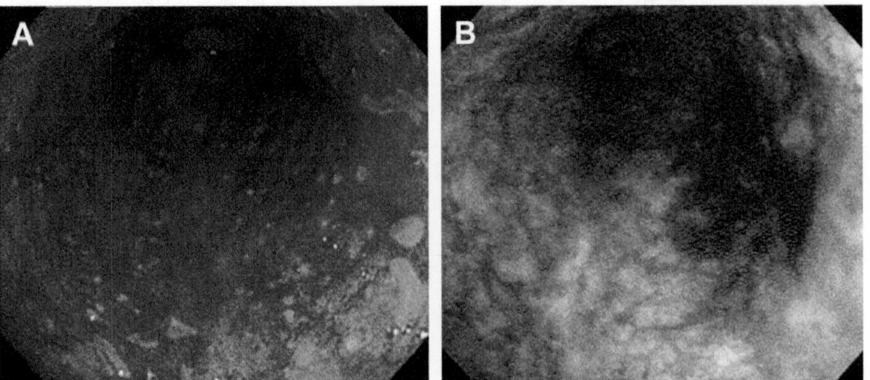

Fig. 7. (*A*) Image of white light of esophagus in a patient with BE. (*B*) AF image, showing blue or purple, suspicion of HGD/esophageal cancer (EC), and greenish color. Biopsy specimens from the blue or purple area revealed EC; those from the greenish area revealed no dysplasia. (*Adapted from* Kara MA, Peters FP, Ten Kate FJ, et al. Endoscopic video autofluorescence imaging may improve the detection of early neoplasia in patients with Barrett's esophagus. Gastrointest Endosc 2005;61(6):679–85; with permission.)

Table 8
Studies evaluating efficacy of autofluorescence imaging in Barrett's esophagus

Study	Study Design	Subjects, Number	Lesions, Number	Histologic Reference Standard	Results
Curvers et al,[69] 2008	Prospective, multicenter (tertiary referral centers)	84	—	HGD, cancer	False-positive rate: 81% False-positive rate after NBI: 26%
Curvers et al,[70] 2010	Crossover, randomized	87	—	HGD, cancer	False-positive rate: 79% False-positive rate after NBI: 48% No difference in overall detection by ETMI and SVE ($P = .15$) Increased targeted detection of HGD/Ca of ETMI compared with SVE ($P<.001$)
Bergman et al, 2010[72]	Multicenter, randomized, crossover	99	—	ND, ID, LGD, HGD, cancer	No difference in overall detection by ETMI and SVE ($P = .54$) Increased targeted detection of HGD/Ca of ETMI compared with SVE ($P = .053$)
Sharma et al,[71] 2012	Prospective tandem	42	—	HGD, cancer	κ for interobserver agreement for AFI patterns = 0.48 False-positive rate: 24% False-positive rate after NBI: 38%
Mannath et al,[75] 2013	Prospective tandem	63	74	HGD, cancer	All-observers: AFI sensitivity 66%, specificity 77%, accuracy 72% AFI + HRE sensitivity 74%, specificity 84%, accuracy 80% κ of AFI for dysplasia (+): 0.41 (moderate) κ of AFI + HRE for dysplasia (+): 0.61 (substantial)
Boerwinkel et al,[73] 2014	3 prospective cohort, 2 randomized crossover trials	371	—	HGD, cancer	The additional diagnostic value of AFI was limited to 2% (5/271) subjects compared with WLE Additional therapeutic value of AFI was 2% (6/371) subjects compared with WLE False-positive rate: 78%
Di Pietro et al,[76] 2015	Cross-sectional prospective, multicenter study	157	—	HGD, cancer	Aneuploidy, p53, and cyclin A had the strongest association with dysplasia AUC 0.97 The 3-biomarker panel applied to AFI-targeted biopsies had a sensitivity and specificity of 100% and 85%, respectively
Di Pietro et al, 2015[74]	Prospective tandem	55	194	BE, dysplasia	Sensitivity and specificity of AFI-targeted pCLE: 96.4% and 74.1%, respectively Sensitivity and specificity of AFI-targeted NBI: 57.1% and 74.1%, respectively Sensitivity and specificity of AFI-targeted pCLE, plus 3 biomarker markers: 89.2% and 88.9%, respectively

Abbreviations: Ca, cancer; ETMI, endoscopic trimodal imaging; HRE, high-resolution endoscopy; ID, indefinite for dysplasia; ND, no dysplasia; SVE, standard video endoscopy.

LABELED BIOMARKER ENDOSCOPY (MOLECULAR IMAGING)

Molecular imaging is an evolving technology for surveillance of BE. Although advanced technologies have been developed to increase the efficiency of dysplasia detection, few of them have shown clear advantage for improved detection in BE. Molecular imaging may enable visualization of the cellular, functional, morphologic, and molecular changes that drives the progression of disease in BE. This could eventually increase the effectiveness of endoscopic surveillance and screening programs. For example, epidermal growth factor, ErbB2, fibroblast growth factor receptors 1 and 2, and c-MET are known transmembrane tyrosine kinase receptors that accelerate epithelial cell growth, proliferation, and differentiation[77–79] (**Fig. 8**). Molecular targets are very small and are difficult to visualize with conventional HD-WLE. Therefore, molecular probes are being developed with labeled markers (fluorescent dyes) as an optical reporters. Several molecular probes have been demonstrated in preclinical models of cancer with in vivo imaging such as lectins, peptides, antibodies, affibodies, and activated enzymes[80–83] (**Fig. 9**). In 1 study, use of lectin (wheat germ agglutinin) with fluorescein-labeled endoscopic visualization shown to bind with high affinity (>5 times) in HGD patients with BE.[80] AFI endoscope was used to image the surgically resected specimens. However, its use in in vivo studies is yet to be established. In another study fluorescein isothiocyanate–labelled peptide, which is specific for HGD/cancer, was visualized with pCLE in vivo. The sensitivity was 75% and specificity of 97% for detection of early neoplasia with a tumor-to-background ratio of 3.8.[81]

Molecular imaging is in a developing stage but has an encouraging future. The development of specific molecular probes is always challenging and requires precise validation. However, with the development of cutting-edge in vivo imaging technology, this could revolutionize the dysplasia detection and optimize the BE surveillance programs. Furthermore, it has the potential to precisely guide treatment with molecularly targeted cytotoxic (and fluorescently labeled) therapy.

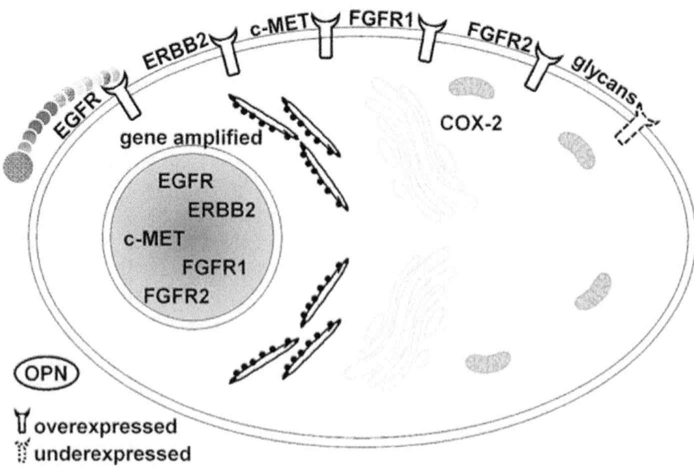

Fig. 8. Molecular imaging targets. Protein targets: epidermal growth factor receptor (EGFR), ERBB2, c-MET, fibroblast growth factor receptor (FGFR). Cell surface glycans are underexpressed with disease progression in EAC and can be detected with lectins. (*From* Sturm MB, Wang TD. Emerging optical methods for surveillance of Barrett's esophagus. Gut 2015;64(11):1816–23; with permission.)

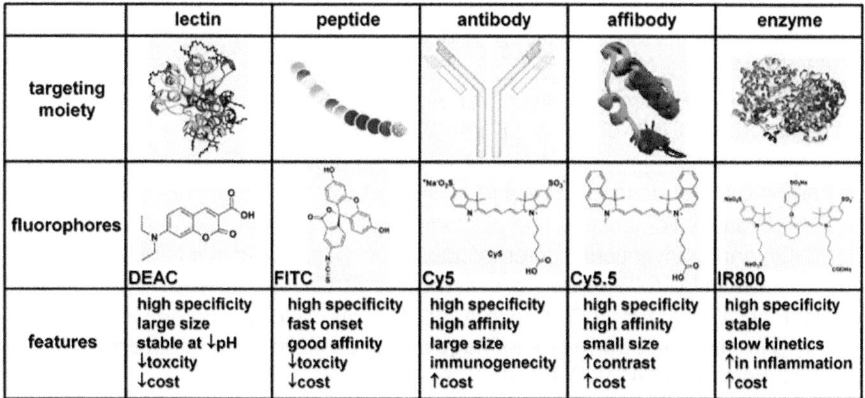

	lectin	peptide	antibody	affibody	enzyme
targeting moiety					
fluorophores	DEAC	FITC	Cy5	Cy5.5	IR800
features	high specificity large size stable at ↓pH ↓toxcity ↓cost	high specificity fast onset good affinity ↓toxcity ↓cost	high specificity high affinity large size immunogenecity ↑cost	high specificity high affinity small size ↑contrast ↑cost	high specificity stable slow kinetics ↑in inflammation ↑cost

Fig. 9. Platforms of molecular probes. Molecular probes have been used on imaging in vivo in preclinical models and in the clinic. Fluorophores used for molecular imaging in BE are shown. DEAC, diethylaminocoumarin, FITC, fluorescein isothiocyanate. (*From* Sturm MB, Wang TD. Emerging optical methods for surveillance of Barrett's esophagus. Gut 2015;64(11):1816–23; with permission.)

SUMMARY

Advances in imaging technologies have demonstrated promise in early detection of dysplasia and cancer in BE. Optical chromoendoscopy (eg, NBI), dye-based chromoendoscopy, and novel technologies such as CLE have provided the opportunity to visualize the cellular and subcellular structures. Currently, only NBI and acetic acid chromoendoscopy have reached benchmarks for clinical use to guide biopsy. New-generation optical tomography (nVLE) has demonstrated significant promise in dysplasia detection in BE given its quick and wide-field cross-sectional HR imaging. Despite having good diagnostic accuracy, VLE remains to be established for routine use in management of BE.[3] In addition the clinical benefits of molecular imaging in BE is yet to be established. Thus, best practice in management of BE should be focused on careful endoscopic examination, resection, or ablation of the entire abnormal lesion, as well as the use of available imaging technique that has good diagnostic accuracy.[84]

REFERENCES

1. Reid BJ, Sanchez CA, Blount PL, et al. Barrett's esophagus: cell cycle abnormalities in advancing stages of neoplastic progression. Gastroenterology 1993;105(1):119–29.
2. Pohl H, Welch HG. The role of overdiagnosis and reclassification in the marked increase of esophageal adenocarcinoma incidence. J Natl Cancer Inst 2005;97(2):142–6.
3. Shaheen NJ, Falk GW, Iyer PG, et al. ACG clinical guideline: diagnosis and management of Barrett's Esophagus. Am J Gastroenterol 2016;111(1):30–50.
4. Vieth M, Ell C, Gossner L, et al. Histological analysis of endoscopic resection specimens from 326 patients with Barrett's esophagus and early neoplasia. Endoscopy 2004;36(9):776–81.
5. Qumseya BJ, Wang H, Badie N, et al. Advanced imaging technologies increase detection of dysplasia and neoplasia in patients with Barrett's esophagus: a meta-analysis and systematic review. Clin Gastroenterol Hepatol 2013;11(12):1562–70.e1–2.

6. Fitzgerald RC, Di Pietro M, Ragunath K, et al. British Society of Gastroenterology guidelines on the diagnosis and management of Barrett's oesophagus. Gut 2014; 63(1):7–42.
7. Muthusamy VR, Kim S, Wallace MB. Advanced Imaging in Barrett's Esophagus. Gastroenterol Clin North Am 2015;44(2):439–58.
8. Gono K, Obi T, Yamaguchi M, et al. Appearance of enhanced tissue features in narrow-band endoscopic imaging. J Biomed Opt 2004;9(3):568–77.
9. Pohl J, May A, Rabenstein T, et al. Comparison of computed virtual chromoendoscopy and conventional chromoendoscopy with acetic acid for detection of neoplasia in Barrett's esophagus. Endoscopy 2007;39(7):594–8.
10. Hoffman A, Korczynski O, Tresch A, et al. Acetic acid compared with i-scan imaging for detecting Barrett's esophagus: a randomized, comparative trial. Gastrointest Endosc 2014;79(1):46–54.
11. Kara MA, Ennahachi M, Fockens P, et al. Detection and classification of the mucosal and vascular patterns (mucosal morphology) in Barrett's esophagus by using narrow band imaging. Gastrointest Endosc 2006;64(2):155–66.
12. Kara MA, Peters FP, Fockens P, et al. Endoscopic video-autofluorescence imaging followed by narrow band imaging for detecting early neoplasia in Barrett's esophagus. Gastrointest Endosc 2006;64(2):176–85.
13. Sharma P, Bansal A, Mathur S, et al. The utility of a novel narrow band imaging endoscopy system in patients with Barrett's esophagus. Gastrointest Endosc 2006;64(2):167–75.
14. Goda K, Kato T, Tajiri H. Endoscopic diagnosis of early Barrett's neoplasia: perspectives for advanced endoscopic technology. Dig Endosc 2014;26(3):311–21.
15. Anagnostopoulos GK, Yao K, Kaye P, et al. Novel endoscopic observation in Barrett's oesophagus using high resolution magnification endoscopy and narrow band imaging. Aliment Pharmacol Ther 2007;26(3):501–7.
16. Song J, Zhang J, Wang J, et al. Meta-analysis of the effects of endoscopy with narrow band imaging in detecting dysplasia in Barrett's esophagus. Dis Esophagus 2015;28(6):560–6.
17. Sharma P, Bergman JJ, Goda K, et al. Development and validation of a classification system to identify high-grade dysplasia and esophageal adenocarcinoma in Barrett's esophagus using narrow-band imaging. Gastroenterology 2016; 150(3):591–8.
18. Pascarenco OD, Coroş MF, Pascarenco G, et al. A preliminary feasibility study: narrow-band imaging targeted versus standard white light endoscopy non-targeted biopsies in a surveillance Barrett's population. Dig Liver Dis 2016; 48(9):1048–53.
19. Wolfsen HC, Crook JE, Krishna M, et al. Prospective, Controlled Tandem Endoscopy Study of Narrow Band Imaging for Dysplasia Detection in Barrett's Esophagus. Gastroenterology 2008;135(1):24–31.
20. Qumseya BJ, Wang H, Badie N, et al. Dysplasia and neoplasia in patients with Barrett's Esophagus: meta-analysis and systematic review. Clin Gastroenterol Hepatol 2013;11(12):1562–70.e1–2.
21. Thosani N, Abu Dayyeh BK, Sharma P, et al. ASGE Technology Committee systematic review and meta-analysis assessing the ASGE Preservation and Incorporation of Valuable Endoscopic Innovations thresholds for adopting real-time imaging–assisted endoscopic targeted biopsy during endoscopic surveillance of Barrett's esophagus. Gastrointest Endosc 2016;83(4):684–98.e7.

22. Curvers W, Baak L, Kiesslich R, et al. Chromoendoscopy and narrow-band imaging compared with high-resolution magnification endoscopy in Barrett's Esophagus. Gastroenterology 2008;134(3):670–9.
23. Curvers WL, Bohmer CJ, Mallant-Hent RC, et al. Mucosal morphology in Barrett's esophagus: interobserver agreement and role of narrow band imaging. Endoscopy 2008;40(10):799–805.
24. Kara MA, Peters FP, Rosmolen WD, et al. High-resolution endoscopy plus chromoendoscopy or narrow-band imaging in Barrett's esophagus: a prospective randomized crossover study. Endoscopy 2005;37(10):929–36.
25. Sharma P, Hawes RH, Bansal A, et al. Standard endoscopy with random biopsies versus narrow band imaging targeted biopsies in Barrett's oesophagus: a prospective, international, randomised controlled trial. Gut 2013;62(1):15–21.
26. Fujimoto JG. Optical coherence tomography for ultrahigh resolution in vivo imaging. Nat Biotechnol 2003;21(11):1361–7.
27. Swanson EA, Huang D, Hee MR, et al. High-speed optical coherence domain reflectometry. Opt Lett 1992;17(2):151–3.
28. Sivak MV Jr, Kobayashi K, Izatt JA, et al. High-resolution endoscopic imaging of the GI tract using optical coherence tomography. Gastrointest Endosc 2000;51(4 I):474–9.
29. Jackle S, Gladkova N, Feldchtein F, et al. In vivo endoscopic optical coherence tomography of the human gastrointestinal tract - Toward optical biopsy. Endoscopy 2000;32(10):743–9.
30. Chen Y, Aguirre AD, Hsiung PL, et al. Ultrahigh resolution optical coherence tomography of Barrett's esophagus: preliminary descriptive clinical study correlating images with histology. Endoscopy 2007;39(7):599–605.
31. Jackle S, Gladkova N, Feldchtein F, et al. In vivo endoscopic optical coherence tomography of esophagitis, Barrett's esophagus, and adenocarcinoma of the esophagus. Endoscopy 2000;32(10):750–5.
32. Isenberg G, Sivak MV Jr, Chak A, et al. Accuracy of endoscopic optical coherence tomography in the detection of dysplasia in Barrett's esophagus: a prospective, double-blinded study. Gastrointest Endosc 2005;62(6):825–31.
33. Cobb MJ, Hwang JH, Upton MP, et al. Imaging of subsquamous Barrett's epithelium with ultrahigh-resolution optical coherence tomography: a histologic correlation study. Gastrointest Endosc 2010;71(2):223–30.
34. Poneros JM, Brand S, Bouma BE, et al. Diagnosis of specialized intestinal metaplasia by optical coherence tomography. Gastroenterology 2001;120(1):7–12.
35. Tao Y, Ahsen OO, Tsai TH, et al. Follow-up of treatment response of radiofrequency ablation of Barrett's esophagus using optical coherence tomography. Gastroenterology 2012;1:S110.
36. Lee HC, Ahsen OO, Liang K, et al. Ultrahigh speed endoscopic optical coherence tomography angiography for visualization of subsurface vasculature in Barrett's esophagus and dysplasia. Gastrointest Endosc 2015;1:AB388.
37. Trindade AJ, Smith MS, Pleskow DK. The new kid on the block for advanced imaging in Barrett's esophagus: a review of volumetric laser endomicroscopy. Therap Adv Gastroenterol 2016;9(3):408–16.
38. Cash BD, Joshi V, Wolfsen HC, et al. Volumetric laser endomicroscopy increases detection of persistent or recurrent Barrett's esophagus and dysplasia in the absence of findings on white light endoscopy. Gastroenterology 2016;1:S257.
39. Evans JA, Poneros JM, Bouma BE, et al. Optical coherence tomography to identify intramucosal carcinoma and high-grade dysplasia in Barrett's esophagus. Clin Gastroenterol Hepatol 2006;4(1):38–43.

40. Sauk J, Coron E, Kava L, et al. Interobserver agreement for the detection of Barrett's esophagus with optical frequency domain imaging. Dis Sci 2013;58(8): 2261–5.
41. Leggett CL, Gorospe EC, Chan DK, et al. Comparative diagnostic performance of volumetric laser endomicroscopy and confocal laser endomicroscopy in the detection of dysplasia associated with Barrett's esophagus. Gastrointest Endosc 2016;83(5):880–8.e2.
42. Trindade AJ, George BJ, Berkowitz J, et al. Volumetric laser endomicroscopy can target neoplasia not detected by conventional endoscopic measures in long segment Barrett's esophagus. Endosc Int Open 2016;4(3):E318–22.
43. Swager AF, Boerwinkel DF, de Bruin DM, et al. Detection of buried Barrett's glands after radiofrequency ablation with volumetric laser endomicroscopy. Gastrointest Endosc 2016;83(1):80–8.
44. Han J, Tsujino T, Samarasena JB, et al. Is volumetric laser endomicroscopy (VLE) helpful in determining complete response of intestinal metaplasia (CRIM) after endoscopic treatment of Barrett's esophagus? Gastrointest Endosc 2016;1: AB551.
45. Cash BD, Joshi V, Wolfsen HC, et al. Volumetric laser endomicroscopy improves detection of persistent or recurrent Barrett's esophagus, dysplasia and Neoplasia following endoscopic treatment. Gastrointest Endosc 2016;1:AB550.
46. Cash BD, Joshi V, Wolfsen HC, et al. Absence of suspicious findings on volumetric laser endomicroscopy strongly predicts histopathologic complete remission of dysplasia and intestinal metaplasia in patients after visual eradication of Barrett's esophagus. Gastrointest Endosc 2016;1:AB123.
47. Wang Z, Lee HC, Ahsen OO, et al. Novel optical coherence tomography image analysis reveals subsquamous glandular structures as strong predictors of poorer response to radiofrequency ablation in Barrett's esophagus. Gastroenterology 2016;1:S434.
48. Rodriguez-Diaz E, Singh SK. Computer-assisted image interpretation of volumetric laser endomicroscopy in Barrett's esophagus. Gastroenterology 2015;1: S91–2.
49. Swager AF, Van Der Sommen F, Zinger S, et al. Feasibility of a computer algorithm for detection of early Barrett's neoplasia using volumetric laser endomicroscopy. Gastroenterology 2016;1:S56.
50. Trindade AJ, Inamdar S, Smith MS, et al. Volumetric laser endomicroscopy in Barrett's esophagus: interobserver agreement for interpretation of Barrett's esophagus and associated neoplasia among high-frequency users. Gastrointest Endosc 2016. [Epub ahead of print].
51. Swager AF, Van Oijen MG, Tearney GJ, et al. How good are experts in identifying endoscopically visible early Barrett's Neoplasia on in vivo volumetric laser endomicroscopy? Gastrointest Endosc 2016;1:AB573.
52. Swager AF, Van Oijen MG, Tearney GJ, et al. Stepwise development of a volumetric laser endomicroscopy prediction score for barrett's Neoplasia using matched VLE-histology images of endoscopic resection specimens. Gastrointest Endosc 2016;1:AB485–6.
53. Leggett CL, Chan DK, Gorospe EC, et al. Diagnostic performance of in-vivo volumetric LASER endomicroscopy for detection of Barrett's esophagus dysplasia. Gastrointest Endosc 2015;1:AB502.
54. Wolfsen HC, Sharma P, Wallace MB, et al. Safety and feasibility of volumetric laser endomicroscopy in patients with Barrett's esophagus (with videos). Gastrointest Endosc 2015;82(4):631–40.

55. Wallace MB, Aranda-Michel EC, Leggett CL, et al. Accuracy and inter-observer agreement of volumetric LASER endomicroscopy (Nvle) for detection of Barrett's esophagus and dysplasia: a prospective multicenter trial. Gastrointest Endosc 2014;1:AB156–7.
56. Leggett CL, Gorospe EC, Anderson M, et al. Optimization of a scoring index for detection of dysplasia in Barrett's esophagus using volumetric laser endomicroscopy. Gastrointest Endosc 2014;1:AB356–7.
57. Neumann H, Kiesslich R, Wallace MB, et al. Confocal laser endomicroscopy: technical advances and clinical applications. Gastroenterology 2010;139(2): 388–92, 392.e1–2.
58. Wallace M, Lauwers GY, Chen Y, et al. Miami classification for probe-based confocal laser endomicroscopy. Endoscopy 2011;43(10):882–91.
59. Kiesslich R, Gossner L, Goetz M, et al. In vivo histology of Barrett's esophagus and associated neoplasia by confocal laser endomicroscopy. Clin Gastroenterol Hepatol 2006;4(8):979–87.
60. Sharma P, Meining AR, Coron E, et al. Real-time increased detection of neoplastic tissue in Barrett's esophagus with probe-based confocal laser endomicroscopy: final results of an international multicenter, prospective, randomized, controlled trial. Gastrointest Endosc 2011;74(3):465–72.
61. Dunbar KB, Okolo Iii P, Montgomery E, et al. Confocal laser endomicroscopy in Barrett's esophagus and endoscopically inapparent Barrett's neoplasia: a prospective, randomized, double-blind, controlled, crossover trial. Gastrointest Endosc 2009;70(4):645–54.
62. Pohl H, Rosch T, Vieth M, et al. Miniprobe confocal laser microscopy for the detection of invisible neoplasia in patients with Barrett's oesophagus. Gut 2008; 57(12):1648–53.
63. Wallace MB, Sharma P, Lightdale C, et al. Preliminary accuracy and interobserver agreement for the detection of intraepithelial neoplasia in Barrett's esophagus with probe-based confocal laser endomicroscopy. Gastrointest Endosc 2010; 72(1):19–24.
64. Bajbouj M, Vieth M, Rösch T, et al. Probe-based confocal laser endomicroscopy compared with standard four-quadrant biopsy for evaluation of neoplasia in Barrett's esophagus. Endoscopy 2010;42(6):435–40.
65. Di Pietro M, Bird-Lieberman EL, Liu X, et al. The combination of autofluorescence imaging and probe-based confocal laser endomicroscopy has an excellent diagnostic accuracy for dysplasia in Barrett's esophagus. Gastrointest Endosc 2013; 1:AB327–8.
66. Canto MI, Anandasabapathy S, Brugge W, et al. In vivo endomicroscopy improves detection of Barrett's esophagus-related neoplasia: A multicenter international randomized controlled trial (with video). Gastrointest Endosc 2014;79(2): 211–21.
67. Kara MA, Peters FP, Ten Kate FJ, et al. Endoscopic video autofluorescence imaging may improve the detection of early neoplasia in patients with Barrett's esophagus. Gastrointest Endosc 2005;61(6):679–85.
68. Costello S, Singh R. Endoscopic imaging in Barrett's oesophagus: applications in routine clinical practice and future outlook. Clin Endosc 2011;44(2):87–92.
69. Curvers WL, Singh R, Song LM, et al. Endoscopic tri-modal imaging for detection of early neoplasia in Barrett's oesophagus: a multi-centre feasibility study using high-resolution endoscopy, autofluorescence imaging and narrow band imaging incorporated in one endoscopy system. Gut 2008;57(2):167–72.

70. Curvers WL, Alvarez Herrero L, Wallace MB, et al. Endoscopic tri-modal imaging is more effective than standard endoscopy in identifying early-stage neoplasia in Barrett's esophagus. Gastroenterology 2010;139(4):1106–14.
71. Giacchino M, Bansal A, Kim RE, et al. Clinical utility and interobserver agreement of autofluorescence imaging and magnification narrow-band imaging for the evaluation of Barrett's esophagus: a prospective tandem study. Gastrointest Endosc 2013;77(5):711–8.
72. Curvers WL, van Vilsteren FG, Baak LC, et al. Endoscopic trimodal imaging versus standard video endoscopy for detection of early Barrett's neoplasia: a multicenter, randomized, crossover study in general practice. Gastrointest Endosc 2011;73(2):195–203.
73. Boerwinkel DF, Holz JA, Kara MA, et al. Effects of autofluorescence imaging on detection and treatment of early neoplasia in patients with Barrett's esophagus. Clin Gastroenterol Hepatol 2014;12(5):774–81.
74. di Pietro M, Bird-Lieberman EL, Liu X, et al. Autofluorescence-directed confocal endomicroscopy in combination with a three-biomarker panel can inform management decisions in Barrett's Esophagus. Am J Gastroenterol 2015;110(11):1549–58.
75. Mannath J, Subramanian V, Telakis E, et al. An inter-observer agreement study of autofluorescence endoscopy in Barrett's esophagus among expert and non-expert endoscopists. Dig Dis Sci 2013;58(2):465–70.
76. di Pietro M, Boerwinkel DF, Shariff MK, et al. The combination of autofluorescence endoscopy and molecular biomarkers is a novel diagnostic tool for dysplasia in Barrett's oesophagus. Gut 2015;64(1):49–56.
77. Sturm MB, Wang TD. Emerging optical methods for surveillance of Barrett's oesophagus. Gut 2015;64(11):1816–23.
78. Cronin J, McAdam E, Danikas A, et al. Epidermal growth factor receptor (EGFR) is overexpressed in high-grade dysplasia and adenocarcinoma of the esophagus and may represent a biomarker of histological progression in Barrett's esophagus (BE). Am J Gastroenterol 2011;106(1):46–56.
79. Varghese S, Lao-Sirieix P, Fitzgerald RC. Identification and clinical implementation of biomarkers for Barrett's esophagus. Gastroenterology 2012;142(3):435–41.e2.
80. Bird-Lieberman EL, Neves AA, Lao-Sirieix P, et al. Molecular imaging using fluorescent lectins permits rapid endoscopic identification of dysplasia in Barrett's esophagus. Nat Med 2012;18(2):315–21.
81. Sturm MB, Joshi BP, Lu S, et al. Targeted imaging of esophageal neoplasia with a fluorescently labeled peptide: first-in-human results. Sci Transl Med 2013;5(184):184ra161.
82. Atreya R, Neumann H, Neufert C, et al. In vivo imaging using fluorescent antibodies to tumor necrosis factor predicts therapeutic response in Crohn's disease. Nat Med 2014;20(3):313–8.
83. Lofblom J, Feldwisch J, Tolmachev V, et al. Affibody molecules: engineered proteins for therapeutic, diagnostic and biotechnological applications. FEBS Lett 2010;584(12):2670–80.
84. Sharma P, Brill J, Canto M, et al. White paper AGA: advanced imaging in Barrett's Esophagus. Clin Gastroenterol Hepatol 2015;13(13):2209–18.

Beyond Dysplasia Grade

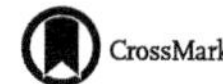

The Role of Biomarkers in Stratifying Risk

Kerry B. Dunbar, MD, PhD[a], Rhonda F. Souza, MD[b,*]

KEYWORDS

- Barrett's esophagus • Biomarker • Dysplasia • In vivo imaging
- Confocal laser endomicroscopy • Fluorescence endoscopy

KEY POINTS

- Gastroenterology society guidelines recommend endoscopic surveillance of Barrett's esophagus using high-definition white-light endoscopy with 4-quadrant random biopsies to detect dysplasia and early cancers.
- The presence of dysplasia is the current gold standard biomarker for cancer risk in Barrett's esophagus.
- Precision medicine and new biomarker development techniques have the potential to improve cancer risk assessment and response to treatment of patients with Barrett's esophagus by identifying specific subtypes based on biomarker expression.
- Immunostaining for p53 is recommended by the British Society of Gastroenterology as an adjunct to histologic assessment of dysplasia in patients with Barrett's esophagus.
- Early proof-of-principal studies demonstrate the promise of fluorescent-tagged molecular biomarkers to enhance the sensitivity and specificity of neoplasia detection during in vivo imaging for patients with Barrett's esophagus.

INTRODUCTION

Barrett's esophagus is an extremely common condition occurring in approximately 5.6% of adult Americans.[1] The risk of esophageal adenocarcinoma for the general population of patients with nondysplastic Barrett's esophagus is low, between 0.12% and 0.33% per year.[2,3] For patients with high-grade dysplasia, the risk of esophageal adenocarcinoma is approximately 6% per year, whereas those patients with low-grade dysplasia (LGD) have a cancer incidence rate that lies between that of nondysplastic Barrett's esophagus and high-grade dysplasia (HGD).[4,5]

Disclosure Statement: This work was supported by the National Institutes of Health (R01-DK63621 and R01-DK103598 to R.F. Souza).

[a] Division of Gastroenterology and Hepatology, Department of Medicine, Esophageal Diseases Center, Dallas VA Medical Center, VA North Texas Health Care System, University of Texas Southwestern Medical Center, CA 111-B1, 4500 South Lancaster Road, Dallas, TX 75216, USA; [b] Center for Esophageal Diseases, Department of Medicine, Baylor University Medical Center and Center for Esophageal Research, Baylor Scott and White Research Institute, 2 Hoblitzelle, Suite 250, 3500 Gaston Avenue, Dallas, TX 75246, USA

* Corresponding author. Rhonda.Souza@BSWHealth.org

Gastrointest Endoscopy Clin N Am 27 (2017) 447–459
http://dx.doi.org/10.1016/j.giec.2017.02.003
1052-5157/17/Published by Elsevier Inc.

Gastrointestinal society guidelines recommend endoscopic surveillance using high-definition white-light endoscopy with 4-quadrant random biopsies obtained every 1 to 2 cm, as a means to detect dysplasia and early cancers in Barrett's esophagus.[3,6,7] However, this strategy has limited effectiveness, as rates of esophageal adenocarcinoma have continued to increase.[8,9] Among the challenges associated with our current cancer preventive strategy are the endoscopist's ability to identify suspicious areas in the entire field of Barrett's mucosa for targeted biopsies and the reliance on the histopathologic diagnosis of dysplasia. To overcome these challenges, new endoscopic imaging techniques are being explored that highlight neoplastic tissue. Some of the new techniques use fluorescent-tagged molecular biomarkers that bind to abnormal tissue and then are visualized during the imaging process. The combination of new imaging techniques and fluorescein-tagged molecular probes has been termed *in vivo molecular imaging*, an emerging technology that has garnered intense interest both for clinicians and scientists.

The following sections highlight the limitations of using dysplasia to stratify cancer risk for patients with Barrett's esophagus, concepts regarding the development and use of biomarkers ex vivo and in vivo, and proof-of-principle studies demonstrating the potential of in vivo imaging using molecular biomarkers to detect early neoplasia in Barrett's esophagus. This review focuses on current concepts supported by recently published key studies.

LIMITATIONS WITH USING DYSPLASIA TO STRATIFY CANCER RISK IN BARRETT'S ESOPHAGUS

Histologic analysis of biopsies to identify dysplasia is the current gold standard for assessing cancer risk in patients with Barrett's esophagus. However, there are several limitations when relying on the grading of dysplasia to risk stratify patients with Barrett's esophagus. Four-quadrant random biopsies may not detect areas of dysplasia, leading to sampling error and missed cases of dysplasia. Assuming adequate biopsies are taken, technical or processing artifact of the tissue can hinder accurate determine of dysplasia.[10] Histologic interpretation of biopsies is more challenging when active inflammation and ulceration are present, which is not uncommon in patients with Barrett's esophagus. Inflammation induces regenerative changes in the Barrett's epithelium, and these regenerative changes can mimic dysplasia. This mimicry can lead to diagnostic uncertainty and may result in a biopsy specimen labeled indefinite for dysplasia, leading to the need for repeat endoscopy with biopsies.[10] This issue of inflammation mimicking dysplasia is the rationale underlying the recommendation in the American College of Gastroenterology's (ACG) guidelines, which advise against taking biopsies in areas of erosive esophagitis until after intensive antisecretory therapy has healed any mucosal injury.[3]

Even without the presence of inflammation, histologic interpretation of dysplasia is challenging. There are no scientifically validated morphologic features to distinguish LGD from HGD, leading to variations in interpretation between pathologists.[10–12] In addition to the difficulties in distinguishing low-grade from high-grade dysplasia, there is also a substantial disagreement among pathologists when distinguishing HGD from intramucosal cancer.[10,13] To compound the problem, there is a high degree of interobserver and intraobserver variability in the diagnosis and grading of dysplasia in Barrett's esophagus, which has been seen in multiple studies.[13,14] In studies in which expert gastrointestinal pathologists reviewed histopathology slides from cases of nondysplastic and dysplastic (both LGD and HGD) Barrett's esophagus, the interobserver agreement for nondysplastic Barrett's esophagus was fair to moderate, with a kappa statistic (K) of 0.2 to 0.58, higher for HGD/carcinoma (K = 0.43–0.65) and lower for LGD (K = 0.11–0.4).[12–14] These findings among expert gastrointestinal pathologists with a research interest in Barrett's esophagus emphasize the limitations of using dysplasia to stratify the risk of cancer in patients with Barrett's esophagus. As dysplasia is an imperfect measure of cancer risk, new techniques are needed to improve the identification of patients who may progress from nondysplastic Barrett's esophagus to cancer.

BIOMARKER DEVELOPMENT: CANCER HALLMARKS

Biomarkers have been used in multiple diseases to assess risk of cancer, predict response to treatment, and estimate prognosis.[15] Many of these biomarkers are derived from cellular and tissue features specific to cancer. In 2000, Hanahan and Weinberg proposed the concept that genetic alterations of different molecular pathways alter normal cellular physiologic function, allowing cells to acquire essential cancer hallmarks that enable them to transform into malignant cells (**Fig. 1**). These essential cancer hallmarks are core physiologic attributes allowing cells to proliferate without exogenous stimulation, resist growth-inhibitory signals, avoid apoptosis, resist cell senescence, develop new vascular supplies (angiogenesis), and invade and metastasize.[16] In 2011, the same investigators proposed 2 additional requisite physiologic hallmarks: cancer cells must reprogram their energy metabolism to support their malignant proliferation and cancer cells must evade destruction by immune cells, including T and B lymphocytes, macrophages, and natural killer cells (see **Fig. 1**).[17] Finally, the acquisition of these cancer attributes is accelerated by 2 enabling features, including genome instability and mutation, which facilitates the genetic alterations essential for tumorigenesis, and tumor-promoting inflammation, which supports the capabilities endowed by the core hallmarks. Many of these cancer

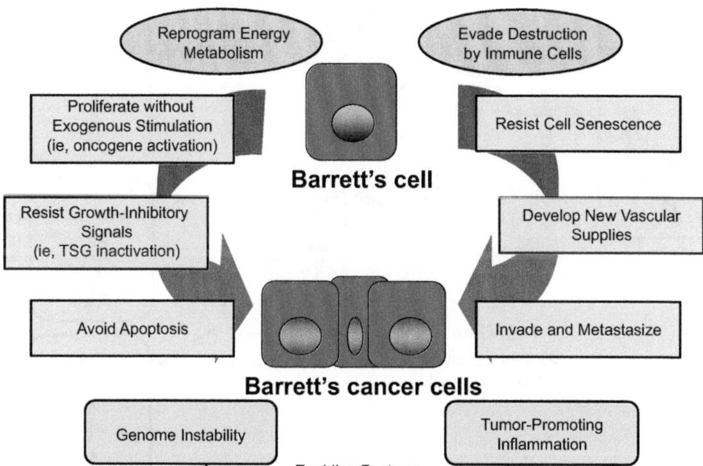

Fig. 1. Cancer hallmarks. The core physiologic attributes of cancer cells are shown in the green boxes. In general, oncogene activation is the way in which cells can proliferate without exogenous stimulation and inactivation of tumor suppressor genes (TSG) is a common way in which cells resist growth-inhibitory signals. The two additional requisite physiologic attributes of cancer cells are shown in the orange circles. The rounded boxes in blue are the enabling features that accelerate the rate at which cells acquire the core and the additional 2 physiologic attributes of cancer cells.

hallmarks have been developed into biomarkers for different diseases. This circumstance is also a factor in Barrett's esophagus, as some of these cancer hallmarks are present in metaplastic Barrett's cells even before they exhibit the histologic features of dysplasia.[18] In the future, molecular biomarkers may become better predictors of neoplastic progression than dysplasia.

BIOMARKER DEVELOPMENT FOR BARRETT'S ESOPHAGUS IN THE PRECISION MEDICINE ERA

The US Precision Medicine Initiative, announced by President Barack Obama during the 2015 State of the Union Address, aspires to improve health by collecting clinical and biomarker data from patients with the same disease and then integrating these findings to reclassify the disease into subtypes (**Fig. 2**).[15,19] The goal of the precision medicine approach is the development of better biomarkers for disease; however, the magnitude of data collected and the speed of analysis have been substantially accelerated by this initiative. The idea is to determine which pieces of data from the large quantity of collected data (ie, histology, RNA, protein, and so forth) are the best predictors of disease risk, treatment response, and/or prognosis, and quickly move these data forward into the biomarker development pipeline.[15]

Classification of tumor subtypes is already underway, with the discovery of mutations and targeted therapies that impact treatment of certain tumor subtypes. For

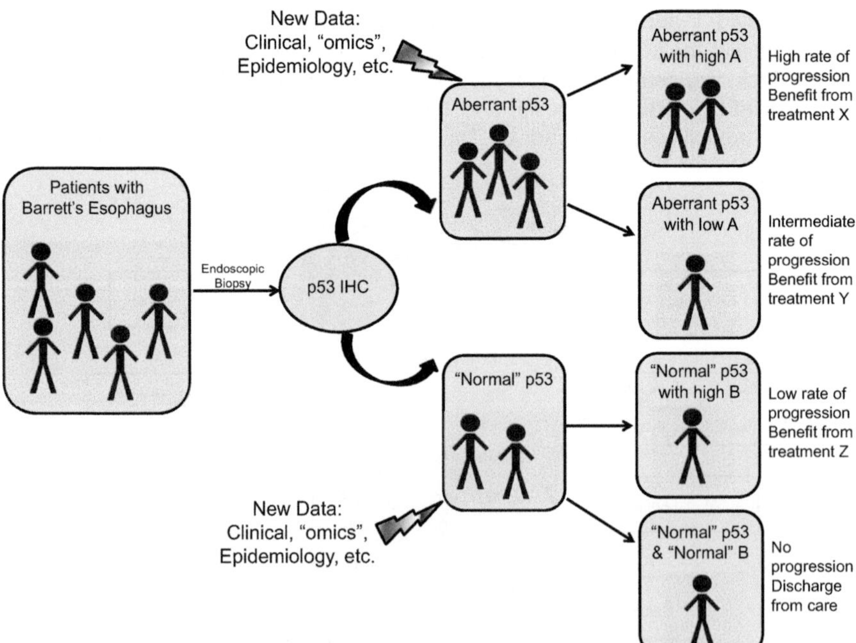

Fig. 2. Theoretic reclassification of Barrett's esophagus based on biomarkers in the era of precision medicine. Patients with Barrett's esophagus would be classified based on molecular subtypes, such as aberrant p53 immunostaining (IHC). Large amounts of data collected from clinical medicine, omics, and epidemiologic associations will be analyzed and synthesized to develop more precise molecular subtypes. These molecular subtypes will not only predict progression to cancer but may also guide treatment decisions for patients with Barrett's esophagus.

example, colorectal cancers with mutant Ras respond to different chemotherapy than colorectal cancers negative for the Ras mutation.[20] Categorization of breast cancers has led to targeted chemotherapy, as tumors with the human epidermal growth factor receptor 2 (HER2) mutation respond to specific chemotherapy targeted to the mutation, whereas other breast cancers do not.[21]

Incredible technological advances have now accelerated biomarker discovery and development. DNA, RNA, proteins, cell metabolites, microbial products, and host cell products are being measured by omics techniques, such as genomics and metabolomics. The profiles derived from these omics techniques can then be used to identify viable biomarkers.[15] Specifically, over the last 10 years, The Cancer Genome Atlas collaborative initiative has performed omic profiling of advanced stage tumors using multiple platforms, such as DNA sequencing for mutations and RNA sequencing for micro-RNA expression, to gain insight into the molecular alterations associated with cancer.[22] This effort has uncovered several hundred genes that are potential drivers of cancer formation. In addition, performance of multiple omics arrays has allowed recategorization of several tumor types. For example, low-grade gliomas are traditionally classified based on histology; but this classification suffers from large intraobserver and interobserver variability and does not adequately predict clinical outcomes.[23] By combining data from multiple omics profiles from low-grade gliomas, a new classification was developed, composed of 3 molecular subtypes strongly associated with overall survival, outperforming histologic classification for prediction of survival.[23] Similar to the study of gliomas, the histologic classification in Barrett's esophagus suffers from the same issues, as histologic classification does not always accurately predict clinical outcomes. Using the precision medicine approach to categorize molecular subtypes of Barrett's esophagus holds promise for the future of biomarker development (see **Fig. 2**).

Using a precision medicine-type approach, Stachler and colleagues[24] performed whole-exome sequencing on DNA extracted from esophageal adenocarcinoma and Barrett's esophagus from the same patient. Using complex bioinformatics analyses, they found that most esophageal adenocarcinomas harbored a p53 mutation and that the same p53 mutation could be detected in the nondysplastic Barrett's metaplasia of patients who progressed to cancer. Interestingly, this study found 2 general pathways for neoplastic transformation in Barrett's esophagus (**Fig. 3**). They found a minority of tumors progressed along the traditional pathway of carcinogenesis, involving the stepwise accumulation of alterations in the p53 and p16 tumor suppressor genes, followed by oncogene activation, and then development of genomic instability. In contrast, most tumors in the study developed through a different pathway, called the genome-doubled pathway. In this pathway, the cell first acquired a p53 mutation that gave that cell a growth advantage and allowed it to expand throughout the mucosa. These p53-mutant cells then underwent whole-genome doubling, an alteration that was primarily detected in areas of dysplasia. Whole-genome doubling was then followed by genomic instability and oncogene amplification, resulting in malignancy. The investigators proposed that the genome-doubled pathway may be a more rapid pathway to cancer development in Barrett's esophagus and may possibly explain the failure of endoscopic surveillance strategies to stem the increasing incidence of esophageal adenocarcinoma.[24] Using the precision medicine approach, perhaps Barrett's esophagus could be stratified into molecular subtypes, based on p53 immunostaining with or without whole-genome doubling. This stratification could potentially improve our ability to risk stratify neoplastic progression and guide treatment decisions for patients with Barrett's esophagus (see **Fig. 2**).

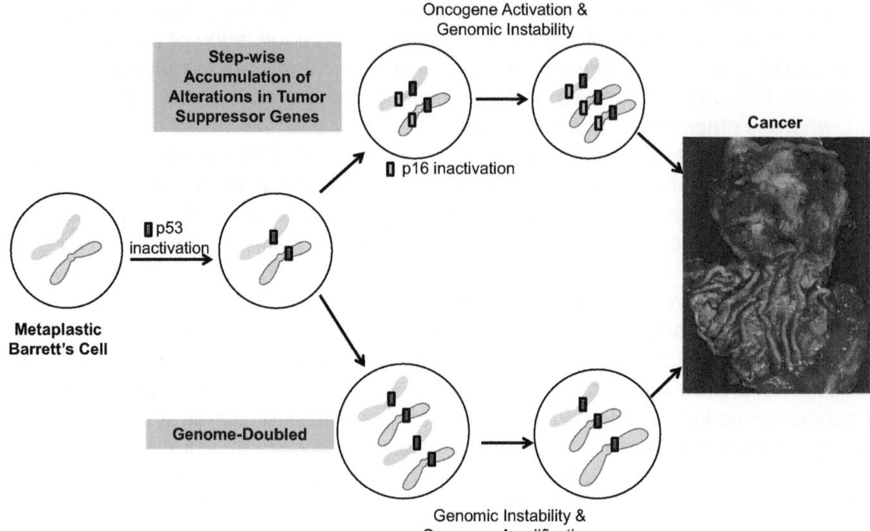

Fig. 3. Two proposed pathways for neoplastic transformation in Barrett's metaplasia. Metaplastic Barrett's cells first acquire a mutation leading to inactivation of p53. In the traditional pathway, there is stepwise accumulation of alterations in tumor suppressor genes, such as p16. This accumulation is followed by the activation of oncogenes and genomic instability, finally resulting in cancer formation. In the genome-doubled pathway, the p53-mutant Barrett's cells undergo whole-genome doubling, followed by genomic instability and oncogene amplification, resulting in cancer formation. It has been proposed that the genome-doubled pathway more rapidly progresses to cancer than the traditional stepwise accumulation of alterations in tumor suppressor genes and oncogenes.

USE OF BIOMARKER PANELS TO ASSESS CANCER RISK IN BARRETT'S ESOPHAGUS

Recently, biomarker studies have focused on panels of biomarkers to attempt to determine the risk of neoplasia in Barrett esophagus patients.[25–27] For each of these studies, the selection of the biomarkers was based on the biology underlying cancer development, as determined by basic and translational research studies. A few of the more promising predictive biomarkers for cancer progression in Barrett's esophagus have been validated in large studies; most with retrospective validation, whereas some studies include both a retrospective validation followed by prospective evaluation in a cohort of patients. Biomarker development and validation is a challenging and lengthy process. The following studies demonstrate the potential for biomarker-based prediction of cancer risk in patients with Barrett's esophagus. However, at this time the guidelines from the ACG and the American Gastroenterological Association recommend against routine use of biomarkers in the management of Barrett's esophagus.[3,28]

Methylation Arrays

One study examined gene methylation arrays in Barrett's esophagus and esophageal adenocarcinoma.[25] Genes with differential methylation were identified and applied to a cohort of samples, including 60 nondysplastic Barrett's esophagus, 9 esophageal adenocarcinomas, and 28 dysplastic Barrett's esophagus. From this retrospective validation, the investigators identified a 4-gene panel that was able to discriminate between nondysplastic Barrett's esophagus and Barrett's-associated neoplasia with a high area under the curve of 0.988. They then prospectively used the 4-gene panel in 61 patients with nondysplastic Barrett's esophagus, 20 patients with HGD/cancer, and 17 patients with LGD to assess the risk of neoplastic progression. They found that the risk of developing dysplasia and cancer was higher in the patients with more methylation.

Mutational Load

Another study examined the mutational load, determined from loss of heterozygosity and microsatellite instability of 10 genomic loci associated with tumor suppressor genes, as a potential biomarker for determining the risk of dysplasia and cancer in Barrett's esophagus.[26] The mutational load score was compared between 23 patients with nondysplastic Barrett's esophagus or those with LGD who progressed to HGD/cancer and 46 patients with nondysplastic Barrett's esophagus or those with LGD who did not progress. The mutational load score was significantly higher in patients who progressed to HGD/cancer than in patients who did not. Using a mutational load score of 1 or more in baseline mucosal biopsies, accuracy for predicting progression to dysplasia and cancer was 89.9%.

Histopathologic Biomarker Classification System

In another study, the investigators developed a 15-feature histopathologic biomarker classification system (p53, p16, cyclooxygenase 2, HER2/neu, and others) to risk stratify patients with Barrett's esophagus.[27] They then tested this biomarker classification system in a validation set of 38 patients who progressed to HGD or cancer and 145 patients who did not progress. Based on study findings, the 15-feature classification system was able to risk stratify patients with Barrett's esophagus into low, intermediate, and high risk for progression over 5 years. The area under the receiver operating characteristic (ROC) curve for prediction of 5-year progression to HGD or cancer was 0.804. The hazard ratio for progression to HGD or cancer in the high-risk versus low-risk group was 9.42.

P53 IMMUNOSTAINING: SO CLOSE AND PERHAPS NOT SO FAR AWAY

Among the potential molecular biomarkers in Barrett's esophagus, immunostaining for p53 protein alterations has advanced the farthest into clinical practice. p53 is a tumor suppressor gene that is activated in response to DNA injury. Activation of p53 decreases cell proliferation, a process that prevents cells with damaged DNA from undergoing mitosis and perpetuating the genomic damage. If the DNA injury is severe and irreparable, then p53 induces cell destruction through apoptosis. p53 is frequently inactivated in several human tumors, including Barrett's-associated cancers.

In response to DNA injury, normal (wild-type) p53 protein rapidly accumulates and then is rapidly degraded, making it difficult to detect p53 protein expression in normal biopsy samples. In contrast, mutant p53 protein is stable and overexpression can be easily detected in tissue samples by immunostaining techniques. In addition to overexpression, mutant p53 can also lead to loss of expression in tissue samples, which can also be evaluated by immunostaining. In a recent case-control study performed in the Netherlands, p53 protein expression was determined by immunostaining in more than 12,000 biopsies from 49 cases of patients with Barrett's esophagus who progressed to HGD or cancer and from 586 control patients whose Barrett's esophagus did not progress to neoplasia.[29] Aberrant p53 expression, defined as overexpression or loss of expression, was identified in 49% of biopsies from progressors compared with 14% in control biopsies from patients that did not progress to HGD or cancer. With aberrant p53 expression, the overall relative risk (RR) of neoplastic progression increased by a factor of 6.2.[29] Aberrant p53 expression in nondysplastic Barrett's esophagus was associated with an increased RR (4.3) of neoplastic progression, whereas an even higher RR (12.2) was seen for LGD.[29]

More recently, p53 immunostaining was prospectively evaluated as a predictor of progression to HGD and esophageal adenocarcinoma.[30] Patients with Barrett's esophagus referred for treatment of HGD or early cancer and patients undergoing Barrett's esophagus surveillance had p53 immunostaining of their Barrett's mucosal biopsies. Patients without a diagnosis of HGD or esophageal adenocarcinoma were then followed for a median of 71 months, and 12% progressed to HGD or cancer during this time.[30] Aberrant p53 expression was significantly higher in the baseline biopsies of those patients who progressed to HGD or cancer (63.6%) than in those who did not progress (7.5%).[30] Multivariate analysis demonstrated that aberrant p53 expression in baseline Barrett's mucosal biopsies was a significant and independent predictor of progression to neoplasia (hazard ratio 17).[30]

Recent studies such as these highlight the promise for biomarkers, in particular aberrant p53 expression, to predict cancer progression in Barrett's esophagus either alone or in combination with histology. In fact, the British Society for Gastroenterology has given a grade B recommendation (nonrandomized, supportive clinical studies) to the use of p53 immunostaining as an adjunct to routine histologic assessment for dysplasia, which may enhance the performance of a diagnosis of dysplasia as a risk stratification biomarker for Barrett's esophagus.[7]

CHALLENGES OF ENDOSCOPIC BARRETT'S ESOPHAGUS SURVEILLANCE AND NEW ADVANCES IN IMAGING

Our current cancer preventive strategy relies on endoscopic surveillance to detect dysplasia. Although there are no data from randomized controlled trials, several observational studies demonstrate that surveillance programs allow detection of Barrett's-associated cancers at an earlier stage and are associated with an increase in survival for patients undergoing surveillance compared with patients not undergoing regular endoscopic surveillance (Reviewed in[3,6]). However, there are numerous challenges with current endoscopic surveillance protocols. Currently, standard endoscopic surveillance uses high-definition white-light endoscopy to visually inspect the mucosa coupled with systematic 4-quadrant biopsies obtained at 1- to 2-cm intervals along the length of the nondysplastic Barrett's metaplasia, with areas of mucosal irregularity sampled separately.[3,28] Thus, it is not surprising that current surveillance programs are expensive, labor intensive, and time consuming both for patients and physicians.[3,6] Studies have found that physician adherence to this surveillance protocol ranges from 30% to 51%, which is problematic.[31,32] Moreover, even if strict adherence to the biopsy protocol is followed, there is still the issue of biopsy sampling error.[33]

To overcome these challenges, newer imaging modalities are being developed that can distinguish dysplasia from the surrounding areas of nondysplastic Barrett's mucosa in vivo so that targeted rather than random biopsies can be obtained. Such a strategy could reduce cost, reduce time, and increase adherence to surveillance protocols. Endoscopic imaging techniques can be classified into 2 basic categories: those that image a wide area of Barrett's mucosa, such as narrow band imaging, and those that image a precise area in great detail, such as confocal laser endomicroscopy (CLE).[34–36] Several of the techniques have been used successfully in patients with Barrett's esophagus for screening, surveillance, and identifying dysplasia and early cancers and have been endorsed by the American Society for Gastrointestinal Endoscopy for detection of dysplasia in Barrett's esophagus.[37] The ideal endoscopic imaging technique would have the ability to survey large areas of Barrett's mucosa but also identify small areas of dysplasia or early cancers. Many of the current endoscopic technologies can accomplish one of these goals but not both requirements.

IN VIVO ENDOSCOPIC MOLECULAR IMAGING USING BIOMARKERS

Some of the most exciting developments in surveillance of Barrett's esophagus stem from the development of biomarker-based endoscopic imaging. Many of these biomarkers are coupled with current endoscopic imaging techniques. In vivo molecular imaging techniques are being developed that use specific biomarker-based contrast enhancement in combination with in vivo imaging. The specificity of these contrast agents is guided by the underlying molecular biology of the tissue of interest, such as imaging agents targeted to neoplastic Barrett's esophagus.[38] Peptides, antibodies, activated enzymes, and lectins are all being developed for use as molecular biomarkers to specifically target regions of neoplasia during in vivo molecular imaging.[39–42] These biomarkers are often tagged with bright, fluorescent dyes that provide a high level of contrast to enhance visualization. Detection of these fluorescent-tagged molecular biomarkers requires an imaging modality that can detect fluorescence. Current modalities include endoscopes with a single blue light excitation channel (ie, autofluorescence-capable endoscopes), endoscopes with a spiral scanning fiber with 3 excitation wavelengths (red, green, and blue), and CLE.[40,43,44]

Lectins

One molecular imaging study examined fluorescent-tagged lectins as a biomarker for Barrett's esophagus. Lectins are carbohydrate-binding proteins that have specificity for particular glycans located on the cell surface. It has been shown that glycan expression is altered in cancers of the pancreas, colon, and breast.[45] Using a lectin protein expression array, Bird-Lieberman and colleagues[42] identified the lectin *Tritiicum vulgare* agglutinin (WGA), from wheat germ, as binding with high affinity to tissue samples of squamous esophagus. When tissue samples of Barrett's metaplasia and dysplasia were analyzed using 2 independent lectin arrays, the binding of WGA decreased as the degree of dysplasia increased. WGA was then fluorescently tagged, incubated with biopsies obtained from patients with nondysplastic and dysplastic (low grade and high grade) Barrett's esophagus at the bedside ex vivo, and then imaged with a fluorescent camera. Compared with nondysplastic Barrett's biopsies, fluorescence intensities were lower in those biopsies containing dysplasia. These findings were further studied using esophagectomy specimens from patients with Barrett's esophagus containing HGD or cancer. The esophageal mucosa was treated with fluorescent-labeled WGA and imaged with a fluorescence endoscope. This imaging demonstrated a reduction in fluorescence intensity in areas of Barrett's-associated dysplasia when compared with nondysplastic Barrett's esophagus or squamous mucosa.[42]

Peptides

A second study identified a short peptide (ASYNYDA) that binds preferentially to neoplastic Barrett's esophagus.[39] This peptide was then fluorescent tagged and used for in vitro, ex vivo, and in vivo imaging. In vitro, confocal fluorescence microscopy demonstrated binding of this peptide to the plasma membrane of esophageal adenocarcinoma cell lines FLO1, OE33, and OE19 but not to the nondysplastic Barrett's cell line Q-hTERT.[39] Ex vivo imaging using a fluorescence-stereomicroscope of Barrett's esophagus with HGD confirmed specificity in binding of the peptide to Barrett's neoplasia, with a significantly higher fluorescence intensity for HGD and esophageal adenocarcinoma than for squamous mucosa and nondysplastic Barrett's mucosa. The investigators then prospectively examined 25 patients with a history of HGD or esophageal adenocarcinoma. The esophageal mucosa was sprayed with the fluorescent peptide and CLE was performed. In vivo imaging of the squamous mucosa showed no binding of the peptide (**Fig. 4**A), and nondysplastic Barrett's mucosa demonstrated some fluorescent signal by peptide binding (**Fig. 4**B, C). In contrast, HGD (see **Fig. 4**D) and esophageal adenocarcinoma showed intense and specific peptide binding to the neoplastic crypts; histology confirmed the presence of neoplasia (**Fig. 4**E). The investigators found a sensitivity of 75% and a specificity of 97% for the fluorescent-tagged peptide to detect HGD and esophageal adenocarcinoma, with an area under the ROC curve of 0.91.[39]

This fluorescent-tagged peptide specific for Barrett's-associated neoplasia was then tested in a prospective study of 50 patients with Barrett's esophagus using a multimodal fluorescence-reflectance endoscope. The patients had been referred for endoscopic therapy for Barrett's mucosa with HGD or early cancer.[41] Imaging was then performed using a wide-field fluorescence-reflectance endoscope modified to match the fluorescence spectrum of fluorescein. Areas of the mucosa were evaluated by combining the fluorescence and reflectance images.[41] After optimizing the target to background ratio of mean fluorescence intensity, the investigators found a sensitivity of 76% and a specificity of 94% for the peptide to detect HGD and esophageal adenocarcinoma, with an area under the ROC curve of 0.884.[41]

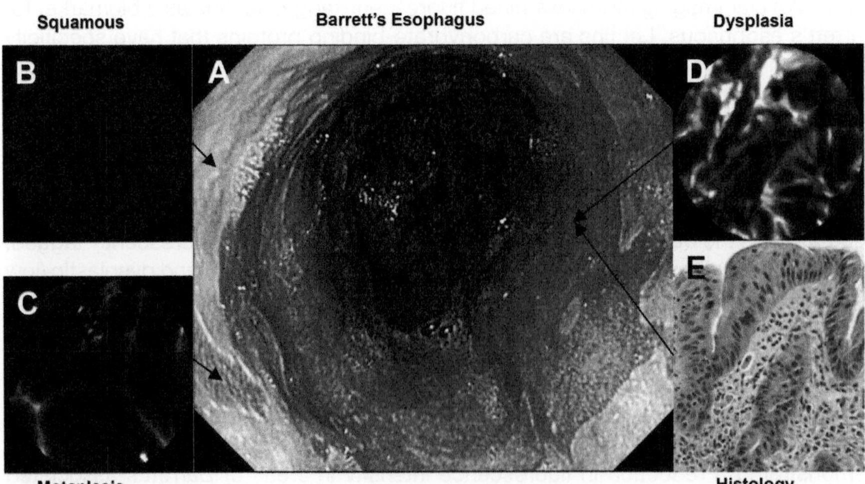

Fig. 4. In vivo molecular imaging using CLE and a fluorescein-tagged molecular peptide in Barrett's esophagus. Representative white-light (*A*) and peptide-based fluorescence images of normal squamous epithelium (*B*), nondysplastic Barrett's metaplasia (*C*), and dysplasia (*D*) obtained using CLE. (*E*) Histology confirms dysplasia in (hematoxylin-eosin, orignial magnificaiton ×20) (*D*). Black arrows indicate the white-light images of the mucosa depicted in panels (*B–E*). (*Courtesy of* Thomas D. Wang, MD, PhD, University of Michigan, Ann Arbor, MI.)

Antibodies

Another potential molecular imaging method for identification of dysplasia in Barrett's esophagus is the use of targeted antibodies. One study in a rat model of Barrett's esophagus and esophageal adenocarcinoma used a fluorescent-labeled anti-HER2 antibody to identify areas of dysplasia and cancer.[46] In ex vivo esophageal specimens treated with an anti-HER2 antibody, the fluorescence intensity of esophageal adenocarcinoma was significantly higher than in normal squamous mucosa or nondysplastic Barrett's mucosa. CLE imaging of rat esophagi was then performed after injection of the fluorescent-labeled anti-HER2 antibody. In vivo fluorescence intensity was higher in esophageal adenocarcinoma than in normal mucosa or nondysplastic Barrett's mucosa demonstrating the future potential for antibody-based molecular imaging in Barrett's esophagus.

SUMMARY

Endoscopic surveillance is currently recommended to detect dysplasia and cancer at an early stage in Barrett's mucosa. Despite its limitations, dysplasia is still the gold standard biomarker to stratify cancer risk in patients with Barrett's esophagus. Among the potential molecular biomarkers, immunostaining for p53 has advanced the farthest into clinical practice, with the British Society of Gastroenterology suggesting its use as an adjunct to the routine histologic assessment for dysplasia. Newer biomarker panels incorporating multiple molecular targets are in development. In vivo molecular imaging, which uses fluorescent-labeled biomarkers, shows promise for use in detecting early neoplasia arising from Barrett's mucosa.

REFERENCES

1. Hayeck TJ, Kong CY, Spechler SJ, et al. The prevalence of Barrett's esophagus in the US: estimates from a simulation model confirmed by SEER data. Dis Esophagus 2010;23(6):451–7.
2. Desai TK, Krishnan K, Samala N, et al. The incidence of oesophageal adenocarcinoma in non-dysplastic Barrett's oesophagus: a meta-analysis. Gut 2012;61(7): 970–6.
3. Shaheen NJ, Falk GW, Iyer PG, et al. ACG clinical guideline: diagnosis and management of Barrett's esophagus. Am J Gastroenterol 2016;111(1):30–50 [quiz: 51].
4. Spechler SJ, Souza RF. Barrett's esophagus. N Engl J Med 2014;371(9):836–45.
5. Rastogi A, Puli S, El-Serag HB, et al. Incidence of esophageal adenocarcinoma in patients with Barrett's esophagus and high-grade dysplasia: a meta-analysis. Gastrointest Endosc 2008;67(3):394–8.
6. Spechler SJ, Sharma P, Souza RF, et al. American Gastroenterological Association technical review on the management of Barrett's esophagus. Gastroenterology 2011;140(3):e18–52 [quiz: e13].
7. Fitzgerald RC, di Pietro M, Ragunath K, et al. British Society of Gastroenterology guidelines on the diagnosis and management of Barrett's oesophagus. Gut 2014; 63(1):7–42.
8. Pohl H, Sirovich B, Welch HG. Esophageal adenocarcinoma incidence: are we reaching the peak? Cancer Epidemiol Biomarkers Prev 2010;19(6):1468–70.
9. Thrift AP, Whiteman DC. The incidence of esophageal adenocarcinoma continues to rise: analysis of period and birth cohort effects on recent trends. Ann Oncol 2012;23(12):3155–62.

10. Naini BV, Souza RF, Odze RD. Barrett's esophagus: a comprehensive and contemporary review for pathologists. Am J Surg Pathol 2016;40(5):e45–66.
11. Curvers WL, ten Kate FJ, Krishnadath KK, et al. Low-grade dysplasia in Barrett's esophagus: overdiagnosed and underestimated. Am J Gastroenterol 2010; 105(7):1523–30.
12. Vennalaganti P, Kanakadandi V, Goldblum JR, et al. Discordance among pathologists in the United States and Europe in diagnosis of low-grade dysplasia for patients with Barrett's esophagus. Gastroenterology 2016;152(3):564–70.e4.
13. Montgomery E, Bronner MP, Goldblum JR, et al. Reproducibility of the diagnosis of dysplasia in Barrett esophagus: a reaffirmation. Hum Pathol 2001;32(4): 368–78.
14. Coco DP, Goldblum JR, Hornick JL, et al. Interobserver variability in the diagnosis of crypt dysplasia in Barrett esophagus. Am J Surg Pathol 2011;35(1):45–54.
15. Vargas AJ, Harris CC. Biomarker development in the precision medicine era: lung cancer as a case study. Nat Rev Cancer 2016;16(8):525–37.
16. Hanahan D, Weinberg RA. The hallmarks of cancer. Cell 2000;100(1):57–70.
17. Hanahan D, Weinberg RA. Hallmarks of cancer: the next generation. Cell 2011; 144(5):646–74.
18. Souza RF, Spechler SJ. Concepts in the prevention of adenocarcinoma of the distal esophagus and proximal stomach. CA Cancer J Clin 2005;55(6):334–51.
19. Collins FS, Varmus H. A new initiative on precision medicine. N Engl J Med 2015; 372(9):793–5.
20. Stintzing S, Stremitzer S, Sebio A, et al. Predictive and prognostic markers in the treatment of metastatic colorectal cancer (mCRC): personalized medicine at work. Hematol Oncol Clin North Am 2015;29(1):43–60.
21. Dawood S, Broglio K, Buzdar AU, et al. Prognosis of women with metastatic breast cancer by HER2 status and trastuzumab treatment: an institutional-based review. J Clin Oncol 2010;28(1):92–8.
22. Campbell JD, Mazzilli SA, Reid ME, et al. The case for a pre-cancer genome Atlas (PCGA). Cancer Prev Res (Phila) 2016;9(2):119–24.
23. Brat DJ, Verhaak RG, Aldape KD, et al. Comprehensive, integrative genomic analysis of diffuse lower-grade gliomas. N Engl J Med 2015;372(26):2481–98.
24. Stachler MD, Taylor-Weiner A, Peng S, et al. Paired exome analysis of Barrett's esophagus and adenocarcinoma. Nat Genet 2015;47(9):1047–55.
25. Alvi MA, Liu X, O'Donovan M, et al. DNA methylation as an adjunct to histopathology to detect prevalent, inconspicuous dysplasia and early-stage neoplasia in Barrett's esophagus. Clin Cancer Res 2013;19(4):878–88.
26. Eluri S, Brugge WR, Daglilar ES, et al. The presence of genetic mutations at key loci predicts progression to esophageal adenocarcinoma in Barrett's esophagus. Am J Gastroenterol 2015;110(6):828–34.
27. Critchley-Thorne RJ, Duits LC, Prichard JW, et al. A tissue systems pathology assay for high-risk Barrett's esophagus. Cancer Epidemiol Biomarkers Prev 2016;25(6):958–68.
28. Spechler SJ, Sharma P, Souza RF, et al. American Gastroenterological Association medical position statement on the management of Barrett's esophagus. Gastroenterology 2011;140(3):1084–91.
29. Kastelein F, Biermann K, Steyerberg EW, et al. Aberrant p53 protein expression is associated with an increased risk of neoplastic progression in patients with Barrett's oesophagus. Gut 2013;62(12):1676–83.
30. Davelaar AL, Calpe S, Lau L, et al. Aberrant TP53 detected by combining immunohistochemistry and DNA-FISH improves Barrett's esophagus progression

prediction: a prospective follow-up study. Genes Chromosomes Cancer 2015; 54(2):82–90.
31. Curvers WL, Peters FP, Elzer B, et al. Quality of Barrett's surveillance in The Netherlands: a standardized review of endoscopy and pathology reports. Eur J Gastroenterol Hepatol 2008;20(7):601–7.
32. Abrams JA, Kapel RC, Lindberg GM, et al. Adherence to biopsy guidelines for Barrett's esophagus surveillance in the community setting in the United States. Clin Gastroenterol Hepatol 2009;7(7):736–42 [quiz: 710].
33. Harrison R, Perry I, Haddadin W, et al. Detection of intestinal metaplasia in Barrett's esophagus: an observational comparator study suggests the need for a minimum of eight biopsies. Am J Gastroenterol 2007;102(6):1154–61.
34. Curvers WL, van den Broek FJ, Reitsma JB, et al. Systematic review of narrow-band imaging for the detection and differentiation of abnormalities in the esophagus and stomach (with video). Gastrointest Endosc 2009;69(2):307–17.
35. Dunbar KB, Canto MI. Confocal laser endomicroscopy in Barrett's esophagus and endoscopically in apparent Barrett's neoplasia: a prospective, randomized, double-blind, controlled, crossover trial. Gastrointest Endosc 2010;72(3):668.
36. Canto MI, Anandasabapathy S, Brugge W, et al. In vivo endomicroscopy improves detection of Barrett's esophagus-related neoplasia: a multicenter international randomized controlled trial (with video). Gastrointest Endosc 2014;79(2): 211–21.
37. Thosani N, Abu Dayyeh BK, Sharma P, et al. ASGE Technology Committee systematic review and meta-analysis assessing the ASGE preservation and incorporation of valuable endoscopic innovations thresholds for adopting real-time imaging-assisted endoscopic targeted biopsy during endoscopic surveillance of Barrett's esophagus. Gastrointest Endosc 2016;83(4):684–98.e7.
38. Sturm MB, Piraka C, Elmunzer BJ, et al. In vivo molecular imaging of Barrett's esophagus with confocal laser endomicroscopy. Gastroenterology 2013;145(1): 56–8.
39. Sturm MB, Joshi BP, Lu S, et al. Targeted imaging of esophageal neoplasia with a fluorescently labeled peptide: first-in-human results. Sci Transl Med 2013;5(184): 184ra161.
40. Sturm MB, Wang TD. Emerging optical methods for surveillance of Barrett's oesophagus. Gut 2015;64(11):1816–23.
41. Joshi BP, Duan X, Kwon RS, et al. Multimodal endoscope can quantify wide-field fluorescence detection of Barrett's neoplasia. Endoscopy 2016;48(2):A1–13.
42. Bird-Lieberman EL, Neves AA, Lao-Sirieix P, et al. Molecular imaging using fluorescent lectins permits rapid endoscopic identification of dysplasia in Barrett's esophagus. Nat Med 2012;18(2):315–21.
43. Lee CM, Engelbrecht CJ, Soper TD, et al. Scanning fiber endoscopy with highly flexible, 1 mm catheterscopes for wide-field, full-color imaging. J Biophotonics 2010;3(5–6):385–407.
44. Miller SJ, Lee CM, Joshi BP, et al. Targeted detection of murine colonic dysplasia in vivo with flexible multispectral scanning fiber endoscopy. J Biomed Opt 2012; 17(2):021103.
45. Fuster MM, Esko JD. The sweet and sour of cancer: glycans as novel therapeutic targets. Nat Rev Cancer 2005;5(7):526–42.
46. Realdon S, Dassie E, Fassan M, et al. In vivo molecular imaging of HER2 expression in a rat model of Barrett's esophagus adenocarcinoma. Dis Esophagus 2015; 28(4):394–403.

Management of Nodular Neoplasia in Barrett's Esophagus

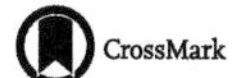

Endoscopic Mucosal Resection and Endoscopic Submucosal Dissection

Kamar Belghazi, MD, Jacques J.G.H.M. Bergman, MD, PhD, Roos E. Pouw, MD, PhD*

KEYWORDS

- Barrett's esophagus • High-grade dysplasia • Early cancer • Endoscopic resection
- Endoscopic mucosal resection • Endoscopic submucosal dissection

KEY POINTS

- Endoscopic resection is an important diagnostic and curative tool in the management of early neoplasia in Barrett's esophagus.
- Endoscopic resection provides an adequate tissue specimen to enable optimal histologic assessment of risk factors for lymph node metastasis.
- Mucosal Barrett's cancer and low-risk submucosal cancers have a minimal risk for lymph node metastasis, and local endoscopic treatment is therefore justified.
- Multiband mucosectomy is currently the most widely used technique for endoscopic resection of early Barrett's neoplasia.

INTRODUCTION

In the past 2 decades, endoscopic therapy has been proven to be an effective, safe, and minimally invasive alternative to surgery for Barrett's esophagus (BE) with early neoplasia (ie, high-grade dysplasia [HGD] or early cancer).[1–5] Endoscopic resection

---

Disclosures: No disclosures (K. Belghazi). Research support for IRB approved studies from GI Solutions Medtronic, Erbe Medical, C2 Therapeutic, Olympus Endoscopy, Fuji Film, Boston Scientific, Ninepoint Medical, Cernostics, Interpase, Lumen-R. Financial support for training programs from GI Solutions Medtronic, Boston Scientific. Honorarium-consultancy-speakers fee from Boston Scientific, GI Solutions Medtronic, Olympus Endoscopy, Fuji Film, WATTS-3d (J.J.G.H.M. Bergman). No disclosures (R.E. Pouw).
Department of Gastroenterology and Hepatology, Academic Medical Center, Meibergdreef 9, Amsterdam 1105 AZ, The Netherlands
* Corresponding author.
E-mail address: r.e.pouw@amc.nl

Gastrointest Endoscopy Clin N Am 27 (2017) 461–470
http://dx.doi.org/10.1016/j.giec.2017.02.004
giendo.theclinics.com

(ER) is considered the cornerstone of endoscopic therapy for early Barrett's neoplasia. The aim of ER is 2-fold: it results in potential curative treatment, but it also serves as a diagnostic tool by providing a specimen for accurate histopathological assessment, which is important to determine further management. The ER technique was developed by the Japanese endoscopist H. Inoue, and he was the first to perform an esophageal endoscopic mucosal resection.[6] ER was adapted by Western endoscopists in the following years. After focal ER of lesions, the remaining Barrett's mucosa carries a risk of approximately 30% of developing metachronous lesions.[2,3,7] Therefore, eradication of the remaining BE is advised.

INDICATIONS FOR ENDOSCOPIC RESECTION

ER only allows for local removal of a lesion, in contrast to surgical resection whereby the esophagus and the regional lymph nodes are removed. Therefore, a prerequisite for endoscopic treatment is adequate selection of patients with a minimal risk of lymph node metastasis. Furthermore, the risk of lymph node metastasis in patients treated endoscopically should be weighed against the risk of morbidity (20%–50%) and mortality (2%–5%) of a surgical esophageal resection.[8–10]

Mucosal Cancer

Endoscopic treatment of BE with HGD or cancer limited to the mucosa (ie, T1m1–m3) has been studied extensively in the past decades and has been shown to be effective and safe.[1–5] One of the largest series of 963 patients treated endoscopically for mucosal esophageal adenocarcinoma demonstrated a long-term complete remission rate of 94%, with only 2 Barrett's cancer–related deaths.[11] In addition, mucosal cancers are associated with a very low risk of lymph node metastasis (<2%).[11] Therefore, ER is considered the treatment of choice for this indication.

Submucosal Cancer

Currently, surgical treatment is in general still considered the gold standard for submucosal Barrett's cancer (ie, T1sm1–sm3) given the supposedly high risk of lymph node metastasis. This recommendation is mainly based on retrospective surgical series showing lymph node metastases in up to 50% of the patients with submucosal cancer.[12–15] However, this risk may be overestimated, because these studies often did not differentiate between different depths of submucosal infiltration because this was not required for patient management. In addition, surgical resection specimens are cut in larger sections than ER specimens, which may lead to underestimation of the infiltration depth associated with risk of lymph node metastasis, because the deepest infiltrating part of a tumor may have been missed. Recent studies on risk of lymph node metastasis based on endoscopic series have shed new light on this indication.

In superficial submucosal cancers (ie, T1sm1, submucosal invasion $\leq$500 μm) without any other histologic risk factors for lymph node metastasis (ie, good to moderate differentiation, no presence of lymphovascular invasion [LVI], and radical resection), the risk of lymph node metastasis appears to be much lower than previously assumed (0%–2%).[16–18] Because the lymph node metastasis risk does not appear to exceed the mortality risk of esophagectomy, endoscopic therapy followed by strict endoscopic follow-up seems to be a valid alternative to surgical resection for this indication.

In high-risk submucosal cancers (ie, submucosal invasion >500 μm, and/or presence of LVI, and/or poor tumor differentiation, and/or irradical resection), the results of endoscopic series show metastasis in 9% to 30% of patients.[18–20] Although the risk is lower than previously assumed, it does exceed the mortality of surgical resection. Therefore, surgical resection is still considered the treatment of choice for patients with high-risk submucosal cancer who are still candidates for surgery. Larger and prospective studies are necessary to establish the role of endoscopic treatment of patients with submucosal Barrett's cancer in the future.

ENDOSCOPIC WORKUP

Patients with HGD or cancer in biopsies, regardless of the presence of a macroscopic abnormality, should be referred to an expert center for Barrett's neoplasia for further workup and treatment. A Dutch study showed that 76% of patients referred for evaluation of HGD or cancer in random biopsies, without visible abnormalities reported during endoscopy, did have a visible abnormality detected during workup endoscopy by an expert endoscopist.[21] This study demonstrates 2 important points: early neoplastic lesions are often difficult to detect and centralization of Barrett's neoplasia care is of high importance. On the other hand, if a visible lesion is detected but biopsies do not show HGD/cancer, one should consider the possibility a false negative histologic result with a low threshold for performing an ER for optimal histologic diagnosis or at least repeat endoscopy with biopsies.

Detection of Early Neoplastic Lesions

Detection of more advanced neoplastic lesions such as nodularities or ulcerating lesions is relatively easy. However, early neoplastic lesions often present as subtle mucosal abnormalities. It is essential to be familiar with the appearance of these kinds of lesions. It is advisable to use the best endoscope available. High-resolution endoscopy, complemented with virtual chromoendoscopy (eg, narrow-band imaging, blue-laser imaging), is the preferred method for evaluation of BE.

The esophagus should be thoroughly inspected. It is important to first clean the esophagus by removing all mucus and saliva. Flushing water is often sufficient; however, the use of acetylcysteine (1%) may be helpful. Afterward, the endoscope should be gradually withdrawn in order to perform a systematic endoscopic inspection. The extent of BE should be documented according to the Prague C&M classification.[22] Then, the inflated esophagus should be gradually deflated. In this way, any irregularities that may have been flattened during inflation will be revealed. Special attention should be paid to the area between 6 and 12 o'clock because most neoplastic lesions are detected here. Also, the transition of the BE into the hiatal hernia should always be assessed in the retrograde position because this area can be less well visualized from the antegrade position.[23]

Macroscopic Appearance of Early Barrett's Neoplasia

As described earlier, mucosal cancer and low-risk submucosal cancers are indications for endoscopic treatment. Removing a visible lesion from a BE with ER is a valuable diagnostic step, because the pathologist will be able to provide accurate information on infiltration depth and other risk factors for submucosal invasion based on the ER specimen. However, knowledge of which lesions are amendable for ER is required for all endoscopists performing ER. The macroscopic appearance of a lesion in a BE should be classified according to the Paris classification.[24] The classification of early lesions is divided into 3 major types of lesions: protruded, flat, and excavated lesions. Protruded lesions (Paris type 0-Is and 0-Ip) are defined as being higher than a closed biopsy forceps (2.5 mm). The flat lesions are subdivided into 3 types: the slightly elevated lesions (Paris type 0-IIa) are less high than a closed biopsy forceps, the completely flat lesions (Paris type 0-IIb), and the slightly depressed lesions (Paris type 0-IIc) are less deep than one cup of an open biopsy forceps. The macroscopic appearance of the lesion appeared to be associated with the infiltration depth in a study by Pech and colleagues.[23] Protruded lesions (Paris type 0-Is and 0-Ip) and slightly depressed lesions (Paris type 0-IIc) significantly more often infiltrated the submucosa (25%–26%) than slightly elevated (Paris type 0-IIa) lesions (9%), or completely flat (Paris type 0-IIb) lesions (0%). None of the Paris type 0-I or type 0-II lesions were associated with a very high risk of submucosal invasion, and diagnostic ER therefore appears indicated and safe for these lesions.[25] For the excavated lesions (Paris type 0-III), no good data are available on the rate of submucosal invasion. The ulceration present in these lesions probably often prohibits safe and radical ER of these lesions.

PRINCIPLES OF ENDOSCOPIC RESECTION

En-bloc Resection Versus Piecemeal Endoscopic Resection

Most conventional ER techniques allow for en-bloc resection of lesions with a maximum diameter of 2 cm. Larger lesions require resection in multiple resections during a so-called piecemeal procedure. Piecemeal resections are technically more demanding and time-consuming, have a higher risk of complications, and are associated with a higher rate of local recurrence if no additional ablation of the Barrett's is performed.[11] Furthermore, one of the downsides of piecemeal ER is that histologic assessment of the radicality of the ER at the lateral margins is almost impossible. However, in early neoplastic lesions in BE, this may be less relevant because eradication of all residual Barrett's tissue is considered part of the current treatment algorithm for BE with neoplasia.

Marking the Target Lesion

After a lesion has been detected, it is important to delineate the lesion before the ER by placing coagulation markers around the lateral margins of the lesion. These markers are necessary because the margins of the lesions may be difficult to recognize during resection, due to lifting of the lesion, bleeding, or coagulation effect. When the ER is finished, the macroscopic radicality of the resection can be easily assessed by checking if all coagulation markers are removed. The different ER techniques are described in later discussion.

ENDOSCOPIC RESECTION TECHNIQUES

Several ER techniques have been described for BE. For cap-based ER, 2 different techniques are available: the lift-suck-cut technique and the ligate-and-cut technique.

Lift-Suck-Cut Technique

The lift-suck-cut technique was the first cap-based ER technique. A transparent ER cap is attached to the tip of an endoscope; the cap has a distal ridge that allows positioning of a crescent-shaped electrocoagulation snare (Olympus Medical Systems Europe GmbH, Hamburg, Germany). This technique is also known as the ER-cap technique.

First, the lesion is lifted by injection of saline into the submucosal layer. Then, the lesion is sucked into the cap, thus creating a pseudopolyp. The pseudopolyp is immediately captured by closing the prepositioned resection snare and removed by using electrocoagulation (**Fig. 1**).

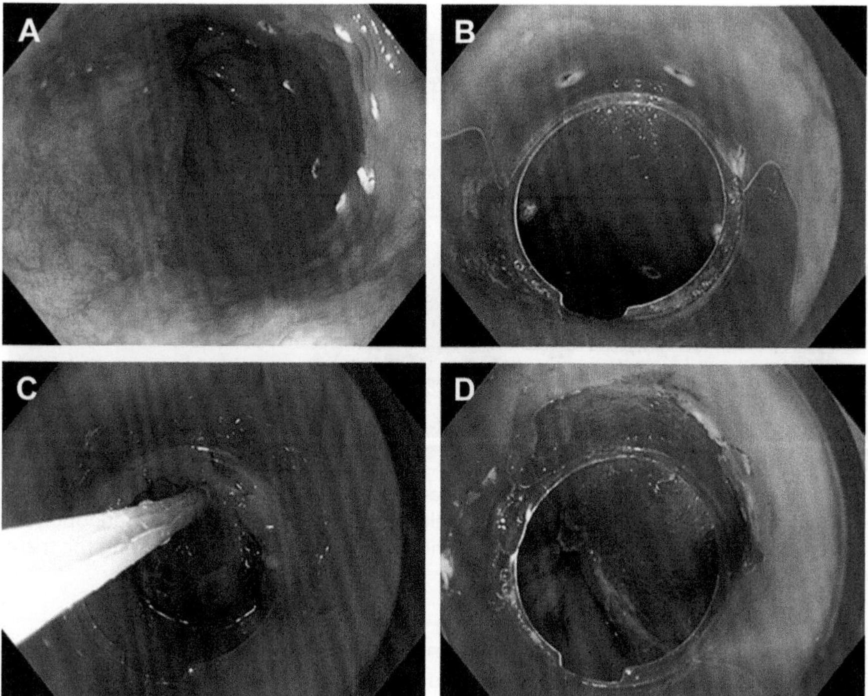

Fig. 1. ER using the ER-cap technique. (*A*) C1M5 BE with a visible lesion at 2 o'clock. (*B*) View through the distal attachment cap on the delineated lesion. (*C*) After submucosal lifting of the lesion, the mucosa is sucked, and into the cap, and by closing the prelooped snare the mucosa is captured and can be resected using electrocautery. (*D*) ER wound.

There are ER caps available with different diameters, and the caps either have an oblique or a straight shape. The largest en-bloc resections (approximately 20 mm) can be achieved by using a large-caliber flexible cap. A disadvantage of this technique is that the procedure is technically demanding, particularly when multiple resections (ie, piecemeal) are required.

Ligate-and-Cut Technique

The ligate-and-cut technique is a more user-friendly alternative to the ER-cap method, and it is currently the most widely used technique for ER of Barrett's lesions. For this technique, a modified variceal band ligator with a control handle is mounted at the proximal end of the working channel. The handle is connected by a tripwire to a transparent cap with 6 rubber bands that are placed on the distal end of the endoscope. The lesion is sucked into the cap followed by the release of a rubber band. No prior submucosal injection is required because the esophageal muscle layer will immediately retract when captured within a rubber band. The created pseudopolyp is subsequently resected using a hexagonal snare (**Fig. 2**). The ligate-and-cut or "multiband-mucosectomy (MBM)" technique can be performed using the Duette System (Cook, Limerick, Ireland), or the recently introduced Captivator device (Boston Scientific).

Several studies have shown that removal of focal lesions can be safely and effectively achieved by ER.[1,3,7,11,26–28] A recent single-center trial with 1000 BE patients with mucosal cancer demonstrated complete eradication of neoplasia in 96% of

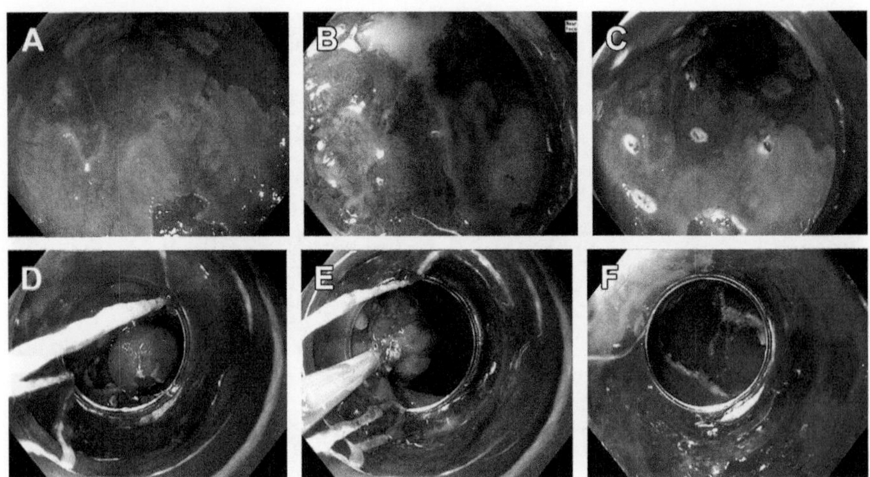

Fig. 2. ER using the MBM technique. (*A, B*) Early neoplastic lesion in a BE with white light endoscopy and narrow band imaging. (*C*) Delineation of the lesion. (*D*) A pseudopolyp is created after release of the rubber band. (*E*) The pseudopolyp is removed by using the snare. (*F*) ER wound.

patients. Major complications developed in 1.5% (n = 15, bleeding n = 14, perforation = 1) but could all be managed conservatively.[11] In early Barrett's neoplasia, MBM achieves comparable success rates for effective piecemeal resection compared with the ER-cap technique, yet the procedure is quicker and cheaper.[28,29] Furthermore, complication rates (ie, perforation or bleeding) are low, and most endoscopists consider the MBM technique easier to learn. Therefore, MBM is considered the technique of choice for piecemeal resection of early Barrett's neoplasia.

Endoscopic Submucosal Dissection

En-bloc resection of lesions larger than 20 mm can be achieved by using the endoscopic submucosal dissection (ESD) technique, which allows proper assessment of the lateral margins. ESD was initially developed in Japan to improve endoscopic treatment of early gastric cancer.[30] The concept of ESD is to incise the mucosa around a lesion, regardless how large, and then remove the lesion in one piece by visual submucosal dissection using an electrosurgical knife instead of blind resection using a snare. The ESD procedure starts with delineating the resection borders by placing coagulation markings followed by lifting with submucosal injection of fluid. A circumferential incision using the electrosurgical knife should be made outside the markings with repeat submucosal lifting when necessary. After the circumferential incision is complete, submucosal dissection of the submucosa should be performed under endoscopic visualization in order to remove the lesion in one piece (**Fig. 3**). The exact approach for ESD of lesions may vary depending on lesion size, localization, and operator preference (eg, complete circumferential incision vs partial incision and stepwise alternation of mucosal incision and submucosal dissection). Common rules are to start with the most difficult accessible part of the lesion and make optimal use of gravity to expose the right dissection plane. Although ESD results in higher en-bloc resection rates, it has disadvantages as well: it is a technically challenging technique; it is associated with a higher complication rate (up to 67%) compared with ER; and it is more time consuming.[31–35] However, to date, only one trial directly compared ER with

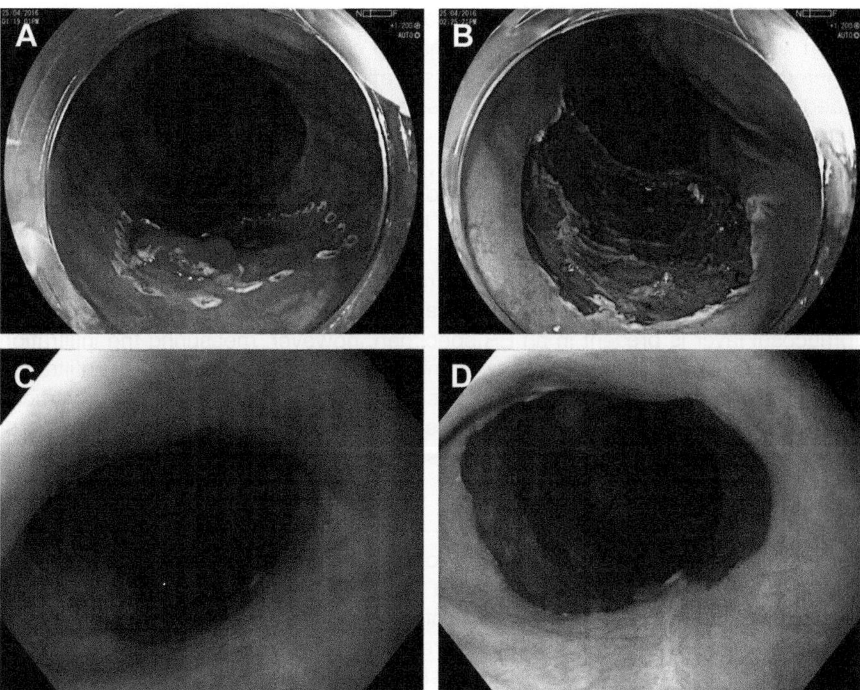

Fig. 3. ESD. (*A*) Delineation of a nodularity in a BE. (*B*) Resection wound after removal by endoscopic submucosal dissection. (*C, D*) Endoscopic submucosal dissection scar with white light endoscopy and narrow band imaging.

ESD in patients with early Barrett's neoplasia.[36] A total of 40 patients were randomized to ESD (n = 20) or ER (n = 20). Histology of the resected specimens showed HGD or cancer in all but 6 cases. Radical resection, defined as margins free of HGD or cancer, was achieved more frequently with ESD (10/17 vs 2/17, P = .01). However, there was no difference in complete remission from neoplasia at 3 months (ESD 15/16 vs ER 16/17, P = 1.0). During a mean follow-up period of 23.1 months, recurrence of cancer was observed in one case in the ESD group. Two severe adverse events were recorded for ESD, both perforations, and none for ER (P = .49). The study concluded that in terms of need for surgery, neoplasia remission, and recurrence, ESD and ER were both highly effective for endoscopic removal of early Barrett's neoplasia. ESD is more time consuming and may cause severe adverse events. However, ESD achieves a higher radical resection rate, but for most Barrett's patients, this bears little clinical relevance, because there is an indication for additional treatment of residual Barrett's mucosa. In their 2015 guideline on ESD, the European Society for Gastroenterology recommends ER with a curative intent for visible lesions in BE. ESD has not been shown to be superior to ER for excision of mucosal cancer, and for that reason, ER should be preferred. ESD may be considered in selected cases, such as lesions larger than 15 mm, poorly lifting tumors, and lesions at risk for submucosal invasion.[37]

HISTOPATHOLOGICAL ASSESSMENT ENDOSCOPIC RESECTION SPECIMENS

ER specimens should be pinned down on paraffin or cork before fixation in formalin, to provide better orientation for the pathologist. After fixation, specimens are routinely cut in 2-mm slices and embedded in paraffin, sectioned, put on glass slides, and stained with hematoxylin and eosin. Esophageal neoplasia is classified according to the internationally accepted Vienna classification.[38] The Vienna classification is divided into 5 categories: category 1: no dysplasia; category 2: indefinite for dysplasia; category 3: low-grade dysplasia; category 4: high-grade dysplasia; category 5: invasive cancer. When invasive cancer is found, the infiltration depth, differentiation grade (good, moderate, poor, or undifferentiated), presence of LVI, and radicality of the resection should be assessed. Infiltration is accurately described for mucosal and submucosal invasion: T1m2: infiltration into the lamina propria; T1m3: infiltration into the muscularis mucosae (T1m3). Infiltration into the submucosa can measured in microns or by subdividing the submucosa into 3 equal parts. Because not the entire submucosal layer is present in an ER specimen, however, measuring the infiltration depth in microns is preferred: T1sm1: infiltration $\leq$500 μm; T1sm2-3: infiltration greater than 500 μm. Radicality of the resection is assessed at the deep (vertical) resection margin in all ER specimens. In the case of en-bloc removed ER specimens, the radicality of the lateral margins is assessed as well.

ENDOSCOPIC TREATMENT ALGORITHM

After endoscopic detection of an early neoplastic lesion in BE, endoscopic assessment of the morphologic appearance of a lesion should guide the decision if ER is feasible. Biopsies can be obtained to confirm the diagnosis of cancer, but are not required. The finding of a visible lesion warrants diagnostic ER to obtain a definite histologic diagnosis. Additional imaging and staging with endoscopic ultrasound (EUS), computerized axial tomography, or PET scan before ER is generally not very useful during workup for early Barrett's neoplasia. EUS is not reliable in the differentiation between mucosal and submucosal cancers, and even discriminating T1 from T2 lesions may be challenging. Given the very low risk of lymph node and distant metastasis associated with early esophageal neoplasia, the yield of finding these with radiological examination is very low. The most important step during workup of early Barrett's neoplasia is therefore diagnostic ER, which provides a large tissue specimen, enabling accurate histologic assessment of risk factors associated with lymph node metastasis. If there are no risk factors, the patient can be managed further endoscopically. If a patient is at high risk for lymph node metastasis based on the outcome of the diagnostic ER, additional staging can still be performed to decide on optimal further treatment. Optimal management for high-risk patients should be discussed during a multidisciplinary team meeting, including a gastroenterologist, a surgeon, and an oncologist.

REFERENCES

1. Ell C, May A, Gossner L, et al. Endoscopic mucosal resection of early cancer and high grade dysplasia in Barrett's esophagus. Gastroenterology 2000;118:670–7.
2. May A, Gossner L, Pech O, et al. Local endoscopic therapy for intraepithelial high-grade neoplasia and early adenocarcinoma in Barrett's oesophagus: acute-phase and intermediate results of a new treatment approach. Eur J Gastroenterol Hepatol 2002;14:1085–91.
3. Peters FP, Kara MA, Rosmolen WD, et al. Endoscopic treatment of high-grade dysplasia and early stage cancer in Barrett's esophagus. Gastrointest Endosc 2005;61:506–14.
4. Pech O, Behrens A, May A, et al. Long-term results and risk factor analysis for recurrence after curative endoscopic therapy in 349 patients with high-grade

intraepithelial neoplasia and mucosal adenocarcinoma in Barrett's oesophagus. Gut 2008;57:1200–6.

5. Ono H, Kondo H, Gotoda T, et al. Endoscopic mucosal resection for treatment of early gastric cancer. Gut 2001;48:225–9.
6. Inoue H, Endo M. Endoscopic esophageal mucosal resection using a transparent tube. Surg Endosc 1990;4:198–201.
7. Ell C, May A, Pech O, et al. Curative endoscopic resection of early esophageal adenocarcinomas (Barrett's cancer). Gastrointest Endosc 2007;65:3–10.
8. Hölscher AH, Vallböhmer D, Bollschweiler E. Early Barrett's carcinoma of the esophagus. Ann Thorac Cardiovasc Surg 2008;14:347–54.
9. Williams VA, Watson TJ, Herbella FA, et al. Esophagectomy for high grade dysplasia is safe, curative, and results in good alimentary outcome. J Gastrointest Surg 2007;11:1589–97.
10. Rice TW. Pro: esophagectomy is the treatment of choice for high-grade dysplasia in Barrett's esophagus. Am J Gastroenterol 2006;101:2177–9.
11. Pech O, May A, Manner H, et al. Long-term efficacy and safety of endoscopic resection for patients with mucosal adenocarcinoma of the esophagus. Gastroenterology 2014;146:652–60.
12. Nigro JJ, Hagen JA, DeMeester TR, et al. Prevalence and location of nodal metastases in distal esophageal adenocarcinoma confined to the wall: implications for therapy. J Thorac Cardiovasc Surg 1999;117:16–23.
13. Stein HJ, Feith M, Bruecher BL, et al. Early esophageal cancer: pattern of lymphatic spread and prognostic factors for long-term survival after surgical resection. Ann Surg 2005;242:566–73.
14. Hölscher AH, Bollschweiler E, Schneider PM, et al. Early adenocarcinoma in Barrett's oesophagus. Br J Surg 1997;84:1470–3.
15. Bollschweiler E, Baldus SE, Schröder W, et al. High rate of lymph node metastasis in submucosal esophageal squamous-cell carcinomas and adenocarcinomas. Endoscopy 2006;38:149–56.
16. Alvarez Herrero L, Pouw RE, van Vilsteren FG, et al. Risk of lymph node metastasis associated with deeper invasion by early adenocarcinoma of the esophagus and cardia: study based on endoscopic resection specimens. Endoscopy 2010;42:1030–6.
17. Manner H, Pech O, Heldmann Y, et al. The frequency of lymph node metastasis in early-stage adenocarcinoma of the esophagus with incipient submucosal invasion (pT1b sm1) depending on histological risk patterns. Surg Endosc 2015;29:1888–96.
18. Schölvinck D, Künzli H, Meijer S, et al. Management of patients with T1b esophageal adenocarcinoma: a retrospective cohort study on patient management and risk of metastatic disease. Surg Endosc 2016;30:4102–13.
19. Boys JA, Worrell SG, Chandrasoma P, et al. Can the risk of lymph node metastases be gauged in endoscopically resected submucosal esophageal adenocarcinomas? A multi-center study. J Gastrointest Surg 2016;20:6–12.
20. Manner H, Wetzka J, May A, et al. Early-stage adenocarcinoma of the esophagus with mid to deep submucosal invasion (pT1b sm2-3): the frequency of lymph-node metastasis depends on macroscopic and histological risk patterns. Dis Esophagus 2016. [Epub ahead of print].
21. Schölvinck DW, van der Meulen K, Bergman JJ, et al. Detection of lesions in dysplastic Barrett's esophagus by community and expert endoscopists. Endoscopy 2017;49(2):113–20.

22. Sharma P, Dent J, Armstrong D, et al. The development and validation of an endoscopic grading system for Barrett's esophagus: the Prague C&M criteria. Gastroenterology 2006;131:1392–9.
23. Pech O, Gossner L, Manner H, et al. Prospective evaluation of the macroscopic types and location of early Barrett's neoplasia in 380 lesions. Endoscopy 2007;39:588–93.
24. The Paris endoscopic classification of superficial neoplastic lesions: esophagus, stomach, and colon: November 30 to December 1, 2002. Gastrointest Endosc 2003;58:S3–43.
25. Peters FP, Brakenhoff KP, Curvers WL, et al. Histologic evaluation of resection specimens obtained at 293 endoscopic resections in Barrett's esophagus. Gastrointest Endosc 2008;67:604–9.
26. Behrens A, May A, Gossner L, et al. Curative treatment for high-grade intraepithelial neoplasia in Barrett's esophagus. Endoscopy 2005;37:999–1005.
27. Larghi A, Lightdale CJ, Ross AS, et al. Long-term follow-up of complete Barrett's eradication endoscopic mucosal resection (CBE-EMR) for the treatment of high grade dysplasia and intramucosal carcinoma. Endoscopy 2007;39:1086–91.
28. Pouw RE, van Vilsteren FGI, Peters FP, et al. Randomized trial on endoscopic resection-cap versus multiband mucosectomy for piecemeal endoscopic resection of early Barrett's neoplasia. Gastrointest Endosc 2011;74:35–43.
29. Alvarez Herrero AL, Pouw RE, van Vilsteren FG, et al. Safety and efficacy of multiband mucosectomy in 1060 resections in Barrett's esophagus. Endoscopy 2011;43:177–83.
30. Miyamoto S, Muto M, Hamamoto Y, et al. A new technique for endoscopic mucosal resection with an insulated-tip electrosurgical knife improves the completeness of resection of intramucosal gastric neoplasms. Gastrointest Endosc 2002;55:576–81.
31. Neuhaus H, Terheggen G, Rutz EM, et al. Endoscopic submucosal dissection plus radiofrequency ablation of neoplastic Barrett's esophagus. Endoscopy 2012;44:1105–13.
32. Kagemoto K, Oka S, Tanaka S, et al. Clinical outcomes of endoscopic submucosal dissection for superficial Barrett's adenocarcinoma. Gastrointest Endosc 2014;80:239–45.
33. Probst A, Aust D, Märkl M, et al. Early esophageal cancer in Europe: endoscopic treatment by endoscopic submucosal dissection. Endoscopy 2015;47:113–21.
34. Höbel S, Dautel P, Baumbach R, et al. Single center experience of endoscopic submucosal dissection (ESD) in early Barrett's adenocarcinoma. Surg Endosc 2015;29:1591–7.
35. Chevaux JP, Piessevaux H, Jouret-Mourin A, et al. Clinical outcome in patients treated with endoscopic submucosal dissection for superficial Barrett's neoplasia. Endoscopy 2015;47:103–12.
36. Terheggen G, Horn E, Vieth M, et al. A randomised trial of endoscopic submucosal dissection versus endoscopic mucosal resection for early Barrett's neoplasia. Gut 2016. [Epub ahead of print].
37. Pimentel-Nunes P, Dinis-Ribeiro M, Ponchon T, et al. Endoscopic submucosal dissection: European Society of Gastrointestinal Endoscopy (ESGE) guideline. Endoscopy 2015;47:829–54.
38. Schlemper RJ, Riddell RH, Kato Y, et al. The Vienna classification of gastrointestinal epithelial neoplasia. Gut 2000;47:251–5.

The Role of Endoscopic Ultrasound in the Management of Patients with Barrett's Esophagus and Superficial Neoplasia

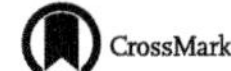

Bashar J. Qumseya, MD, MPH[a], Herbert C. Wolfsen, MD[b,*]

KEYWORDS

- Endoscopy • Esophageal cancer • Advanced imaging • Endosonography

KEY POINTS

- Endoscopic ultrasound (EUS) is safe and widely available.
- Evidence suggests that EUS can accurately change the management strategy in 14% of patients referred for evaluation of Barrett neoplasia.
- EUS has suboptimal specificity and a high rate of overstaging early tumors.
- EUS is especially useful to exclude advanced disease and nodal involvement.
- Cost-effectiveness of EUS for this indication has not been established.

INTRODUCTION

Esophageal adenocarcinoma (EAC) continues to be a major cause of cancer mortality in Western populations. The incidence of EAC seems to be increasing.[1–3] Although several risk factors have been identified for EAC, Barrett esophagus (BE), which is intestinal metaplasia of squamous esophageal mucosa, is the only treatable factor. The risk of progression to EAC among patients with BE varies by degree to dysplasia.[4] As with most cancers, local staging of neoplasia is of critical importance and dictates treatment options and patient outcomes. The current staging of EAC follows the TNM staging (**Table 1**).[5] Superficial cancers are those arising in the mucosa (T1m) or submucosa (T1sm). Current practice includes endoscopic mucosal resection (EMR) or endoscopic submucosal dissection (ESD) for patients with superficial neoplasia (T1m) and some

Disclosure Statement: Dr. H.C. Wolfsen receives research funding from NinePoint Medical.
[a] Division of Gastroenterology and Hepatology, Archbold Medical Group, Florida State University, 112 Mimosa Drive, Thomasville, GA 31792, USA; [b] Division of Gastroenterology and Hepatology, Mayo Clinic, 4500 San Pablo Road, Jacksonville, FL 32224, USA
* Corresponding author.
E-mail address: herbert.wolfsen@mayo.edu

Gastrointest Endoscopy Clin N Am 27 (2017) 471–480
http://dx.doi.org/10.1016/j.giec.2017.03.001
1052-5157/17/

Table 1
TNM classification for staging esophageal cancer

	Primary Tumor (T)
TX	Primary tumor cannot be assessed
T0	No evidence of primary tumor
Tis	High-grade dysplasia
T1	Tumor invades lamina propria, muscularis mucosae, or submucosa
T1a or T1m	Tumor invades lamina propria or muscularis mucosae
T1b or T1sm	Tumor invades submucosa
T2	Tumor invades muscularis propria
T3	Tumor invades adventitia
T4	Tumor invades adjacent structures
T4a	Resectable tumor invading pleura, pericardium, or diaphragm
T4b	Unresectable tumor invading other adjacent structures, such as the aorta, vertebral body, and trachea
	Regional Lymph Nodes (N)
NX	Regional lymph node(s) cannot be assessed
N0	No regional lymph node metastasis
N1	Metastasis in 1–2 regional lymph nodes
N2	Metastasis in 3–6 regional lymph nodes
N3	Metastasis in 7 or more regional lymph nodes
	Distant Metastasis (M)
M0	No distant metastasis
M1	Distant metastasis

T1sm (**Fig. 1**). This is followed by radiofrequency ablation (RFA) to eradicate the remaining BE segment.[6–9] Such therapy, referred to as endoscopic eradication therapy (EET), has been shown efficacious and safe in management of those superficial cancer patients.[10–13] EET, however, is not risk-free. There are risks to EMR and ESD, including perforation, bleeding, and stricture formation.[14] Thus, among patients with advanced disease, T1sm or beyond or N1 or beyond, EMR and ESD are not indicated. Instead, these patients are normally referred to surgeons for consideration of esophagectomy with or without neoadjuvant chemoradiotherapy. Accurate staging for disease is, therefore, essential. Cross-sectional imaging with modalities, such as CT and MRI, are limited in their ability to stage EAC at local levels, especially in early stages.[15] Therefore, EUS has been proposed and used as a better diagnostic test for this indication.[6–9] This review discusses the usefulness of EUS in identifying those patients and better examining the role of EUS for this frequently encountered clinical scenario. Given the availability of several studies on the topic, best evidence-based recommendations are used to inform the discussion and conclusions.

MANAGEMENT GOALS

Defining the exact management goals for EUS in patients with BE is paramount to this discussion. In the performance of EUS for patients with BE, the authors and

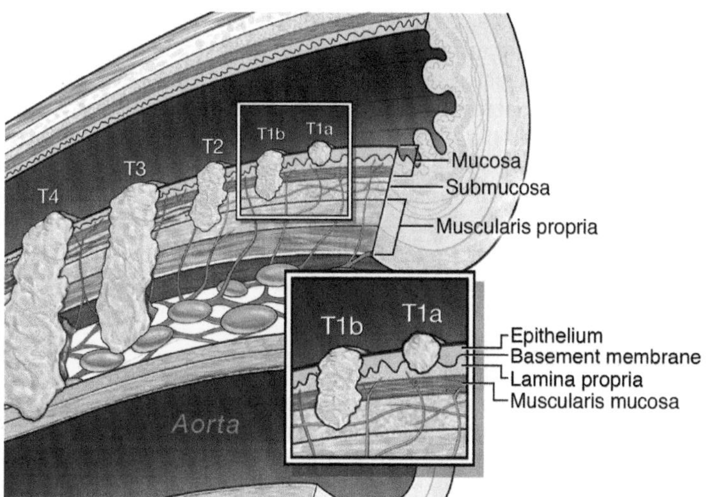

Fig. 1. Schematic representation of staging of esophageal cancer. (*Courtesy of* Mayo Clinic Foundation, Rochester, MN; with permission.)

colleagues believe that the main goal is the accurate identification of advanced disease. If a patient has superficial disease, then EMR is indicated and potentially provides curative treatment. If a patient has advanced disease, however, the only curative option may be esophagectomy. In such patients, EMR is not indicated and may increase risk of morbidity from adverse outcomes like perforation or bleeding. Therefore, being able to stratify patients based on their disease stage is essential. Accurate identification of advanced disease deals with 2 specific issues:

1. Definition of advanced disease
2. Test characteristics, which include sensitivity, specificity, and accuracy

Definition of Advanced Disease

EAC is staged based on the TNM classification (see **Table 1**). The difference between mucosal (T1m) and submucosal (T1sm) disease is subtle and requires high image resolution (**Fig. 2**). Cross-sectional imaging modalities, such as CT and MRI, do not have the sufficient imaging resolution to stage EAC at the T1 to T1sm levels.

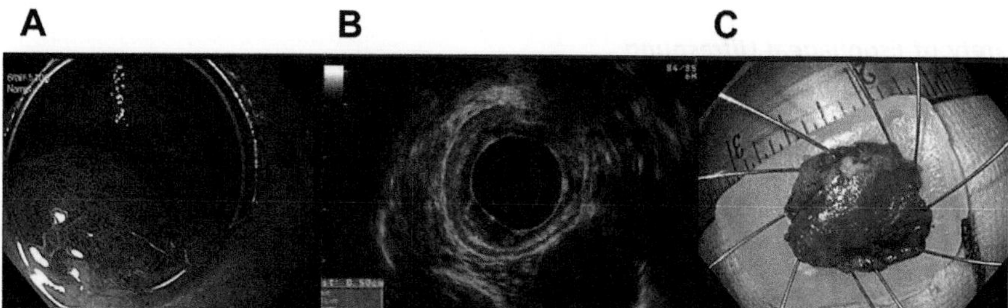

Fig. 2. Patient with BE and a nodule with high-grade dysplagia: (*A*) endoscopic view of the nodule with narrow-band imaging; (*B*) corresponding endosonographic view; and (*C*) tissue embedded on paraffin after EMR of the lesion.

For this reason, EUS, which has a higher resolution, has been used to stage EAC for years. Most experts agree that neoplasia invasive into the submucosa, or involvement of lymph nodes, classifies as advanced disease. In those patients, EMR is not curative, and esophagectomy with or without neoadjuvant chemoradiotherapy is the only curative option. There continues to be some debate on the classification of T1sm. Some expert pathologists can subdivide the submucosa into 3 zones. Sm1 is defined at the upper third of the submucosa within less than 500 μm. In patients with T1sm1, EMR may be curative.[16] This approach has been mostly accepted in several European centers. In the United States, most centers refer patients to surgery on finding T1sm. For the purposes of this review, advanced disease is defined as disease at or beyond T1sm or N1.

Test Characteristics

The accuracy of EUS in diagnosing advanced disease depends on the test characteristics. These includes sensitivity, specificity, and positive and negative predictive values. The tests' positive and negative predictive values largely depend on the prevalence of the disease in the population. Hence, in a tertiary referral center where the prevalence of advanced disease is high, EUS may have better positive predictive values compared with a community practice setting where the prevalence may be lower. Therefore, the authors and colleagues prefer to discuss sensitivity and specificity, because these parameters are not dependent on the prevalence of the disease and may be more reflective of overall test performance. Accuracy provides an overall measure of the proportion of cases in which EUS correctly diagnosed disease among all patients who underwent the procedure. Additionally, a measure of false-positive results, which is termed the false discovery rate (FDR), is discussed. This test helps estimate the risk of overstaging among patients undergoing EUS. Those test characteristics are essential to understanding of the role of EUS in this patient population.

EVALUATION

EUS was first introduced in the 1980s for staging of pancreatic cancers. Since then, EUS has shown superior results in the staging of cancer compared with CT and MRI. One of the main advantages of this technology is the ability to image the esophageal lumen at a high resolution of 7.5 MHz to 12.5 MHz. Whether EUS should be used in the management algorithm of patients with BE depends on multiple variables, including safety, availability, cost-effectiveness, and accuracy. Although accuracy is the most important of those factors, the other factors are addressed in brief before assessing the issue of accuracy.

Safety of Esophageal Ultrasound

EUS is not a risk-free test. The risk of esophageal perforation from cervical intubation has been reported to be approximately 0.3% to 0.6%.[17,18] In a survey of 86 physicians of 43,000 procedures, perforation was reported in 0.03% (n = 16).[19] Of those, 15 perforations were reported with the use of radial EUS scopes, and 12 procedures involved trainees. There was 1 EUS procedure–related death reported. Although EUS procedural safety data are scarce, they point to EUS as a safe test with rare but serious adverse events, especially when performed by experienced endosonographers. In comparison, EMR may be associated with a much higher risk of adverse outcomes. In a recent meta-analysis, the authors and colleagues showed that performing even focal EMR prior to RFA increases the risks of adverse outcomes by 4.4-fold compared with RFA alone.[14] Additionally, most perforations reported in the EET literature are associated with the use of EMR, not RFA. Therefore, this increased risk of adverse outcomes from EMR compared with EUS should be part of the discussion on whether EUS should be replaced by EMR.

Availability of Esophageal Ultrasound

In addition to its safety profile, EUS is increasingly available to clinicians. Since its introduction in the 1980s, EUS seems to be one of the fastest growing areas of gastrointestinal endoscopy.[20] Again, specific data on availability are lacking; anecdotal evidence comes from the number of advanced endoscopy training positions, which has steadily increased. This additional training has resulted in the availability of EUS capability in many if not most community gastroenterology practices.

Cost-Effectiveness of Esophageal Ultrasound in Barrett Esophagus

Despite its increasing availability and relative safety, the cost-effectiveness of EUS in patients with BE neoplasia has not be clearly reported. The authors and colleagues believe that EUS could be cost-effective if done at the same setting of the initial upper endoscopy. This may be especially true in populations where EAC is more prevalent. Nevertheless, detailed cost-effectiveness analyses are needed to better understand this issue.

Accuracy of Esophageal Ultrasound in Barrett Esophagus

Of all the factors discussed, the accuracy of EUS in the detection and staging of advanced disease is the most critical issue to consider. The performance of EUS for this indication has been reported in many studies. Some of the best evidence on the topic comes from a meta-analysis that the authors and colleagues published in 2014.[21] The primary outcome of this study was the proportion of patients with BE suspected dysplasia or neoplasia who were accurately diagnosed with advanced disease on EUS. This was defined as disease into or beyond the submucosa (≥T1sm) or nodal involvement (≥N1). This is a clinically relevant outcome because it gives a quantitative perception of the difference EUS can make in this patient population. A total of 11 studies were included with more than 650 patients. Results from EUS were compared with EMR or pathology reports. The study showed that 14% of all-comers would be accurately diagnosed with advanced disease on EUS. The number needed to treat for this analysis was 7.[21] These data suggest that EUS may make an important difference in the diagnosis, staging, and management of BE patients with suspected neoplasia. The study also showed pooled sensitivity of 56%, however. The low sensitivity means that EUS can miss advanced disease (understaged). The pooled specificity was higher at 89%. Although this value is high, it still shows that 1of 10 patients may be misdiagnosed with advanced disease when they did not have it (overstaged).

Looking more specifically at the accuracy of EUS in T staging of esophageal cancer, Puli and colleagues[22] conducted a meta-analysis of 49 studies with more than 2500 patients. For T1 staging, EUS had a pooled specificity of 99.4%.They reported lower sensitivity for earlier stages (81% for T1), however, compared with later stages (92% for T4). Thus, EUS performs well overall for T staging but better in later stages.

The most recent data on this topic come from the Florida campus of Mayo Clinic. Bartel and colleagues[23] presented the experience using EUS in patients referred for evaluation of BE dysplasia and neoplasia. Patients who had advanced disease (T3 or more) were excluded from this study. In the evaluation of 335 patients, there was a sensitivity of 50% for EUS at the T1sm level. The authors and colleagues main concern, however, was the rate of overstaging. Of 335 patients, 8.5% (n = 19) were overstaged by EUS. Most of these cases (12/19) were staged at T1sm when patients had T1m. Only 1% (n = 3) of patients were staged at T2 when they had T1sm.

The authors and colleagues recently updated a previous meta-analysis to include the Mayo Clinic study[23] and another study by Thota and colleagues,[24] with the intention of better understanding the issue of EUS overstaging. The authors and colleagues focused on the FDR, which gives an estimate of the rate of overstaging; of all people who have advanced disease on EUS, how many have a false-positive test? Mathematically, FDR is the number of false-positive results divided by the number of all patients who tested positive. Using 11 studies[24–33] and 895 patients, a pooled FDR of 37% (23%–53%) was reported. This means that for each 10 patients who are diagnosed with advanced disease based on EUS, approximately 4 of them do not have advanced disease (false-positive results). The pooled accuracy of EUS in this analysis was low, at 76% (95% CI, 63%–85%). The pooled sensitivity was 54% (46%–62%), and specificity was 91% (89%–93%). These data are intriguing and show that EUS is fraught with significant overstaging at the T1sm level.

More data were recently published on the performance of EUS in staging of esophageal squamous cell carcinoma (SCC). Although SCC is different from EAC, the performance of EUS in SCC can be informative on the performance of EUS in the esophagus overall. Luo and colleagues[34] looked at 44 studies with a total of more than 2800 patients. They showed that EUS had a pooled sensitivity of 84% at the T1a level and 83% at T1b. The specificity was 91% at T1a and 89% at the T1b level. Thus, EUS seems to have better overall sensitivity for SCC compared with EAC. Although the reasons behind this trend are not clear, this shows that EUS has the potential to achieve good performance characteristics in esophageal tumors even at the T1a–T1b level.

Having explored the performance of EUS in T staging, another subset of patients in whom EUS may be useful—patients with flat BE form, is considered. These patients are not considered candidates for EMR or ESD because they lack mucosal irregularities. Flat, featureless BE, however, may still harbor advanced disease. The authors and colleagues previously cited meta-analysis looked at the issues of patient who have flat, non-nodular BE. The evidence showed that EUS could accurately detect advanced disease in the absence of suspicious endoscopic findings (ie, nodules, ulcers, or strictures). Specifically, in this setting, EUS detected advanced disease in 4% of cases in which no evidence of advanced disease was suspected on white light endoscopy with or without narrow band imaging. In this analysis, the number needed to treat was 25.

Lastly, the accuracy of EUS for nodal staging needs to be addressed. Although EUS had suboptimal accuracy for staging of superficial EAC, the evidence for nodal staging shows much better performance. In the authors and colleagues analysis of 5 studies,[25,28–30,35] EUS had a pooled sensitivity for nodal disease of 71% and a specificity of 94%.[21] Similarly, the meta-analysis by Puli and colleagues[22] showed that the sensitivity increased to 96% when fine-needle aspirate of suspicious lymph nodes was performed. Therefore, EUS with or without fine-needle aspirate is critically important for the exclusion of nodal disease.

DISCUSSION

Debate on the use of EUS for diagnosis and staging of BE dysplasia and neoplasia continues. Many experts question the usefulness and reliability of EUS in this patient group.[33,36,37] With the increasing use of EMR, it can be seen how EMR could serve as a diagnostic and therapeutic tool in BE patients with suspected neoplasia. This review has explored the benefits and risks of performing EUS for BE patients with suspected neoplasia. Although data are scarce, the authors and colleagues argue that EUS is a safe and increasingly available diagnostic test and have shown that EUS can detect advanced disease in an important subset of patients who are referred for BE with high-grade dysphagia or EAC.

Despite its obvious advantages, the main concern with EUS is the suboptimal diagnostic performance. The overall accuracy of the test is only approximately 76%. This means that 1 in 4 patients is inaccurately staged with EUS (understaged or overstaged). Understaging in this scenario is less of a concern. If patients are staged at T1a but have T1b or T2, they still undergo EMR for visible lesions, per current guidelines. Therefore, the staging based on EMR histology is accurate. More concerning is the rate of overstaging as measured by FDR. If patients are staged at T2 but they have T1m, they may end up undergoing an unnecessary esophagectomy. Such cases are devastating and should be avoided. The authors and colleagues have reported that the FDR was as high at 37%. This is not 37% of patients, but 37% of all positive tests are overstaged at the T1sm level. Based on the specificity of 91%, the rate of false staging is expected to be approximately 9% of all patients. Therefore, overstaging is a problem for EUS and a great hindrance to its use in this patient population.

The 91% sensitivity the authors and colleagues reported, however, is much less impressive that the 99% specificity reported by Puli and colleagues[22] for T staging of EUS in EAC. Note that the 2 numbers represent slightly different outcomes, which could partly explain the difference. Puli and colleagues looked at the specificity of T1 staging. On the other hand, the authors and colleagues reviewed the specificity of staging advanced disease versus nonadvanced disease (as defined earlier). But Puli and colleagues[22] help understand that EUS does better in later staging.

EUS seems to perform similarly in patients with SCC with a specificity of approximately 90% at the T1m to T1sm level.[34] EUS seemed more sensitive in SCC, however. The reasons behind this apparent difference are unclear but are unlikely relevant to the discussion of BE with superficial neoplasia.

EUS has suboptimal specificity and high FDR, but are there any particular patients in whom EUS may be more helpful? The answer is yes. Patients may present with EAC with seemingly flat BE that lacks high-risk stigmata. In those cases, EMR is not done. The evidence suggests that EUS may be helpful because approximately 4% of all-comers have been found with advanced disease, despite the lack of nodularity, ulceration, or stricture. Although this rate is low, the authors and colleagues argue that EUS should be done, if available at the same setting, to exclude advanced disease. The cost-effectiveness of this approach is unproved and requires further studies.

SUMMARY

As discussed, the use of EUS in patients with BE has several advantages but some potential pitfalls as well. EUS seems increasingly more available with a good safety profile in experienced hands. Evidence suggests that EUS can detect advanced disease in a significant number of patients, is excellent for excluding nodal disease, and may detect advanced disease in the absence of nodule, stricture, or ulcers in some patients. EUS is hindered, however, by a suboptimal specificity and high FDR at the T1m–T1sm level, which contributes to significant overstaging and overtreatment. On the basis on this analysis of EUS accuracy, the authors and colleagues propose an evidence-based algorithm that may help clinicians in their work-up and management of patients with BE (**Fig. 3**).

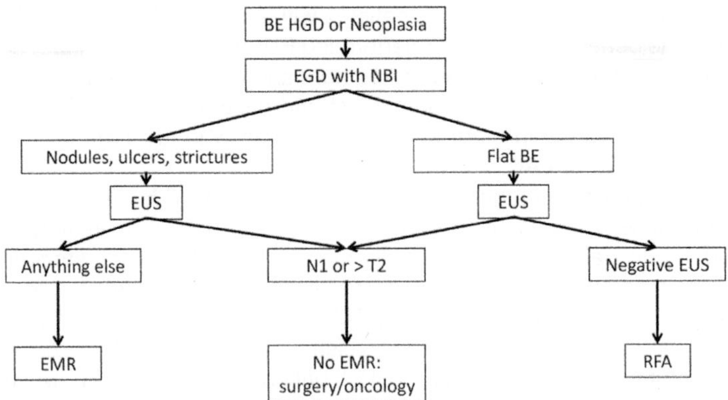

Fig. 3. Suggested algorithm for the use of EUS in patients with BE EGD, upper endoscopy; HGD, high-grade dysplasia.

REFERENCES

1. Rastogi A, Puli S, El-Serag HB, et al. Incidence of esophageal adenocarcinoma in patients with Barrett's esophagus and high-grade dysplasia: a meta-analysis. Gastrointest Endosc 2008;67:394–8.
2. Drewitz DJ, Sampliner RE, Garewal HS. The incidence of adenocarcinoma in Barrett's esophagus: a prospective study of 170 patients followed 4.8 years. Am J Gastroenterol 1997;92:212–5.
3. Vizcaino AP, Moreno V, Lambert R, et al. Time trends incidence of both major histologic types of esophageal carcinomas in selected countries, 1973-1995. Int J Cancer 2002;99:860–8.
4. Shaheen NJ, Falk GW, Iyer PG, et al, American College of Gastroenterology. ACG clinical guideline: diagnosis and management of Barrett's Esophagus. Am J Gastroenterol 2016;111:30–50 [quiz: 51].
5. Shi G, Luo Z, Fu M, et al. Evaluation of the value of 7th editions of UICC-AJCC esophageal and gastric cancer TNM staging systems for prognostic prediction of adenocarcinoma of esophagogastric junction (Siewert type II). Zhonghua Zhong Liu Za Zhi 2014;36:916–21 [in Chinese].
6. Lin JL. T1 esophageal cancer, request an endoscopic mucosal resection (EMR) for in-depth review. J Thorac Dis 2013;5:353–6.
7. Koike T, Nakagawa K, Iijima K, et al. Endoscopic resection (endoscopic submucosal dissection/endoscopic mucosal resection) for superficial Barrett's esophageal cancer. Dig Endosc 2013;25(Suppl 1):20–8.
8. Peters JH, Watson TA. Endoscopic mucosal resection of Barrett's esophagus and early esophageal cancer. J Gastrointest Surg 2011;15:1299–302.
9. Ell C, May A, Pech O, et al. Curative endoscopic resection of early esophageal adenocarcinomas (Barrett's cancer). Gastrointest Endosc 2007;65:3–10.
10. Caillol F, Godat S, Autret A, et al. Neoplastic Barrett's oesophagus and long-term follow-up after endoscopic therapy: complete histological eradication of Barrett associated with high-grade dysplasia significantly decreases neoplasia relapse. Surg Endosc 2016;30:5410–8.
11. Wani S, Komanduri S, Muthusamy VR. Endoscopic eradication therapy in Barrett's Esophagus-Related neoplasia: setting the bar right to optimize patient outcomes. Gastroenterology 2016;150:772–4.

12. Dunbar KB. Endoscopic eradication therapy for mucosal neoplasia in Barrett's esophagus. Curr Opin Gastroenterol 2013;29:446–53.
13. Qumseya B, David W, Woodward TA, et al. Safety of esophageal EMR in elderly patients. Gastrointest Endosc 2014;80:586–91.
14. Qumseya BJ, Wani S, Desai M, et al. Adverse events after radiofrequency ablation in patients with barrett's esophagus: a systematic review and meta-analysis. Clin Gastroenterol Hepatol 2016;14:1086–95.e6.
15. Iyer R, Dubrow R. Imaging of esophageal cancer. Cancer Imaging 2004;4:125–32.
16. Liu L, Hofstetter WL, Rashid A, et al. Significance of the depth of tumor invasion and lymph node metastasis in superficially invasive (T1) esophageal adenocarcinoma. Am J Surg Pathol 2005;29:1079–85.
17. Eloubeidi MA, Tamhane A, Lopes TL, et al. Cervical esophageal perforations at the time of endoscopic ultrasound: a prospective evaluation of frequency, outcomes, and patient management. Am J Gastroenterol 2009;104:53–6.
18. Eisen GM, Baron TH, Dominitz JA, et al. Complications of upper GI endoscopy. Gastrointest Endosc 2002;55:784–93.
19. Das A, Sivak MV Jr, Chak A. Cervical esophageal perforation during EUS: a national survey. Gastrointest Endosc 2001;53:599–602.
20. Hawes RH. The evolution of endoscopic ultrasound: improved imaging, higher accuracy for fine needle aspiration and the reality of endoscopic ultrasound-guided interventions. Curr Opin Gastroenterol 2010;26:436–44.
21. Qumseya BJ, Brown J, Abraham M, et al. Diagnostic performance of EUS in predicting advanced cancer among patients with Barrett's esophagus and high-grade dysplasia/early adenocarcinoma: systematic review and meta-analysis. Gastrointest Endosc 2015;81:865–74.e2.
22. Puli SR, Reddy JB, Bechtold ML, et al. Staging accuracy of esophageal cancer by endoscopic ultrasound: a meta-analysis and systematic review. World J Gastroenterol 2008;14:1479–90.
23. Bartel MJ, Wallace T, Gomez R, et al. The role of EUS in patients with suspected Barrett's esophagus with high-grade dysplasia or early esophageal adenocarcinoma: impact on endoscopic therapy. Gastrointest Endosc 2016. http://dx.doi.org/10.1016/j.gie.2016.11.016.
24. Thota PN, Sada A, Sanaka MR, et al. Correlation between endoscopic forceps biopsies and endoscopic mucosal resection with endoscopic ultrasound in patients with Barrett's esophagus with high-grade dysplasia and early cancer. Surg Endosc 2017;31(3):1336–41.
25. Buskens CJ, Westerterp M, Lagarde SM, et al. Prediction of appropriateness of local endoscopic treatment for high-grade dysplasia and early adenocarcinoma by EUS and histopathologic features. Gastrointest Endosc 2004;60:703–10.
26. Larghi A, Lightdale CJ, Memeo L, et al. EUS followed by EMR for staging of high-grade dysplasia and early cancer in Barrett's esophagus. Gastrointest Endosc 2005;62:16–23.
27. Mino-Kenudson M, Brugge WR, Puricelli WP, et al. Management of superficial Barrett's epithelium-related neoplasms by endoscopic mucosal resection: clinicopathologic analysis of 27 cases. Am J Surg Pathol 2005;29:680–6.
28. Shami VM, Villaverde A, Stearns L, et al. Clinical impact of conventional endosonography and endoscopic ultrasound-guided fine-needle aspiration in the assessment of patients with Barrett's esophagus and high-grade dysplasia or intramucosal carcinoma who have been referred for endoscopic ablation therapy. Endoscopy 2006;38:157–61.

29. Prasad GA, Buttar NS, Wongkeesong LM, et al. Significance of neoplastic involvement of margins obtained by endoscopic mucosal resection in Barrett's esophagus. Am J Gastroenterol 2007;102:2380–6.
30. Thomas T, Gilbert D, Kaye PV, et al. High-resolution endoscopy and endoscopic ultrasound for evaluation of early neoplasia in Barrett's esophagus. Surg Endosc 2010;24:1110–6.
31. Pouw RE, Heldoorn N, Alvarez Herrero L, et al. Do we still need EUS in the workup of patients with early esophageal neoplasia? A retrospective analysis of 131 cases. Gastrointest Endosc 2011;73:662–8.
32. Fernandez-Sordo JO, Konda VJ, Chennat J, et al. Is Endoscopic Ultrasound (EUS) necessary in the pre-therapeutic assessment of Barrett's esophagus with early neoplasia? J Gastrointest Oncol 2012;3:314–21.
33. Bulsiewicz WJ, Dellon ES, Rogers AJ, et al. The impact of endoscopic ultrasound findings on clinical decision making in Barrett's esophagus with high-grade dysplasia or early esophageal adenocarcinoma. Dis Esophagus 2014;27:409–17.
34. Luo LN, He LJ, Gao XY, et al. Endoscopic ultrasound for preoperative esophageal squamous cell carcinoma: a meta-analysis. PLoS One 2016;11:e0158373.
35. Pech O, May A, Gunter E, et al. The impact of endoscopic ultrasound and computed tomography on the TNM staging of early cancer in Barrett's esophagus. Am J Gastroenterol 2006;101:2223–9.
36. Gerke H. Endoscopic mucosal resection for early esophageal cancer: skip EUS and cut to the chase. Gastrointest Endosc 2011;73:669–72.
37. Savoy AD, Wallace MB. EUS in the management of the patient with dysplasia in Barrett's esophagus. J Clin Gastroenterol 2005;39:263–7.

Radiofrequency Ablation of Barrett's Esophagus

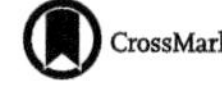

Patient Selection, Preparation, and Performance

Gene K. Ma, MD, Gregory G. Ginsberg, MD*

KEYWORDS

• Barrett's esophagus • Dysplasia • Neoplasia • Radiofrequency ablation

KEY POINTS

- Radiofrequency ablation is a safe and effective thermal ablative therapy for dysplastic and nondysplastic Barrett's esophagus.
- Before performance of radiofrequency ablation, careful endoscopic planning should occur and potential contraindications should be assessed for.
- Successful performance of radiofrequency ablation requires an understanding of the different tools available and a systematic approach to safe and effective application.

INTRODUCTION

The goal of ablation therapy is to eliminate dysplastic or metaplastic epithelium associated with Barrett's esophagus (BE) through the use of thermal techniques, cryotherapy, or photodynamic therapy. Following ablation of dysplasia and specialized intestinal metaplasia (IM), in the setting of effective acid reflux suppression, normal squamous epithelium replaces the ablated tissue. In many/most cases, ablation therapy is used adjunctively after endoscopic resection of visible lesions.

Radiofrequency ablation (RFA) is a safe and effective means of thermal ablative therapy for BE that has become a widely adopted treatment of dysplastic and, to a lesser extent, nondysplastic BE. RFA uses direct contact alternating electrical current to generate thermal energy to produce precise, reproducible, and reliable superficial tissue necrosis, permitting neo-squamous mucosal regeneration and minimizing the risk for fibro-reactive stricture. RFA can be performed with circumferential and focal delivery devices (Covidien, Sunnyvale, CA).

The authors have nothing to disclose.
Division of Gastroenterology and Hepatology, Department of Medicine, University of Pennsylvania, 3400 Civic Center Boulevard, PCAM South Pavilion, 7th Floor, Philadelphia, PA 19104, USA
* Corresponding author.
E-mail address: Gregory.Ginsberg@uphs.upenn.edu

Gastrointest Endoscopy Clin N Am 27 (2017) 481–490
http://dx.doi.org/10.1016/j.giec.2017.02.010

giendo.theclinics.com

Patient Selection

Indications and contraindications for radiofrequency ablation

Several categories of patients with BE may qualify for eradication therapy for BE (**Box 1**). Patients with BE with high-grade dysplasia or greater have been shown to benefit from RFA as a monotherapy for bland, flat BE. RFA should not be used for primary eradication therapy for raised or nodular dysplastic BE. RFA should be used adjunctively in patients with nodular BE following endoscopic resection of all raised or nodular regions. Selected patients with low-grade dysplasia (LGD), who have multifocal LGD, or who have demonstrated persistence of LGD, confirmed by an expert gastrointestinal pathologist, may also be candidates for RFA. Highly selected patients with BE without dysplasia can be considered for RFA if they are at perceived increased risk for development of esophageal adenocarcinoma (EAC), such as those with a strong family history of EAC. In the future, incorporation of biomarkers as part of the prognostic workup for those with BE may identify patients who can derive the most benefit from RFA eradication therapy even in the absence of dysplasia.

Relative contraindications to performance of RFA for BE are listed in **Box 1**. These relative contraindications come from observational accounts and are extrapolated from other BE ablation experiences, including photodynamic therapy. As such, these relative contraindications should be considered when weighing the potential risks and benefits of RFA for individual patients. Ongoing anticoagulation therapy may promote increased risk of bleeding following mucosal ablation. Therefore, temporary cessation of anticoagulation therapy should be considered on an individualized basis when planning RFA. The authors have not observed a need to alter antiplatelet therapy in the peri-procedure period. Ablation therapy in patients who have undergone prior radiation therapy to the esophagus has been associated with delayed healing, persistent ulceration, and increased risk for bleeding, stricture, and fistula.[1] The presence of esophageal varices poses the potential for increased risk of delayed bleeding, and superficial necrosis may unroof high-pressure dilated veins in the submucosa. Preexisting stricture within the treatment segment may impede satisfactory tissue contact with

Box 1
Indications and contraindications for radiofrequency ablation of Barrett's esophagus

Indications

High-grade dysplasia or greater
- In conjunction with endoscopic resection
- Bland, flat BE

Low-grade dysplasia
- Multifocal
- Confirmed persistence

BE without dysplasia
- Family history of esophageal adenocarcinoma

Relative contraindications

Anticoagulation therapy

Prior radiation to esophagus

Esophageal varices

Peptic stricture

Active esophagitis

the ablation device to achieve eradication and will be associated with increased risk for symptomatic postablation dysphagia. Active esophagitis attributed to ongoing acid and even nonacid gastroesophageal reflux is a predictor of ineffective restoration of neo-squamous epithelium. This condition may be observed in patients who are medication noncompliant, those on insufficient acid-suppression therapy, obese patients, active cigarette smokers, those with large sliding hiatal hernia with intrathoracic stomach, patients who are have undergone prior Billroth II gastrectomy or partial esophagectomy, patients with connective tissue disorders affecting the esophagus, and those with true allergy or intolerance to proton-pump inhibitor therapy.

Discussion of Risks and Benefits with Patients

The anticipated benefits of BE eradication therapy should be considered in the context of the potential risks. Patients should be engaged in a candid discussion to make them fully informed and active decision makers when considering RFA as a treatment of BE. The alternatives of continued surveillance and operative resection should be acknowledged. An understanding of the need for compliance with lifelong acid-suppression therapy, multiple treatment sessions and interval posteradication surveillance should be effectively conveyed. Endoscopic eradication therapy is effective in long-term eradication of all IM and all dysplasia in 80% and 90% of patients, respectively.[2] Focal residual/recurrent IM or dysplasia may be detected in up to 20% to 30% of patients with meticulous posteradication endoscopic surveillance. Most recurrence can be effectively treated with adjunctive endoscopic therapy. Failure to comply with prescribed eradication and posteradication surveillance regimens may permit development of advanced esophageal adenocarcinoma.

A systematic review and meta-analysis of adverse events after RFA in patients with BE noted the most common adverse event after RFA is development of a stricture in 5.6% of patients (**Table 1**).[3] Clinically significant bleeding (1.0%) and perforation (0.6%) were found to be less common. Notably, these data were pooled from studies that included both use of RFA alone and RFA used with endoscopic mucosal resection (emr). The benefits of RFA as it relates to its efficacy and durability is discussed by Bashar J. Qumseya and colleagues (See, The role of endoscopic ultrasound in the management of patients with Barrett esophagus and superficial neoplasia).

PREPARATION

Once a decision has been made to proceed with RFA, preparation begins with endoscopic planning. It is necessary that patients are on sufficient acid-suppression therapy to permit effective resquamation of the ablated mucosa. In the Ablation of Intestinal Metaplasia trial by Shaheen and colleagues,[4] patients received a high-dose proton pump inhibitor (PPI; esomeprazole 40 mg 2 times daily) for the duration of the trial. Two studies examined the role of esophageal acid exposure in eradication of intestinal metaplasia and found improved outcomes with reduced esophageal acid

Table 1
Risks associated with radiofrequency ablation of Barrett's esophagus

Risks	Incidence (95% CI)
Stricture	5.6% (4.2%–7.4%)
Bleeding	1.0% (0.8%–1.3%)
Perforation	0.6% (0.4%–0.9%)

Abbreviation: CI, confidence interval.

exposure before and after RFA, respectively.[5,6] The authors have gravitated to high-dose twice-daily PPI to best ensure adequate supportive pharmacotherapy for a minimum of 2 weeks before initiating RFA and continued until complete eradication in achieved. In some patients, the dosing can be reduced to once daily indefinitely.

The planning endoscopy can be done independently or concurrently with initiation of endoscopic eradication therapy depending on the reliability of preceding endoscopic and histopathologic data. Planning endoscopy promotes a detailed endoscopic examination using high-definition white-light and narrow-band imaging to document an accurate depiction of the extent and configuration of specialized intestinal metaplasia and the detection of any suspected nodular dysplasia that should be addressed with endoscopic resection. A systematic examination using high-definition white-light and narrow-band imaging allows for identification of macroscopic abnormalities. Anatomic landmarks, including the presence of hiatal hernia and localization of the top of the gastric folds, should be documented. The Prague classification is used to document the extent of BE in terms of its maximum circumferential length and maximum overall length (**Fig. 1**). Longer BE length correlates with increased

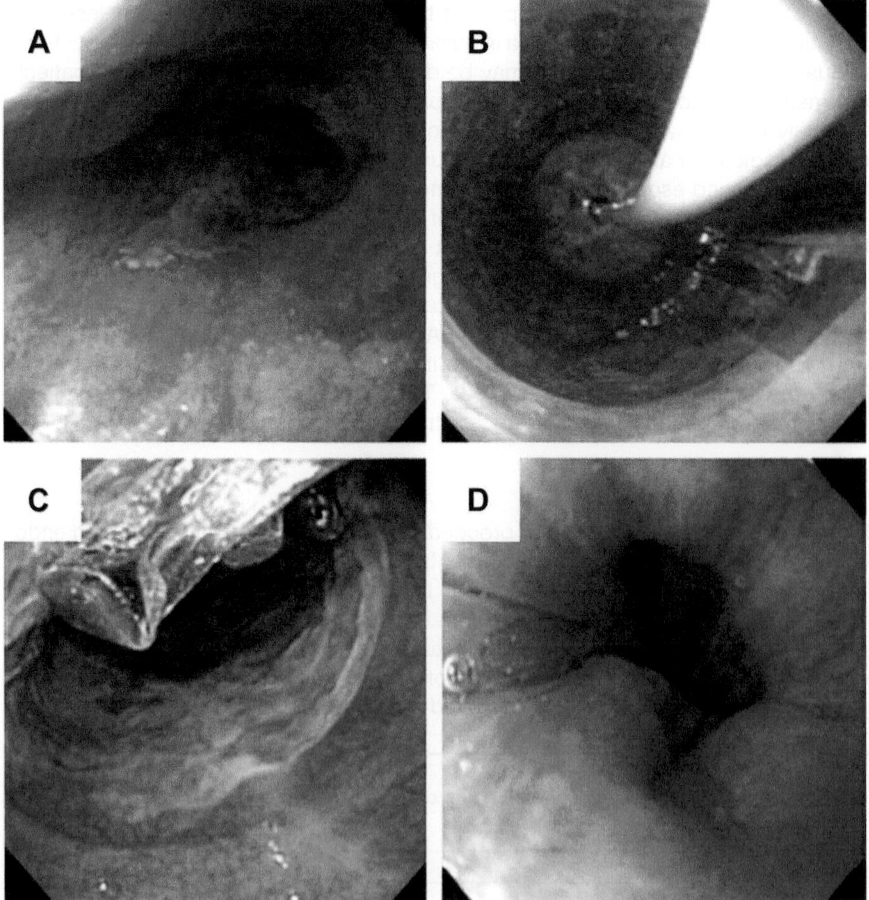

Fig. 1. Circumferential RFA of BE. (*A*) Endoscopic appearance of BE before treatment. (*B*) Balloon ablation catheter inflated within esophagus. (*C*) Endoscopic appearance after ablation. (*D*) Surveillance endoscopy 12 weeks after treatment.

number of treatment sessions to achieve complete eradication.[7] Once nodular lesions have been addressed, the BE configuration dictates the selection of tools for optimizing RFA. Generally, circumferential RFA is used for BE that is circumferential and greater than 2 cm in length, whereas focal RFA is used for shorter segments of BE.

RFA is generally performed as an outpatient procedure with patients in the left lateral decubitus position as for a standard upper endoscopy and using sedation with analgesia or monitored anesthesia care. Prophylactic antimicrobials are not necessary.

The equipment that is used for the RFA system (Barrx-HALO, Medtronic Corp., Minneapolis, MN) includes an energy generator, a sizing balloon for HALO 360 treatments, and a treatment delivery balloon (HALO 360, Medtronic Corp., Minneapolis, MN) for circumferential therapy. This equipment is used to treat circumferential segments of BE 3 cm or greater in length. A variety of flexible RFA plates (HALO 90, 90 Ultra, 60, Medtronic Corp., Minneapolis, MN) can be affixed externally to the tip of the endoscope for direct-contact targeted therapy under endoscopic guidance to treat the esophagogastric junction and limited circumferential and noncircumferential BE. Lastly, a small-surface, through-the-scope contact probe (Channel RFA, Medtronic Corp., Minneapolis, MN) has been developed, intended for small-volume targeted therapy and for treating within stenotic segments.

The principle of radiofrequency electrode technology is to deliver high power (approximately 300 W) in a short period of time (<300 milliseconds) and to use energy density control. When the HALO 360 balloon is used, the idea is to have uniform wall tension, which is achievable with a balloon. In addition, tight electrode spacing (<250 μm) leads to more superficial tissue injury. The concept is that this will allow precise, reliable, and reproducible depth of the penetration to ablate the epithelium and muscularis mucosa with limited injury to the submucosa. Depths of ablation are generally in the range of 500 to 700 μm (**Table 2**).[8]

PERFORMANCE

Circumferential Radiofrequency Ablation

The Barrx Standard HALO 360 ablation catheter is a 6-cm long balloon tip catheter that delivers a 3-cm long circumferential RFA electrode band. The Standard HALO 360 was available in 21-mm to 31-mm diameter catheters. Catheter diameter selection was guided by a dedicated sizing balloon. In 2016, the Express HALO 360 was released as a self-sizing 8-cm length balloon with a 4-cm long circumferential RFA electrode. The Express catheter will replace the Standard catheter and sizing balloon. The HALO 360 ablation catheters are introduced over a guidewire and positioned

Table 2
Equipment list

Required	Optional
Endoscope	Clear cap for debris removal
HALO Flex Generator	Sizing catheter for circumferential ablation
Ablation catheter HALO 360 HALO 360 Express HALO 90 HALO 90 Ultra HALO 60 Channel RFA	N-acetylcysteine solution

under adjacent endoscopic visualization. The process of circumferential RFA may be completed systematically as follows:

Endoscopic inspection

As described earlier, a careful mapping of the extent and location of intestinal metaplasia as well as any dysplasia should be performed before RFA therapy. On the day of the planned RFA therapy, careful endoscopic inspection should again be performed to confirm prior measurements in terms of the location of the gastroesophageal junction (GEJ) and the Prague classification measurements (ie, circumferential extent of BE and maximal extent of BE; see **Fig. 1**A). The presence of ulcers, strictures, or nodularity should also be assessed as these may warrant delay of RFA therapy until these issues have been addressed. RFA of areas with ulceration or erosions may increase the risk of complications. Areas of nodularity may prevent appropriate contact of the balloon ablation catheter to the adjacent mucosa thereby leading to incomplete ablation and/or buried glands. N-acetylcysteine solution applied to the intended ablation segment via a spray tip catheter as a mucolytic agent was promoted in the seminal studies of RFA safety and efficacy. However, there is no clear evidence that the use of N-acetylcysteine improves outcomes and many centers (the authors' included) have abandoned this practice. The application of N-acetylcysteine does add some increased time and cost to the procedure. Moreover, N-acetylcysteine may promote bronchospasm if aspirated.

Sizing balloon

After completing endoscopic assessment, a guidewire is then passed through the endoscope into the gastric antrum. The endoscope is then removed maintaining the guidewire in place. The sizing balloon is first calibrated using a manufacturer-provided plastic sheath. Once calibration is complete, the sizing balloon is inserted over the guidewire and positioned to 12 cm above the GEJ based on previously documented endoscopic measurements. The sizing balloon is inflated by depressing the inflation foot pedal, and the localized esophageal diameter is shown on the generator display. The diameter is recorded, and this process is repeated at 1-cm increments until the GEJ has been reached. A sharp increase in a size measurement may indicate entry of the sizing balloon into the stomach. The sizing balloon is then withdrawn while the guidewire is left in place. The smallest-diameter ablation catheter recommended should be selected for ablation.

The intent of the sizing catheter was to optimize uniform contact between the RFA electrode and the esophageal mucosa. An ablation balloon that was too small or too large (owing to failure of complete expansion) would leave gaps in contact that would result in nonuniform ablation. Many experienced operators came to forgo the use of the sizing balloon once they were able to readily eyeball the optimal treatment balloon diameter. More meaningfully, the Express HALO 360 RFA catheter obviates the sizing-balloon process altogether.

First ablation

The ablation catheter is inserted over the guidewire to the approximate position of the proximal margin of the ablation target. This catheter is guided by distance measures on the catheter shaft that correlate with the proximal aspect of the RFA electrode. The endoscope is then inserted alongside the ablation catheter to allow precise positioning. Under direct visualization, the proximal edge of the ablation balloon is positioned 1 cm proximal to the proximal extent of the intestinal metaplasia. The inflation pedal is then pressed to inflate the balloon (see **Fig. 1**B). Suction with the endoscope is used to deflate the esophageal lumen to best ensure adequate contact of the balloon surface to the esophageal mucosa. The ablation foot pedal is pressed to deliver energy at 12 J/cm^2, and the balloon is then automatically deflated (see **Fig. 1**C). The balloon catheter can then be advanced to the next area designated for treatment. The balloon catheter should not be advanced or retracted if it is inflated or if there is resistance. The balloon should be positioned so that less than 1 cm of overlapping treatment occurs. The ablation procedure is then repeated until the GEJ has been reached. The endoscope and balloon catheter are then removed. The manufacturer's recommendation for the Express RFA balloon catheter is 10 J/cm^2, 1 application, clean, and repeat the application.

Removal of debris

The initial ablation results in a film of coagulative necrotic debris on the treated esophageal surface as well as on the surface of the RFA electrode. It is common practice to clear this debris from both surfaces to optimize the second application. Once the balloon catheter is removed from patients, the balloon is reinflated and the surface gently wiped clean of any adherent debris. The endoscope tip is fitted with a clear cap, and the endoscope is reinserted; this assemblage is used to mechanically scrape adherent debris proximally to distally from the ablated area of the esophagus. The guidewire is then reinserted, and the endoscope is withdrawn and the cap removed. There is emerging evidence that omission of the cleaning phase may reduce procedural time while maintaining efficacy both for circumferential and focal RFA.[9–11] Further research with longer follow-up time is necessary to determine the feasibility of such an approach, as these studies had short-term follow-up (2–3 months) and reported the possibility of increased stricture formation when omitting the cleaning phase in focal RFA. A randomized comparative trial is underway to compare 3 modes of circumferential RFA with the Express HALO 360.

Second ablation

The ablation catheter and the endoscope are then inserted once again as described during the first ablation step. Treatment is applied once again as described earlier to encompass the initially treated segments.

Focal Radiofrequency Ablation

Focal RFA, principally using the HALO 90 catheter, is used in numerous settings as primary, secondary, adjunctive, and salvage therapy for dysplastic BE. As primary therapy, it is used for complete eradication in patients with noncircumferential BE and, to a lesser extent, short-segment (<3 cm) circumferential BE. It is used for secondary ablation, following initial HALO 360 RFA, for focal areas of residual BE and circumferentially at the esophagogastric junction at the first post-HALO 360 RFA follow-up endoscopy. It is used as adjunctive ablation therapy for focal residual BE following EMR. Lastly, it is used to ablate focal areas of residual/recurrent BE identified at posteradication surveillance endoscopies. The selection of specific focal RFA catheter should be individualized to the extent and configuration of the treatment area in the context of reasonable inventory and accessory budgets permit. The authors find that the standard HALO 90 suffices in most instances. Focal RFA follows many of the same principles as circumferential RFA and may be completed as follows:

Endoscopic inspection

Careful endoscopic inspection is performed in the same manner as described for circumferential RFA. N-acetylcysteine solution is often used to clear the esophageal mucosa of any debris or mucus; however, as mentioned earlier in the circumferential RFA procedure section, the practice is not embraced by many.

Choice of catheter

Three focal RFA catheters are currently available: HALO 90, HALO 90 Ultra, and HALO 60. One of the primary differences between these catheters is the area treated with each application. The HALO 60 treats 150 mm^2 (electrode dimensions: 10 mm × 15 mm), the HALO 90 treats 260 mm^2 (electrode dimensions: 13 mm × 20 mm), and the HALO 90 Ultra treats 520 mm^2 (electrode dimensions: 13 mm × 40 mm). The HALO 90 is used most frequently for focal RFA. The HALO 60 probe may be useful for smaller target areas or for treatment at the GEJ where the gastric folds may prevent apposition of larger probes to the mucosa. The HALO 90 Ultra probe requires only one treatment for each ablation step and also treats a larger area per application, which can shorten procedure time.

First ablation

By convention, the focal RFA catheter is attached to the scope tip such that the ablation device is in the 12-o'clock position. Oro-esophageal intubation with the device-mounted endoscope is performed carefully and under direct visualization. The endoscope is advanced to the target area. The scope tip is deflected to promote optimal apposition of the RFA electrode surface to the targeted BE mucosa. The ablation foot pedal is depressed to deliver 12-J/cm^2 to the target area. For the HALO 90 and 60 RFA catheters, after completion of the first application, the position of the ablation catheter is maintained and the ablation foot pedal is pressed a second time. The HALO 90 Ultra probe is recommended for only one application for each ablation step.

Removal of debris

After all target areas have been treated with the first ablation, the front ridge of the probe itself is used to scrap the white coagulum of necrotic surface debris. The ablation device is then removed and its surfaced cleaned to remove any adherent debris.

Second ablation

The endoscope and ablation catheter are reinserted, and the probe is connected back to the generator. A second set of ablations is then performed to all targeted areas in the same manner as was completed during the first ablation step.

Three-hit, no clean alternative

An alternative to the aforementioned routine is to simply apply 3 applications to each treatment site. This approach more reliably synchronizes the applications to the target tissue and promotes efficiency, in as the cleaning phase and second set of application are eliminated.[9–11] This approach has been evaluated at 12 and 15 J/cm^2. The authors' routine is to use 12 J/cm^2.

Channel radiofrequency ablation device

The channel device is a through-the-scope, malleable, small-surface contact RFA probe that fits through the working channel of a standard diagnostic endoscope (2.8 mm or larger accessory channel diameter). The electrode array is 15.7 mm long and 7.5 mm wide and has approximately the same active electrode surface area as the Barrx 60 device. The recommended treatment regimen consists of 2 double applications of energy at 12 J/cm^2 with cleaning or 3 applications of 12 J/cm^2.

POSTTREATMENT CARE

After RFA, acid suppressive therapy must be sustained to allow the ablation zone to heal and regenerate with neo-squamous epithelium. The authors recommend a light diet on the day of the procedure and for patients to advance to their regular diet as tolerated. Patients may experience posttreatment chest discomfort for 12 to 72 hours after the procedure. The authors prescribe a 50% lidocaine and 50% Magnesium hydroxide, Aluminum hydroxide (Maalox) elixir for topical analgesia as well as a liquid narcotic suspension for pain management. Transient dysphagia is not uncommon after RFA, particularly when done adjunctively to prior wide-area endoscopic resection. The authors typically perform repeat endoscopy with dilation for patients who experience persistent dysphagia at 1 week following treatment. Follow-up endoscopies are scheduled at 12-week intervals until all BE is eradicated. Thereafter, the authors perform endoscopy at 6-month intervals for the first 2 years and then annually thereafter with careful visual inspection using high-definition white-light (HDWL) and narrow band imaging (NBI) and targeted biopsies of any suspicious surface or subsurface abnormalities as well as routine biopsies from the glandular side of the neosquamocolumnar junction.

SUMMARY

RFA is a safe and effective thermal ablative therapy for dysplastic BE and, to a lesser extent, nondysplastic BE. Before the utilization of RFA, there must be an appropriate indication, assessment of potential contraindications, discussion of risks and benefits with patients, and careful endoscopic planning. The ease of performance of the procedure along with its efficacy and low rate of adverse events have established RFA as a reliable technique for endoscopic management of dysplastic BE.

REFERENCES

1. Sanfilippo NJ, Hsi A, DeNittis AS, et al. Toxicity of photodynamic therapy after combined external beam radiotherapy and intraluminal brachytherapy for carcinoma of the upper aerodigestive tract. Lasers Surg Med 2001;28(3):278–81.
2. Small AJ, Sutherland SE, Hightower JS, et al. Comparative risk of recurrence of dysplasia and carcinoma after endoluminal eradication therapy of high-grade dysplasia versus intramucosal carcinoma in Barrett's esophagus. Gastrointest Endosc 2015;81(5):1158–66.e1-4.
3. Qumseya BJ, Wani S, Desai M, et al. Adverse events after radiofrequency ablation in patients with Barrett's esophagus: a systematic review and meta-analysis. Clin Gastroenterol Hepatol 2016;14(8):1086–95.e6.
4. Shaheen NJ, Sharma P, Overholt BF, et al. Radiofrequency ablation in Barrett's esophagus with dysplasia. N Engl J Med 2009;360(22):2277–88.
5. Akiyama J, Marcus SN, Triadafilopoulos G. Effective intra-esophageal acid control is associated with improved radiofrequency ablation outcomes in Barrett's esophagus. Dig Dis Sci 2012;57(10):2625–32.
6. Krishnan K, Pandolfino JE, Kahrilas PJ, et al. Increased risk for persistent intestinal metaplasia in patients with Barrett's esophagus and uncontrolled reflux exposure before radiofrequency ablation. Gastroenterology 2012;143(3):576–81.
7. Guarner-Argente C, Buoncristiano T, Furth EE, et al. Long-term outcomes of patients with Barrett's esophagus and high-grade dysplasia or early cancer treated with endoluminal therapies with intention to complete eradication. Gastrointest Endosc 2013;77(2):190–9.
8. Fleischer DE, Sharma VK. Endoscopic ablation of Barrett's esophagus using the Halo system. Dig Dis 2008;26(4):280–4.
9. van Vilsteren FG, Phoa KN, Alvarez Herrero L, et al. Circumferential balloon-based radiofrequency ablation of Barrett's esophagus with dysplasia can be

simplified, yet efficacy maintained, by omitting the cleaning phase. Clin Gastroenterol Hepatol 2013;11(5):491–8.e1.
10. van Vilsteren FG, Phoa KN, Alvarez Herrero L, et al. A simplified regimen for focal radiofrequency ablation of Barrett's mucosa: a randomized multicenter trial comparing two ablation regimens. Gastrointest Endosc 2013;78(1):30–8.
11. Kunzli HT, Scholvinck DW, Phoa KN, et al. Simplified protocol for focal radiofrequency ablation using the HALO90 device: short-term efficacy and safety in patients with dysplastic Barrett's esophagus. Endoscopy 2015;47(7):592–7.

Radiofrequency Ablation of Barrett's Esophagus

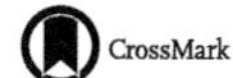

Efficacy, Complications, and Durability

Kavel Visrodia, MD, Liam Zakko, MD, Kenneth K. Wang, MD*

KEYWORDS

- Radiofrequency ablation • Barrett's esophagus • Esophageal adenocarcinoma
- Dysplasia • Neoplasia

KEY POINTS

- Radiofrequency ablation in combination with endoscopic mucosal resection effectively induces reconstitution of (neo)squamous epithelium and reduces the risk of disease progression in patients with dysplastic Barrett's esophagus.
- Radiofrequency ablation has an excellent safety profile, although benign stricturing may occur in approximately 6% to 10% of patients and is usually responsive to endoscopic dilation.
- Despite effective radiofrequency ablation, the risk of recurrent intestinal metaplasia or Barrett's-related neoplasia, including invasive adenocarcinoma, is not negligible and necessitates postablation surveillance.

INTRODUCTION

Barrett's esophagus (BE) is defined as a metaplastic change in the normal esophageal squamous epithelium to an intestinalized columnar epithelium, likely in response to chronic acid-related inflammation. BE may progress through increasingly neoplastic stages beginning with nondysplastic BE (NDBE), followed by BE with low-grade dysplasia (LGD), then BE with high-grade dysplasia (HGD), then intramucosal carcinoma (IMC), and ultimately invasive adenocarcinoma. The prognosis for advanced esophageal adenocarcinoma (EAC) remains dismal with a 5-year survival of less than 20%.[1] Therefore, as the only known precursor to EAC, BE has been the longstanding focus of potential therapies that aim to decrease the risk of malignant progression.

Disclosures: The authors report no conflicts of interest.
Division of Gastroenterology and Hepatology, Department of Internal Medicine, Mayo Clinic, 200 First Avenue, Southwest, Rochester, MN 55905, USA
* Corresponding author.
E-mail address: wang.kenneth@mayo.edu

Gastrointest Endoscopy Clin N Am 27 (2017) 491–501
http://dx.doi.org/10.1016/j.giec.2017.03.003
giendo.theclinics.com

During the last decade, radiofrequency ablation (RFA) has risen to become a first-line option for treating neoplastic BE (LGD, HGD, or IMC following endoscopic resection of nodular lesions). RFA involves applying radiofrequency energy directly to Barrett's epithelium. The high-frequency (typically 350–500 kHz) energy limits the damage to mucosa (and does not involve submucosa or muscularis propria), decreasing the possibility of stricture formation. Energy is delivered circumferentially in the tubular esophagus using a balloon-based 360° catheter that is 3 cm in length, or focally for small/residual areas of intestinalized epithelium using an endoscope-mounted device. More recent technologic advancements include a self-sizing balloon catheter (eliminating the fairly time consuming need for sizing of the esophagus in 1-cm increments) and a through-the-biopsy-channel RFA probe that allows treatment of areas without needing to withdraw the endoscope. Following RFA treatment and appropriate acid suppression, reconstitution of (neo)squamous epithelium can ensue. Typically, two to three RFA treatment sessions are necessary to attain the goal of complete eradication of intestinal metaplasia (CE-IM), as determined by systematic biopsies in the region of initial BE involvement. In some cases, IM may persist after complete eradication of dysplasia (CE-D). Although early studies established the role of RFA in the management of BE, a growing body of literature on long-term outcomes has developed from larger cohorts with longer patient follow-up after treatment. In this article, we provide an updated review of RFA efficacy, complications, and durability.

EFFICACY

Initial Clinical Trials

Initial reports of clinical trials investigating RFA for the treatment of BE appeared in 2007, when Sharma and colleagues[2] reported their findings from a prospective multicenter study titled Ablation of Intestinal Metaplasia (AIM-I) Trial. Seventy patients with NDBE measuring 2 to 6 cm were enrolled for circumferential balloon-based RFA. Initial studies like this were often limited to patients with BE measuring less than 8 cm because of concerns regarding pain control. RFA was applied at an energy density of 10 J/cm^2 (as established during a prior dosimetry phase). A second treatment was applied at 4 months for persistent IM. At 12 months, and after a mean 1.5 treatment sessions per patient, 70% of patients achieved CE-IM, whereas another 25% had persistent, but partial ($\geq$50%) improvement in length of BE.

The investigators hypothesized that treatment efficacy may be enhanced with the incorporation of a forthcoming focal RFA device developed to target anatomically challenging regions, including the flaring gastroesophageal junction in the setting of a hiatal hernia. These devices would also allow treatment of 25% or less of the circumference of the esophagus and up to 3 cm in length with a single application. Subjects were therefore later invited for a follow-up endoscopy and ablation with a focal device if endoscopically or histologically indicated.[3] It should be noted that a higher energy level for focal device was used (and is currently recommended) as compared with the circumferential probe (12 J/cm^2 vs 10 J/cm^2), although the improved efficacy for higher dosimetry has not been conclusively demonstrated. A total of 62 of 70 (89%) participated in the study extension and underwent an additional mean 1.9 treatment sessions focal RFA. At 30 months, CE-IM was achieved in a remarkable 98% of available patients.

Subsequent studies aimed to evaluate the efficacy of RFA in BE with increasing neoplasia, where the opportunity for reducing risk of malignant progression remains greatest. In a prospective multicenter study by Ganz and colleagues,[4] 142 patients with BE and HGD underwent circumferential balloon-based ablation, of which 92 returned for at least one follow-up biopsy. After a median 12 months and median one ablation session, 90% of patients did not have any remaining histologic evidence of HGD (80% CE-D), but only 54% achieved CE-IM. As in the AIM-I Trial, efficacy may have been improved with inclusion of focal ablation.

The efficacy of RFA in neoplastic BE was firmly established in a landmark study by Shaheen and colleagues[5] known as the AIM Dysplasia Trial and published in 2009. This was a multicenter, sham-controlled trial in which 127 patients with neoplastic BE (LGD or HGD) measuring up to 8 cm were randomized to receive either RFA or sham procedure. After initial circumferential balloon-based ablation, patients returned in preset intervals for endoscopic evaluation with biopsies and up to three adjunctive focal ablations as indicated. The primary outcomes were eradication of dysplasia and IM at 12 months. A total 121 patients completed the study protocol. Based on intention-to-treat analysis, 91% of patients with LGD and 81% of patients with HGD in the ablation group achieved CE-D compared with 23% and 19% of those in their respective control arms. Overall, 78% of patients in the ablation group achieved CE-IM as compared with only 2.3% in the control group ($P<.001$). Moreover, subjects receiving ablation had a lower risk of disease progression (3.6% vs 16.3%; $P = .03$). This included risk of progression to esophageal cancer (1.2% vs 9.3%; $P = .045$), which notably was based on few occurrences, all of which were in patients with baseline HGD.

Patients with a history of early esophageal cancer were largely excluded from early RFA study protocols. Although endoscopic mucosal resection (EMR) can be used to curatively treat IMC, it is recognized that the risk of metachronous HGD or cancer arising from residual BE remains substantial.[6,7] Therefore, RFA therapy has naturally been extended to this high-risk cohort of patients. In a cohort of 54 patients with HGD and/or early stage cancer treated with EMR followed by RFA, 98% achieved CE-IM, and only three had recurrent dysplasia or carcinoma during a median 60-month follow-up, and all events were managed endoscopically.[8] Several studies have since reported findings supporting the efficacy of RFA in this high-risk population.[8–10] Thus, RFA is a first-line option for treating background Barrett's epithelium after nodular IMC has been successfully resected.[11]

The role of RFA in the management of patients with LGD was not immediately apparent from early studies including the AIM Dysplasia Trial, which was not powered to detect a difference in the risk of progression from LGD to HGD or cancer.[5] This issue was recently addressed by Phoa and colleagues[12] in a multicenter, randomized, clinical trial (SURF Study) in which 136 patients with BE and confirmed LGD were randomized to receive ablation or endoscopic surveillance (every 6 months the first year, and annually thereafter). A total of 88% of patients in the ablation group achieved CE-IM compared with 0% in the surveillance group. After 3-year follow-up, one patient in the ablation group (1.5%) progressed to HGD or cancer, whereas 18 patients in the surveillance group (26.5%) did, for an absolute risk reduction of 25%. The study had a higher rate of progression to HGD or cancer than previously published rates, which may limit its generalizability to other populations. This high rate of progression may have been caused by the use of centralized experienced pathologists, a process previously described to select for higher risk of progression in patients with BE with LGD.[13,14] Therefore, consideration of RFA therapy is warranted in patients with BE with LGD, particularly if an expert pathologist confirms the diagnosis.[11]

Large Registries and Meta-analyses

A growing body of data outside clinical trials continues to demonstrate the efficacy of RFA for treatment of neoplastic BE. However, the real-world success of RFA treatment may be mitigated because of various clinical factors. In a multicenter United Kingdom registry, 335 patients with neoplastic BE (72% HGD, 24% IMC, 4% LGD) were treated with RFA, and 86% achieved CE-D, whereas 62% achieved CE-IM.[15] These registry results reflect more advanced baseline histology, inclusion of complex disease that failed prior photodynamic therapy (8%), and more extensive BE (mean baseline length, 5.8 cm) compared with clinical trial data. In an updated publication from the same registry, however, the rates of CE-D and CE-IM improved in the latter of two time periods (2008–2010 and 2011–2013) from 56% to 83% and 77% to 92%, respectively.[16] This was perhaps related to better lesion recognition and more frequent endoscopic resection (48% to 60%) before initiating RFA, emphasizing the importance of combination therapy in the treatment of BE.

Abstract data from a large United States RFA Patient Registry comprised of 148 institutions (113 community-based, 35 academic-affiliated) also support the efficacy of RFA.[17] Of 1027 patients with BE and LGD, HGD, or IMC who completed RFA treatment, the rates of CE-IM were 67%, 61%, and 73%, and the rates of CE-D were 90%, 82%, and 85%, respectively. RFA efficacy was independent of treatment center (community-based vs academic-affiliated institution).

In a meta-analysis of 18 studies including 3802 patients with BE and progressive neoplasia, the pooled percentage of patients achieving CE-IM and CE-D was 78% (95% confidence interval [CI], 70%–86%) and 91% (95% CI, 87%–95%).[18] However, substantial heterogeneity was noted at 96% and 78%, respectively. Patients with HGD were significantly less likely to achieve CE-IM (relative risk, 0.92; 95% CI, 0.87–0.98) or CE-D (relative risk, 0.94; 95% CI, 0.91–0.97). Progression to EAC occurred in 0.2% of patients during treatment and 0.7% during 1.5-years follow-up. These data overwhelmingly support the efficacy of RFA therapy in eradicating IM and neoplasia.

Predictors of Response

Several other studies have identified statistically significant predictors of poor response to RFA therapy. In one study, active reflux esophagitis, endoscopic resections scar, narrow esophagus, and duration of neoplasia were associated with poor initial response to circumferential RFA.[19] In other studies, increasing BE length, age, and incomplete healing between treatment sessions were associated with longer times to achieving CE-IM.[9,20] A history of fundoplication does not seem to impact the efficacy of RFA.[21] Data do suggest a correlation between endoscopist RFA volume and rate of CE-IM.[22,23] The number of treatment sessions required to achieve CE-IM seems to attenuate after treatment of approximately 30 patients.[23]

COMPLICATIONS

RFA has a favorable safety profile, particularly in comparison with alternative techniques, such as photodynamic therapy and widespread endoscopic resection. This has undoubtedly contributed to its rise in the BE treatment algorithm.

Stricture

Perhaps the most concerning complication of RFA is benign stricture formation, because perforation, major bleeding and need for hospitalization are extremely rare. Initial animal and human studies showed limited mucosal penetration without submucosal injury or stricturing at 10 J/cm^2 to 12 J/cm^2 energy doses.[24,25] In the AIM Dysplasia Trial, 84 patients in the ablation group underwent a mean of 3.5 RFA treatments and five (6.0%) developed esophageal stricture (defined as endoscopic narrowing with or without dysphagia).[5] All strictures were successfully dilated (mean, 2.6 sessions per patient). There were three serious events potentially associated with ablation, including upper gastrointestinal bleeding in a patient on antiplatelet therapy for heart disease, overnight hospitalization for new-onset chest pain 8 days after RFA, and overnight hospitalization for chest pain and nausea immediately following RFA.

Several large RFA series have continued to assess the safety of RFA, particularly stricture formation. In a recent large meta-analysis of 37 studies involving 9200 patients, the pooled rate of adverse events related to RFA was 8.8%. This was mainly in the form of strictures (5.6%), bleeding (1%), or perforation (0.6%).[26] Risk factors for developing complications included advanced pretreatment histology and increasing BE length. These clinical findings require more treatment sessions to achieve eradication, likely explaining the increase in complications. In one study, the development of strictures (8.2%; 20 of 244) was also associated with nonsteroidal anti-inflammatory drug use, history of antireflux surgery, and active erosive esophagitis.[9] The median time to stricture formation was 63 days after initial treatment. Most affected patients were free of dysphagia. All strictures were short (<1 cm) and responsive to endoscopic dilation (median, 1; maximum, 4), findings confirmed in other series.[15,20]

Safety of Endoscopic Mucosal Resection with Radiofrequency Ablation

Whether EMR increases the risk of RFA complication is of considerable concern given the utility of EMR in treating nodular BE before RFA therapy. In the previously discussed meta-analysis, the rate of complications was compared among studies based on inclusion of EMR in their treatment protocol (26 studies including EMR vs 6 studies treating with RFA alone).[26] Although not statistically significant, a trend toward a higher rate of adverse events was found in the RFA + EMR group (10.3% vs 7.5%; $P = .28$). Furthermore, a subset analysis of three studies in which outcomes were reported separately for these two treatment groups (RFA + EMR vs RFA alone) showed a significantly increased rate of adverse events among patients receiving EMR (22.2% [95% CI, 16.4%–29.4%] vs 5% [95% CI, 2.9%–8.3%]; $P = .015$). Although evidence is limited, endoscopists should take these data into account when counseling patients before performing EMR and RFA.

Chest Discomfort

Patients may commonly experience chest discomfort immediately postprocedurally. This discomfort may persist up to a few days following therapy. In the AIM Dysplasia Trial, the degree of chest discomfort on Day 1 was higher in the ablation group versus the control group with median scores of 23 versus 0 (based on a 100-point visual analog scale).[5] By Day 8, however, the median chest discomfort score returned to 0. This is likely related to the extent of ablation, because the median Day 1 score following focal RFA was 0. Symptomatic therapy is usually provided using viscous lidocaine and other forms of topical analgesia. Nonetheless, patients with persistent or atypical postprocedural symptoms may require further evaluation in the form of electrocardiogram, chest radiograph, laboratory testing, and/or extended observation depending on the clinical circumstances.

DURABILITY

The risk of recurrent IM or dysplasia after eradication is becoming increasingly understood as data from larger RFA treatment cohorts with longer follow-up become available. This remains an important topic because of its implications for determining optimal postablation surveillance and risk of malignant progression.

Initial Clinical Trials

In the AIM-I Trial, 50 of 60 patients achieving CE-IM returned 2.5 years later (5 years total after initial RFA) for endoscopic assessment.[3,27] CE-IM was maintained in 92% (46 of 50) of patients, and 8% (4 of 50) had recurrent focal IM, most within 1 cm of the squamocolumnar junction. All patients with recurrence responded to focal ablation and reachieved CE-IM. In the AIM Dysplasia Trial, 119 of 127 patients underwent RFA (including 35 sham crossover patients), and were followed for a mean 3.05 years from initial RFA.[28] Based on Kaplan-Meier estimate, greater than 75% of patients maintained CE-IM, and more than 85% of HGD patient and 90% of LGD patients were free of dysplasia (ie, maintained CE-D) during the mean follow-up without any additional therapy. Hence, a minority of patients experience recurrence of IM or dysplasia.

Large Registries and Meta-analyses

Subsequent large series and meta-analyses have affirmed similar rates of BE recurrence. In 2013, Orman and colleagues[29] identified six studies comprised of 540 patients that reported on durability of RFA outcomes. IM was found to recur in 13% (95% CI, 9%–18%). In a more recent meta-analysis of 21 RFA studies and 3186 patients with 5741 patient-years of follow-up, there were 603 recurrences. The pooled incident ratios of recurrent IM, dysplasia, and HGD/EAC after RFA were 9.5% (95% CI, 6.7%–12.3%), 2.0% (95% CI, 1.3%–2.7%), and 1.2% (95% CI, 0.8%–1.6%) per patient-year, respectively. Finally, data from the US RFA Registry showed that IM recurred in 334 of 1634 (20%) patients after achieving CE-IM during 2.4 years of follow-up (**Fig. 1**).[30] Most (86%) of these cases were nondysplastic or indefinite for dysplasia. Most (94%) were identical to or less severe than baseline degree of dysplasia.

Predictors of Recurrence

Predictors of recurrent IM are similar to those for predicting poor response to therapy. These include increasing age, BE segment length, and degree of baseline dysplasia.[29–31] Moreover, being nonwhite and requiring more treatment sessions has also been associated with increased likelihood of recurrence.[30]

Location of Recurrence

Recurrence is often minute (mean, 0.5–0.6 cm) and close to the squamocolumnar junction.[20,30] There are data to suggest that dysplastic recurrences may be more common in the gastric cardia.[20,31] In one study, 17 (33%) recurrences were isolated to the cardia (all LGD or HGD) within 1 cm of the gastroesophageal junction, but only visible in four (24%) cases.[31] These data support the inclusion of gastric cardia in post-RFA surveillance biopsy protocols. It should be noted that detection of IM (without dysplasia) in the gastric cardia is not uncommon in patients with chronic reflux and therefore is disregarded in many RFA studies. Studies including gastric cardia IM in their outcomes may therefore report increased rates of recurrence.[20,32]

Implications for Management and Cancer Risk

Recurrent IM with or without dysplasia can usually be treated endoscopically. In one meta-analysis, 97% of recurrences were endoscopically managed.[29] Rarely, however, invasive adenocarcinoma may occur. In a series of 218 patients achieving CE-IM, 52 (24%) patients experienced recurrent IM or BE-related neoplasia, including four

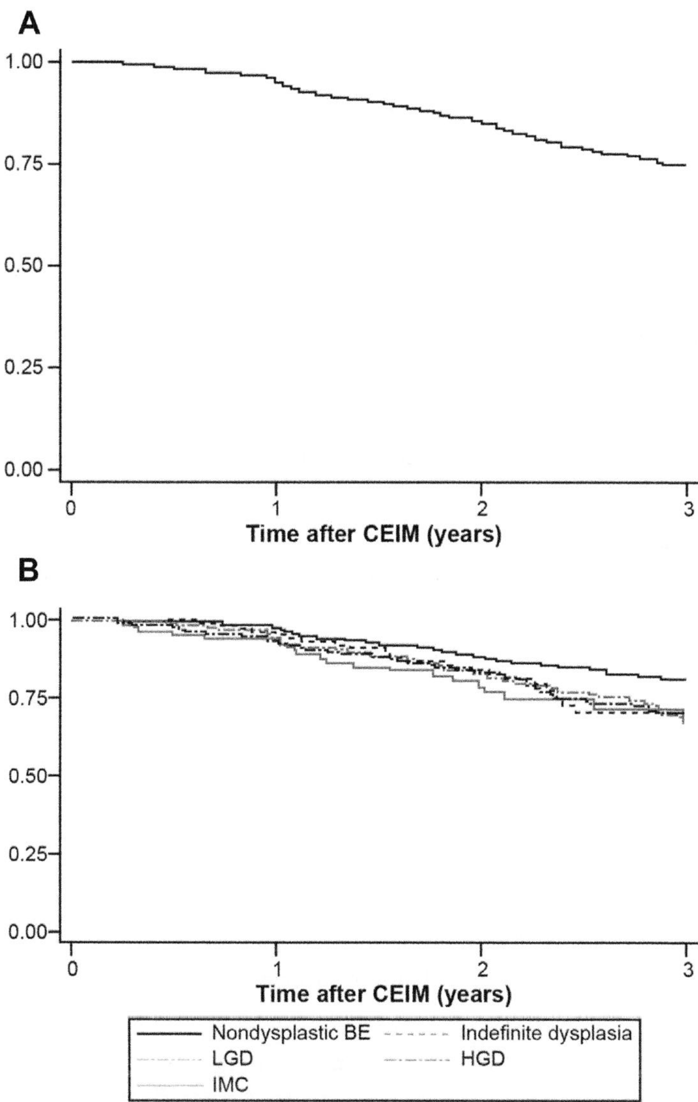

Fig. 1. Kaplan-Meier plots of IM recurrence (*A*) among all subjects treated with RFA and achieving CEIM (n = 1634), and (*B*) among the same subjects categorized by pretreatment histology. (*From* Pasricha S, Bulsiewicz WJ, Hathorn KE, et al. Durability and predictors of successful radiofrequency ablation for Barrett's esophagus. Clin Gastroenterol Hepatol 2014;12:1840–7.e1.)

(1.8%) with invasive adenocarcinoma requiring surgical management.[31] Moreover, in a large series from the US RFA Registry of 4982 patients ever receiving RFA, 100 (2%) developed EAC and nine patients (0.2%) died from EAC during a mean 2.7 ± 1.6 years follow-up (**Fig. 2**).[33] Although these data are reassuring, it should be noted that nearly half (47%) of the registry patients had NDBE at baseline, which represents a group less likely to develop recurrences, whereas most incident EAC cases (83 of 100) were among patients with baseline HGD (n = 990). The cancer incidences in NDBE, LGD,

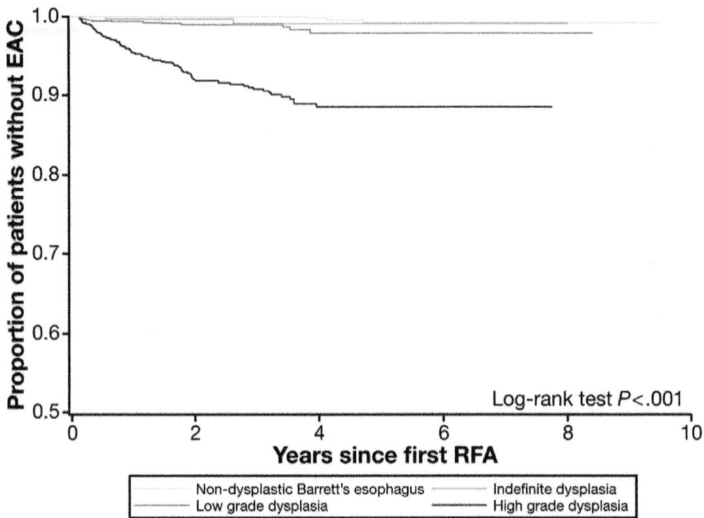

Fig. 2. Kaplan-Meier plots of EAC incidence categorized by pretreatment histology (n = 4698). (*From* Wolf WA, Pasricha S, Cotton C, et al. Incidence of esophageal adenocarcinoma and causes of mortality after radiofrequency ablation of Barrett's esophagus. Gastroenterology 2015;149:1752–61.e1.)

and HGD were 0.5, 4.3, and 30.3 per 1000 person-years, respectively; all rates are significantly lower compared with respective historical control subjects. Nonetheless, these data reinforce a real risk for recurrent neoplasia and need for postablation surveillance. Finally, based on current data, the risk of recurrence seems to stay relatively constant during follow-up precluding the discontinuation of endoscopic surveillance even in patients with sustained CE-IM.

Subsquamous Intestinal Metaplasia

An observation following RFA therapy, as with other BE ablative techniques, is the detection of subsquamous (or "buried") metaplasia. This is believed to occur during

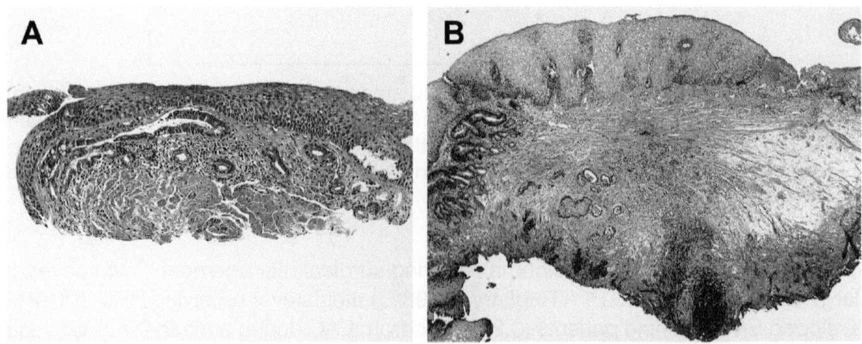

Fig. 3. Photomicrographs of esophageal biopsies revealing subsquamous ("buried") (*A*) metaplasia and (*B*) intramucosal adenocarcinoma after RFA treatment. (hematoxylin-eosin, original magnification ×20). (*Courtesy of* Dr Thomas Smyrk and Dr Tsung-Teh Wu, Department of Pathology, Mayo Clinic, Rochester, MN.)

reconstitution of squamous epithelium, which may overgrow incompletely treated IM (**Fig. 3**A). However, it can also be seen in patients with untreated BE.[34] Concern for this finding stems from reports of dysplasia and carcinoma developing from buried metaplasia after successful ablation (**Fig. 3**B).[35,36] Complicating this matter further is whether standard biopsies are of adequate depth to detect buried metaplasia.[34] Advanced imaging technologies may be of benefit in the future for detecting and assessing buried metaplasia. Volume laser endomicroscopy has been suggested as a method to detect subsquamous disease. Volume laser endomicroscopy can image the submucosa more efficiently than prior techniques, such as confocal laser endomicroscopy.[37] However, at this time the clinical significance and optimal detection of buried metaplasia remains undefined.

SUMMARY

The advent of RFA has broadened the options for gastroenterologists managing patients with BE. Most patients attain CE-IM or CE-D with a significantly reduced risk for progression of BE to EAC. The risk of recurrent IM or BE-related neoplasia, however, is not negligible. Therefore, postablation surveillance remains necessary. Fortunately, most recurrences can be managed endoscopically. RFA therapy may be complicated by benign stricture, which typically responds to endoscopic dilation; more serious adverse events are rare. While ongoing research better defines predictors of response and develops enhanced imaging to detect recurrence, RFA is currently an effective and safe option for treating BE with neoplasia.

REFERENCES

1. Hur C, Miller M, Kong CY, et al. Trends in esophageal adenocarcinoma incidence and mortality. Cancer 2013;119:1149–58.
2. Sharma VK, Wang KK, Overholt BF, et al. Balloon-based, circumferential, endoscopic radiofrequency ablation of Barrett's esophagus: 1-year follow-up of 100 patients. Gastrointest Endosc 2007;65:185–95.
3. Fleischer DE, Overholt BF, Sharma VK, et al. Endoscopic ablation of Barrett's esophagus: a multicenter study with 2.5-year follow-up. Gastrointest Endosc 2008;68:867–76.
4. Ganz RA, Overholt BF, Sharma VK, et al. Circumferential ablation of Barrett's esophagus that contains high-grade dysplasia: a U.S. multicenter registry. Gastrointest Endosc 2008;68:35–40.
5. Shaheen NJ, Sharma P, Overholt BF, et al. Radiofrequency ablation in Barrett's esophagus with dysplasia. N Engl J Med 2009;360:2277–88.
6. Pech O, Behrens A, May A, et al. Long-term results and risk factor analysis for recurrence after curative endoscopic therapy in 349 patients with high-grade intraepithelial neoplasia and mucosal adenocarcinoma in Barrett's oesophagus. Gut 2008;57:1200–6.
7. Prasad GA, Wu TT, Wigle DA, et al. Endoscopic and surgical treatment of mucosal (T1a) esophageal adenocarcinoma in Barrett's esophagus. Gastroenterology 2009;137:815–23.
8. Phoa KN, Pouw RE, van Vilsteren FG, et al. Remission of Barrett's esophagus with early neoplasia 5 years after radiofrequency ablation with endoscopic resection: a Netherlands cohort study. Gastroenterology 2013;145:96–104.
9. Bulsiewicz WJ, Kim HP, Dellon ES, et al. Safety and efficacy of endoscopic mucosal therapy with radiofrequency ablation for patients with neoplastic Barrett's esophagus. Clin Gastroenterol Hepatol 2013;11:636–42.

10. Pouw RE, Wirths K, Eisendrath P, et al. Efficacy of radiofrequency ablation combined with endoscopic resection for Barrett's esophagus with early neoplasia. Clin Gastroenterol Hepatol 2010;8:23–9.
11. Shaheen NJ, Falk GW, Iyer PG, et al. ACG clinical guideline: diagnosis and management of Barrett's esophagus. Am J Gastroenterol 2016;111:30–50 [quiz: 51].
12. Phoa KN, van Vilsteren FG, Weusten BL, et al. Radiofrequency ablation vs endoscopic surveillance for patients with Barrett esophagus and low-grade dysplasia: a randomized clinical trial. JAMA 2014;311:1209–17.
13. Duits LC, Phoa KN, Curvers WL, et al. Barrett's oesophagus patients with low-grade dysplasia can be accurately risk-stratified after histological review by an expert pathology panel. Gut 2015;64:700–6.
14. Curvers WL, ten Kate FJ, Krishnadath KK, et al. Low-grade dysplasia in Barrett's esophagus: overdiagnosed and underestimated. Am J Gastroenterol 2010;105:1523–30.
15. Haidry RJ, Dunn JM, Butt MA, et al. Radiofrequency ablation and endoscopic mucosal resection for dysplastic Barrett's esophagus and early esophageal adenocarcinoma: outcomes of the UK National Halo RFA registry. Gastroenterology 2013;145:87–95.
16. Haidry RJ, Butt MA, Dunn JM, et al. Improvement over time in outcomes for patients undergoing endoscopic therapy for Barrett's oesophagus-related neoplasia: 6-year experience from the first 500 patients treated in the UK patient registry. Gut 2015;64:1192–9.
17. Shaheen NJ, Bulsiewicz WJ, Rothstein RI, et al. Eradication rates of Barrett's esophagus using radiofrequency ablation (RFA): results from the U.S. RFA registry. Gastrointest Endosc 2012;75:AB460.
18. Orman ES, Li N, Shaheen NJ. Efficacy and durability of radiofrequency ablation for Barrett's esophagus: systematic review and meta-analysis. Clin Gastroenterol Hepatol 2013;11:1245–55.
19. van Vilsteren FG, Alvarez Herrero L, Pouw RE, et al. Predictive factors for initial treatment response after circumferential radiofrequency ablation for Barrett's esophagus with early neoplasia: a prospective multicenter study. Endoscopy 2013;45:516–25.
20. Gupta M, Iyer PG, Lutzke L, et al. Recurrence of esophageal intestinal metaplasia after endoscopic mucosal resection and radiofrequency ablation of Barrett's esophagus: results from a US multicenter consortium. Gastroenterology 2013;145:79–86.e1.
21. Shaheen NJ. Prior fundoplication does not improve safety or efficacy outcomes of radiofrequency ablation: results from the US RFA registry closing discussant. J Gastrointest Surg 2013;17:29.
22. Fudman DI, Lightdale CJ, Poneros JM, et al. Positive correlation between endoscopist radiofrequency ablation volume and response rates in Barrett's esophagus. Gastrointest Endosc 2014;80:71–7.
23. Pasricha S, Cotton C, Hathorn KE, et al. Effects of the learning curve on efficacy of radiofrequency ablation for Barrett's esophagus. Gastroenterology 2015;149:890–6.e2.
24. Dunkin BJ, Martinez J, Bejarano PA, et al. Thin-layer ablation of human esophageal epithelium using a bipolar radiofrequency balloon device. Surg Endosc 2006;20:125–30.
25. Ganz RA, Utley DS, Stern RA, et al. Complete ablation of esophageal epithelium with a balloon-based bipolar electrode: a phased evaluation in the porcine and in the human esophagus. Gastrointest Endosc 2004;60:1002–10.

26. Qumseya BJ, Wani S, Desai M, et al. Adverse events after radiofrequency ablation in patients with Barrett's esophagus: a systematic review and meta-analysis. Clin Gastroenterol Hepatol 2016;14:1086–95.e6.
27. Fleischer DE, Overholt BF, Sharma VK, et al. Endoscopic radiofrequency ablation for Barrett's esophagus: 5-year outcomes from a prospective multicenter trial. Endoscopy 2010;42:781–9.
28. Shaheen NJ, Overholt BF, Sampliner RE, et al. Durability of radiofrequency ablation in Barrett's esophagus with dysplasia. Gastroenterology 2011;141:460–8.
29. Krishnamoorthi R, Singh S, Ragunathan K, et al. Risk of recurrence of Barrett's esophagus after successful endoscopic therapy. Gastrointest Endosc 2016;83:1090–106.e3.
30. Pasricha S, Bulsiewicz WJ, Hathorn KE, et al. Durability and predictors of successful radiofrequency ablation for Barrett's esophagus. Clin Gastroenterol Hepatol 2014;12:1840–7.e1.
31. Guthikonda A, Cotton CC, Madanick RD, et al. Clinical outcomes following recurrence of intestinal metaplasia after successful treatment of Barrett's esophagus with radiofrequency ablation. Am J Gastroenterol 2017;112(1):87–94.
32. Vaccaro BJ, Gonzalez S, Poneros JM, et al. Detection of intestinal metaplasia after successful eradication of Barrett's esophagus with radiofrequency ablation. Dig Dis Sci 2011;56:1996–2000.
33. Wolf WA, Pasricha S, Cotton C, et al. Incidence of esophageal adenocarcinoma and causes of mortality after radiofrequency ablation of Barrett's esophagus. Gastroenterology 2015;149:1752–61.e1.
34. Gray NA, Odze RD, Spechler SJ. Buried metaplasia after endoscopic ablation of Barrett's esophagus: a systematic review. Am J Gastroenterol 2011;106:1899–908 [quiz: 1909].
35. Titi M, Overhiser A, Ulusarac O, et al. Development of subsquamous high-grade dysplasia and adenocarcinoma after successful radiofrequency ablation of Barrett's esophagus. Gastroenterology 2012;143:564–6.e1.
36. Haidry RJ, Banks M, Gupta A, et al. Sub-squamous columnar neoplasia after successful radiofrequency ablation for Barrett's related neoplasia is rare but highlights requirement for long term follow up in these patients. Gut 2014;63:A56.
37. Swager AF, Boerwinkel DF, de Bruin DM, et al. Detection of buried Barrett's glands after radiofrequency ablation with volumetric laser endomicroscopy. Gastrointest Endosc 2016;83:80–8.

Cryotherapy for Barrett's Esophagus

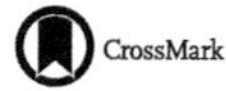

Marcia Irene Canto, MD, MHS

KEYWORDS

- Endoscopic cryotherapy • Cryoablation • Barrett's esophagus
- Esophageal neoplasia • Esophageal cancer

KEY POINTS

- Current cryotherapy systems allow endoscopic application of freezing energy to esophageal tissue by either "spray" or contact balloon method, with resulting mucosal necrosis evolving over several days.
- The accumulating albeit small number of studies suggests that cryotherapy is a safe and effective technique for eradication of Barrett's esophagus and associated neoplasia, with or without prior endoscopic mucosal resection of lesions. It may successfully eradicate Barrett's esophagus even in patients who have prior failed therapy, including radiofrequency ablation.
- The data supporting the use of endoscopic cryotherapy in clinical practice are limited to retrospective cohort studies and a prospective registry study. Prospective large clinical trials are needed.

BACKGROUND

Cryotherapy (also known as cryoablation or cryosurgery) involves freezing to destroy unwanted tissues in situ. It has been used for a variety of neoplastic diseases, including solid organ cancers (prostate,[1,2] kidney,[3–5] liver[6–8]), cervical neoplasia,[9,10] and endobronchial tumors.[11]

Thermal injury or destruction involving freezing is quite different from ablation using high-energy heat, which results in immediate coagulation necrosis. Cryotherapy results in both immediate and delayed tissue injury and necrosis. The proposed mechanisms for cryotherapy effects begin with rapid intracellular and extracellular freezing, resulting in cell necrosis.[12,13] The direct freezing results in cell membrane interruption and protein denaturation. Vascular flow is also compromised, leading to the complete

Financial Disclosures: Research grant, C2 Therapeutics, Cosmo Pharmaceuticals; speaker, Cook Medical; consulting, Pentax.
Division of Gastroenterology and Hepatology, The Johns Hopkins Hospital, Johns Hopkins Medical Institutions, Johns Hopkins University School of Medicine, 1800 Orleans Street, Blalock 407, Baltimore, MD 21287, USA
E-mail address: mcanto@jhmi.edu

Gastrointest Endoscopy Clin N Am 27 (2017) 503–513
http://dx.doi.org/10.1016/j.giec.2017.03.004

cessation of blood flow. Freezing also leads to delayed effects, including self-induced apoptosis (cell death). In addition, immune-mediated toxicity may lead to cell death in cancer cells. The anti-inflammatory response occurs in areas with sublethal injury.[4] The thaw phase of cryotherapy has also been proposed as critical for cryotherapy injury.[14] Hence, freeze and thaw cycles of cryoablation have been typically applied to solid tumors and epithelial tissues.

Endoscopic cryotherapy provides a unique challenge for therapeutic eradication of neoplastic tissue. The degree and duration of freezing influence cell death. However, the vascular flow within the gastrointestinal wall results in tissue warming, resulting in melting of ice and variability in tissue effects. This tissue warming may influence the optimization of cryogen dosimetry and consistency of cryogen application, particularly with spray cryotherapy systems, which are known to potentially result in variable freezing temperature and duration of ice.

ENDOSCOPIC CRYOTHERAPY SYSTEMS: TECHNICAL AND PROCEDURAL ISSUES

There are 3 systems for endoscopic cryotherapy that are approved by the US Food and Drug Administration and commercially available for clinical use in the gastrointestinal tract. These systems are summarized in **Table 1**. In 1999, the first reports of endoscopic cryotherapy systems developed for delivery of liquid nitrogen (LN)[15,16] or carbon dioxide (CO_2) gas[16] were published. More than 10 years later, the third cryotherapy system (cryoballoon focal ablation system or CbFAS) was developed.[17] The LN and nitrous oxide cryotherapy systems cause direct freezing as the liquid evaporates at its boiling point, which is −196 degrees Celsius for liquid nitrogen and −89°C for nitrous oxide. CO_2 gas cryotherapy is based on the Joules Thompson principle, whereby compressed gas expansion results in a drop in temperature to −80°C.

The LN system involves the release of LN through an endoscopic catheter resulting in gaseous expansion (CSA Medical, Lexington, MA, USA). The system consists of the console that contains a LN holding tank (**Fig. 1**A) and a slim flexible disposable

Table 1
Comparison of 3 endoscopic cryotherapy systems

	CryoSpray/TruFreeze (CSA Medical)	Polar Wand (GI Supply)	Cryoballoon Focal Ablation System (C2 Therapeutics)
Delivery of cryogen	CryoSpray (noncontact)	CryoSpray (noncontact)	Contact
Cryogen	LN	CO_2	Nitrous oxide
Tissue temperature	−196°C	−80°C	−85°C
Dosimetry	For 3-cm BE length: 20 s × 2–3 cycles (3 cm length) or 10 s × 4 cycles	For 3–5 cm of BE: 6–8 × 15 s freeze-thaw cycle	1 ablation 8–10 s, multifocal ablations depending on BE extent
Gas evacuation	Orogastric tube	Endoscope-mounted catheter	No additional catheter
System	Console with nitrogen tank, disposable 7-F spray catheter, & 20-F decompression tube	Console with CO_2 tank, disposable 3-F polyethylene catheter, and suction catheter	Lightweight handle, disposable balloon catheters, small cryogen cartridges

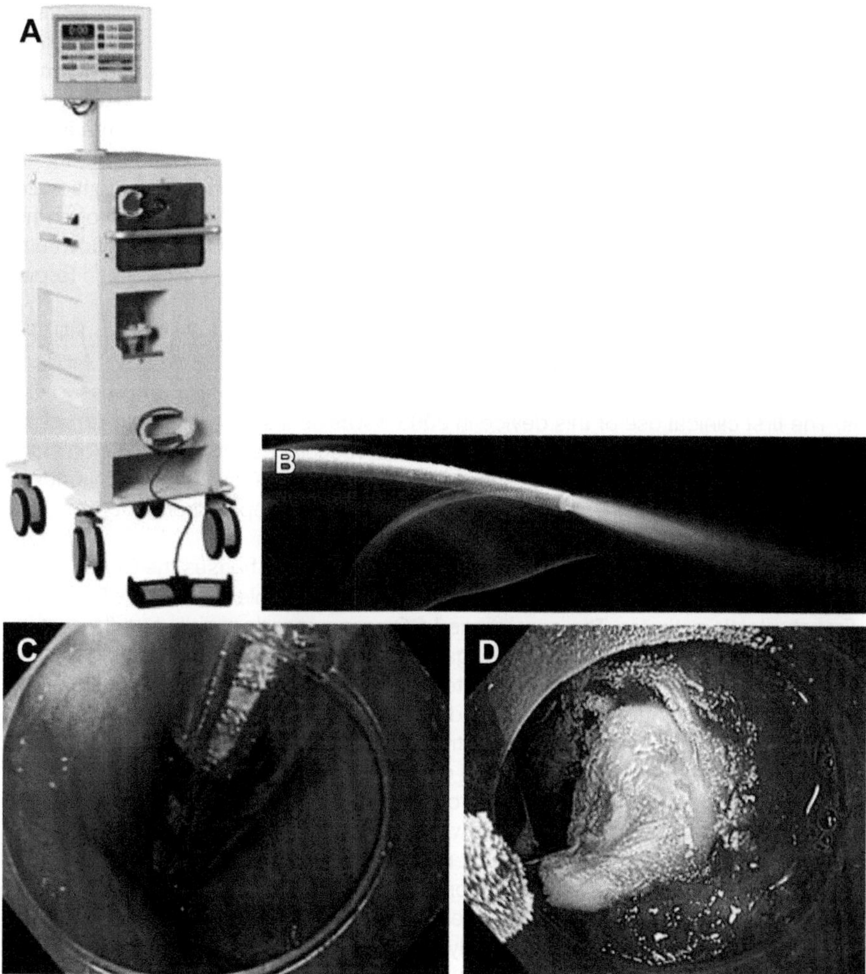

Fig. 1. LN CryoSpray (TruFreeze, CSA Medical). (*A*) Console with built-in suction and pedal (LN tank stored and not shown). (*B*) External view of flexible slim catheter showing LN spray. (*C, D*) Endoscopic view of esophageal mucosa after LN cryospray. (*Courtesy of* [*A, B*] CSA Medical, Inc, Lexington MA; and *From* [*C, D*] Shaheen NJ, Greenwald BD, Peery AF, et al. Safety and efficacy of endoscopic spray cryotherapy for Barrett's esophagus with high-grade dysplasia. Gastrointest Endosc 2010;71(4):682; with permission.)

multilayered stainless steel–reinforced 7-French catheter that is coated with a polymer (**Fig. 1**B). The release of LN and heating of the catheter are controlled by a dual foot pedal. Although previously described as a low-pressure cryotherapy system because the flow rate from the tip of the catheter is low (2–4 psi), the immediate expansion of LN into a gaseous state can generate about 8 L of nitrogen gas, thereby requiring constant orogastric tube decompression. The second-generation LN spray cryotherapy device introduced in 2007 (Cryospray Ablation System, CSA Medical, MD) (see **Fig. 1**A) replaced the first-generation system (CryoSpray) to improve flexibility of the catheter and provide improved laminar flow and decreased intraluminal pressures. The current commercially available third generation system is the truFreeze device introduced in 2012. The LN spray results in very cold tissue freeze, with estimated temperature of −196°C. The technique of LN cryospray involves passing the catheter through the endoscope channel and placing the tip approximately 1 to 2 cm from the mucosal surface. A plastic cap on the tip of the endoscope has been used to decrease "splashback" onto the scope lens, and maintain a distance from the mucosa. After visible ice forms, the catheter tip is moved with the endoscope to "spray" the esophageal mucosa to expand the area of frozen mucosa, typically from distal to proximal. A hemi-circumferential zone of ice is created and the Barrett's esophagus (BE) is frozen for the predetermined time (cryogen dose) (**Fig. 1**C). The dosing of LN cryogen has varied. Studies have typically reported 10 to 20 seconds of solid freeze, followed by a minimum 45 seconds of thaw and reperfusion, repeated for 2 to 4 cycles.[18] Repeat treatments are typically performed after 4 to 8 weeks.

The second type of cryotherapy device (Polar Wand, GI Supply, Camp Hill, PA, USA), which was developed at the Johns Hopkins Hospital in Baltimore, Maryland, originally used nitrogen gas, but second-generation devices apply compressed CO_2 gas. The first clinical use of this device in 2003[19] was as a salvage therapy for refractory gastrointestinal bleeding due to gastric antral vascular ectasia, watermelon stomach, and radiation proctitis. It was subsequently used for BE.[20] Although this device was in use for more than 10 years, the manufacturer has stopped production and provides limited support for existing devices.

The Polar Wand device consists of a portable console that houses the CO_2 tank and suction canister. The CO_2 is released from a 0.005-inch hole at the tip of a flexible 3-French plastic catheter. The compressed CO_2 gas expands rapidly at a flow rate of approximately 6 to 8 L/min. Excess CO_2 gas is removed simultaneously during cryogen delivery with a slim plastic suction catheter attached to the tip of the endoscope. The CO_2 is released from the catheter placed close to the esophageal mucosa, resulting in ice formation, which can be applied to treat the entire BE area. The ice rapidly thaws, and the thaw phase is not timed. Several cycles of freezing and thawing per treatment session are typically administered. In a porcine animal model, increasing duration and number of freeze cycles are associated with increased depth of cryotherapy injury in the esophagus and stomach.[21] The average depth of tissue injury (measured from mucosal surface) due to a single application of 15 seconds of CO_2 cryotherapy in porcine esophagus ranged from 1.2 to 2.5 mm, depending on the number of freeze-thaw applications. With the cryogen dose commonly used in patients (15 seconds × 6–8 cycles), injury could be seen in the submucosa, but this did not lead to transmural necrosis. At 2 weeks, there was complete regeneration of the tissue. In patients, cryotherapy treatments are typically repeated every 4 to 8 weeks until eradication is achieved.[20]

Cryoballoon Ablation

The third and the newest type of endoscopic cryotherapy system is the CbFAS (C2 Therapeutics, Redwood, CA, USA), which was first reported in 2011[17] (see **Table 1**). The CbFAS consists of a small hand-held device (controller) containing liquid nitrous oxide within a small cartridge (**Fig. 2**A). The heat generated in the controller keeps the cryogen in liquid state while the tissue temperature converts the liquid to nitrous oxide gas within a low pressure–compliant 30-mm-long oval-shaped balloon (**Fig. 2**B). The 3.7-mm disposable balloon catheter is passed through a therapeutic endoscope channel, or "side car" accessory, that can be attached externally alongside a standard endoscope[17] (see **Fig. 2**A). The ablation is performed under endoscopic guidance with the endoscope looking through the proximal portion of the transparent balloon. Mucosal freezing is achieved by delivery of liquid nitrous oxide, which is contained in a small portable cartridge placed in the battery-powered "gunlike" controller. The latter has a trigger that opens the valve and allows the nitrous oxide gas to escape

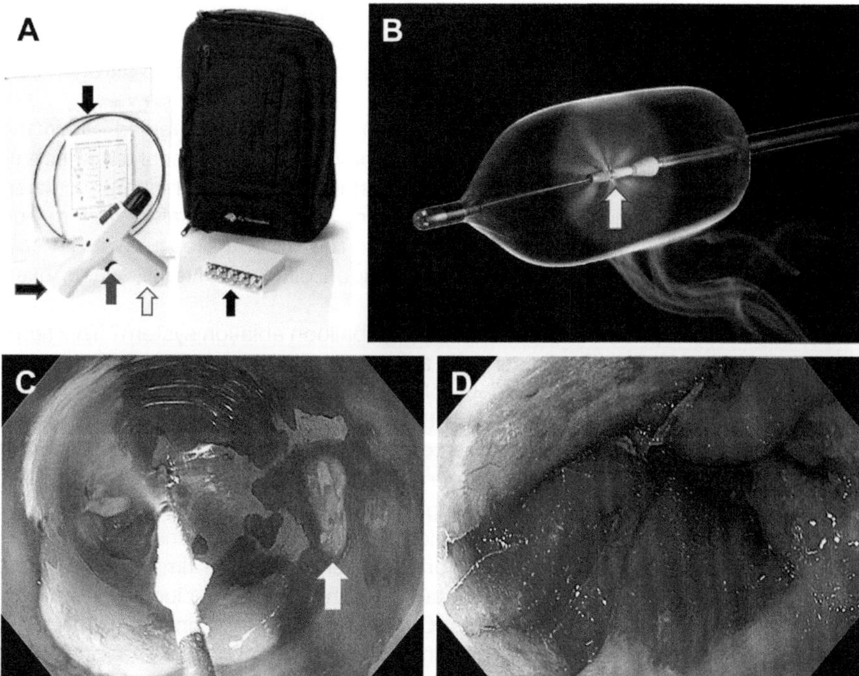

Fig. 2. CbFAS (C2 Therapeutics). (*A*) Controller (*left image*) with handle that holds the nitrogen cartridge (*yellow arrow*), trigger (*red arrow*), and attachment site (*black right arrow*) for the balloon catheter (*black down arrow*). The catheter is attached to a reusable lightweight portable handle, which controls the delivery of liquid nitrous oxide stored in a small cartridge. (*B*) External view of focal cryoballoon ablation catheter (30 mm) with diffuser (*arrow*) and nitrous oxide spray. (*C*) Endoscopic view of focal cryoballoon ablation through the balloon using a high-definition endoscope showing the cryogen released from the diffuser within the balloon and resulting ice patch. The active ablation is the fourth one applied in a clockwise circumferential fashion, with the first ice patch melting (*arrow*). (*D*) Endoscopic view of the distal esophageal and gastric cardia mucosa with red color change and edema immediately after cryoablation. (© *Therapeutic images. Used by permission. The use of any C2 Therapeutics photo or image does not imply C2 Therapeutics' review or endorsement of any article or publication.*)

through a small opening on the diffuser within the center of the balloon. The balloon at the end of the catheter is inflated and simultaneously cooled by the gas expansion. The cryogen makes contract with the balloon and freezes targeted mucosa in contact with the balloon resulting in focal ablations (discrete ice patches) of approximately 2 cm^2 (**Fig. 2**C).[17] With the balloon deflated, the immediate post-cryoablation mucosal effects can be seen as dark red color change, which can be visualized distinctly from untreated areas (**Fig. 2**D).

The current focal cryoballoon ablation system allows targeting of an area in the BE with a 1-second "prepuff" of cryogen, by rotating the handle in a clockwise or counterclockwise direction. This turns the diffuser within the balloon and allows aiming of the cryogen. Delivery of a preset cryogen energy dose (measured in total seconds of application of cryogen) can follow the aiming by pressing the trigger on the controller. The cryogen is automatically delivered according to a preset dose (seconds), which eliminates the need to count the number of seconds of energy delivered. The cryogen dose currently used for BE is 10 seconds per ablation site based on animal and human BE dosimetry studies.[22–24] Multiple ablations (multifocal cryoablation) can be applied, including all visible BE mucosa (see **Fig. 2**C). The balloon catheter and nitrogen cartridges are discarded, and the handle is recycled.

In contrast to the other 2 types of cryotherapy, the gas is contained within the balloon and exits back into the catheter, thereby obviating an additional tube decompression. The balloon pressure remains relatively stable during the ablation, regulated by the software in the controller to a maximum of 3.5 psi. As a safety feature, the balloon deflates if the pressure exceeds 4.5 psi. The balloon pressure is very low compared with standard through-the-scope balloon dilation systems, which exert pressures of 44 (3 atm) to 147 psi (10 atm).

What might be the potential benefits of the cryoballoon ablation system? This technique is still under study, and clinical trials are ongoing (clinicaltrials.gov). Compared with cryospray techniques, cryoballoon ablation might lead to more consistent and effective application of cryogen because the nitrous oxide gas is contained within the balloon and the entire cryogen dose is completely delivered to a target site without gas escaping into the lumen. In addition, the cryogen dose can be preprogrammed but also adjusted during the procedure. A single ice patch per site without freeze-thaw cycling appears to be sufficient for complete ablation of the BE mucosa.[22,23] This might improve the efficiency of ablation and shorten procedure time. Furthermore, there are economic and practical advantages to the CbFAS, including portability, and minimal storage space requirements. Capital expense is eliminated (without the need for a generator or console), and only the costs of the disposables are budgeted. Importantly, small portable nitrogen cartridges replace the large gas tanks that need tank replacement and refilling, which is quite appealing for the staff of the endoscopy unit.

EFFICACY FOR ERADICATION OF DYSPLASIA AND INTESTINAL METAPLASIA

Endoscopic cryotherapy using LN has been used to successfully eradicate previously unablated neoplastic BE[25–27] as well as persistent or recurrent disease after other treatments.[25,28] A pilot clinical study by Johnston and colleagues[29] in 2005 described 11 patients with BE ranging from nondysplastic to multifocal high-grade dysplasia (HGD). Complete eradiation of intestinal metaplasia (CE-IM) was achieved initially in 100% of patients, and after 6 months, 78% of patients.[29]

Subsequent studies reported encouraging treatment outcomes in patients with neoplastic BE (**Table 2**). A single-center cohort study by Dumot and colleagues[30] in 2009 investigated 30 patients who were ineligible for or refused esophagectomy. After treatment, 68% of the patients with HGD and 80% of the patients with intramucosal adenocarcinoma had downgrading of their worst pathologic dysplasia grade at a median follow-up of 12 months. The first large multicenter retrospective cohort study reported by Shaheen and colleagues[27] in 2010 included 9 academic and community centers. Ninety-eight subjects with BE and HGD (including residual disease post-endoscopic mucosal resection [EMR]) were treated with LN cryospray. In the 60 evaluable patients who completed treatments, 58 (97%) had complete eradication of all dysplasia (CE-D), whereas 87% had CE-IM. A study by Ghorbani and colleagues[31] in 2015 reported outcomes of LN cryospray in BE HGD (n = 57) and low-grade dysplasia (LGD) (n = 23) patients (about two-thirds long segment) enrolled in a prospective multicenter registry and treated every 2 to 3 months until complete eradication was achieved. Eighty of the 96 subjects (83%) completed treatment and were followed for 2 years. The eradication rate for LGD patients

Table 2
Comparison of efficacy of cryotherapy for eradication of Barrett's esophagus and associated early esophageal adenocarcinoma

Study	Patient Population	Number of Treatments	Average BE Length (cm)	CE-HGD 1 y (%)	CE-D 1 y (%)	CE-IM 1 y (%)
LN cryotherapy Shaheen et al,[27] 2010	60 HGD	4	5	97	87	57
LN cryotherapy Gosain 2010	32 HGD	3.1–5	3	94	98	81
LN cryotherapy Ghorbani et al,[31] 2015	96 (57 HGD, 23 LGD)	3.5 HGD 2.9 LGD	4.1 HGD 5.1 LGD	91	81 HGD 91 LGD	65 HGD 61 LGD
LN cryotherapy Ramay et al,[32] 2017	50 (46 HGD, 4 T1a ECA)	3	3.5	98	90	60
CO_2 cryotherapy Canto et al,[25] 2015[a,b]	64 (54 HGD, 10 T1a ECA, 4 T1b ECA)	<2 cm: 2 2–8 cm: 4 >8 cm: 7	5.3	94[c]	84[b]	55
Cryoballoon Canto et al,[22] 2016[a,b,d]	40 (13 LGD, 23 HGD, 4 T1a ECA)	2.4	4.1	95	90	71

[a] Includes treatment-naïve and previously ablated resistant BE patients.
[b] Includes patients with esophageal cancer.
[c] 100% for treatment-naïve patients; 91% patients with prior ablation.
[d] Preliminary data, abstract form; data on 21 evaluable patients completed treatment and follow-up.

was 91%, with CE-IM in 61%. In BE HGD patients, the CE-D rate was 81%, and CE-IM was 65%.

Very limited data are available on the efficacy of CO_2 cryotherapy. One single-center retrospective cohort study by Canto and colleagues[25] reported 64 patients with dysplastic BE (20 treatment naive, 44 rescue treatment) who were treated and followed up (median time 4.2 years). At 1 year, the overall complete response rates were 77% for cancer (10/13), 89% for dysplasia (57/64) (CE-D), 94% for HGD (60/64, notably 100% for treatment naive, 91% for rescue treatment), and 55% CE-IM (35/64).

The CbFAS has been used for endoscopic ablation of BE[5] with promising early results.[6] In a multicenter international trial, a single dose of cryogen delivered to the target BE mucosa resulted in full squamous regeneration and was seen in 47 treated areas (6 [60%] of the 6-second areas; 23 [82%] of the 8-second areas; 18 [100%] of 10-second areas).[24] Preliminary data from a single-center prospective single-arm clinical trial including treatment-naïve and previously ablated BE with LGD, HGD, and ImCA (intramucosal adenocarcinoma) are encouraging (**Table 3**). One-year CE-D and CR-IM (complete response for intestinal metaplasia) for neoplastic BE with or without prior EMR are 95% and 71%, respectively. Clinical trials using the CbFAS as a focal and multifocal ablative technique for dysplastic BE ablation are ongoing in the United States and Europe.

SAFETY OF CRYOTHERAPY

Liquid Nitrogen CryoSpray

The adverse event profiles for the 2 established cryotherapy systems are summarized in **Table 3**. Overall, the safety profile for cryotherapy is very good. The serious adverse event rate is 0% to 3%, primarily due to rare perforation and bleeding. The incidence

Table 3
Comparison of safety of cryotherapy for eradication of Barrett's esophagus

Study	SAE Rate	Pain Requiring Narcotics	Strictures Requiring Dilation	Perforation	Bleeding
LN cryotherapy Dumot et al,[30] 2009 N = 30	1 (3%)	3 (10%)	0	1[a]	0
LN cryotherapy Shaheen et al,[27] 2010 N = 60	1 (1%)	2 (3%)	3 (5%)	0	1 (1%)[b]
LN cryotherapy Gosain et al,[26] 2013 N = 32	0	0	3 (9%)	0	0
LN cryotherapy Ghorbani et al,[31] 2015 N = 96 (registry)	1 (2%)	0	0	0	1 (1%)[c]
CO_2 cryotherapy Canto et al,[25] 2015 N = 68	1 (1.5%)	0	1 (1.5%)	1[d]	0

Abbreviation: SAE, serious adverse event.
[a] Patient with Marfan syndrome.
[b] Rectal bleeding leading to hospitalization but no intervention.
[c] Associated with NSAID use.
[d] Microperforation not requiring surgery.

of postablation strictures requiring dilation is low (0%–9%). Bleeding is rare (only 2 patients admitted to the hospital, 1 related to nonsteroidal anti-inflammatory drug [NSAID] use). Remarkably, there is minimal postablation narcotic-requiring pain reported by published studies (3%–10%), and pain is typically short lived.

In 2009, Dumot and colleagues[30] reported an open-label trial including 30 high-risk patients with BE HGD. There was a gastric perforation in a Marfan syndrome patient and lip ulcer related to freezing.

Shaheen and colleagues[27] reported 1 of the 60 patients in the cryospray registry who progressed to intramucosal adenocarcinoma requiring esophagectomy.

Carbon Dioxide Cryotherapy

CO_2 cryotherapy is also well tolerated with no narcotic-requiring pain, stricture, or bleeding (see **Table 3**). One microperforation (minute air under diaphragm) associated with abdominal pain leading to hospitalization but not surgery was noted in the study by Canto and colleagues. Bradycardia was treated with atropine in 1 of the 68 patients during the sedated ablation procedure.

Cryoballoon Ablation

There are limited published data detailing the safety of the CbFAS. In the pilot feasibility trial by Scholvinck and colleagues,[24] no major adverse events occurred in 39 patients. Six patients experienced a minor mucosal balloon trauma requiring no intervention. The cryoablation balloon device was subsequently modified to decrease maximum balloon pressure. Mild pain not requiring narcotic analgesics was reported by 27% of patients immediately after cryoablation and by 14% after 2 days. No strictures were evident at follow-up, but only 2 sites were focally ablated (see **Table 3**).

Preliminary data from the single-center prospective clinical trial at Johns Hopkins Hospital presented in abstract form (35 evaluable patients in the safety cohort) also suggest a favorable pain profile. There was transient pain in 8 of 25 (23%), mostly noted immediately after the procedure in the recovery area of the endoscopy unit, resolving within 48 hours. The median 24-hour 0 to 10 Likert pain score was 2 (range 0–3), with no pain requiring medications beyond 48 hours. Three patients of the 35 reported in the preliminary analysis had inflammatory strictures, but only one required dilation (2.8% incidence). No patient had a persistent or symptomatic stricture after completion of cryoablation, including 9 with preexisting post-EMR/radiofrequency ablation (RFA) strictures.

DURABILITY

Overall, limited data on the durability of cryotherapy for BE eradication are available (see **Table 2**). In a recent follow-up article from a retrospective cohort study of 60 BE patients treated with LN cryospray, Ramay and colleagues[32] reported 3- and 5-year outcomes for 50 and 40 patients, respectively. Initial CE-D and CE-IM were achieved in 90% and 60%, respectively. Dysplasia eradication rates were stable with CE-D of 94% and 88% at 3 and 5 years. Over time and repeated cryotherapy sessions, the CE-IM rate improved. By 5 years, 75% of BE patients still had negative biopsies. However, these long-term data are limited by patient lost to follow-up, introducing possible selection bias, and retrospective study design.

Recurrent disease is a challenge for all BE endoscopic eradication treatments. Recurrent BE neoplasia can be detected in short- and long-term surveillance periods. In the study by Gosain and colleagues[26] of BE HGD patients treated with LN cryotherapy, 6 of 32 (19%) patients who did not have intramucosal cancer at baseline and completed treatments developed recurrent HGD, with median time to recurrence of 6 months (range 3–18 months). Delayed recurrences of neoplasia beyond 1 year are also noted. In the 5-year study by Greenwald and colleagues, the overall recurrence of BE HGD was 18% (7/39), with median time to recurrence of 13.1 months (interquartile range 6.4–50.2). Repeat LN cryotherapy was successful in all but 1 of the 7 patients (86%). This patient progressed to cancer despite treatment. The incidence rates of dysplasia, HGD, and esophageal adenocarcinoma after initial CE-IM were 4.0% and 1.4% per person-year for the 5-year cohort.[32] These rates compare favorably with RFA recurrence rates.

Intestinal metaplasia (IM) recurrences after successful LN cryotherapy are noted between 12.2%[26] and 41%[32] of the time. The location of IM and HGD recurrences are generally in the "hot zone" involving the distal esophagus and gastroesophageal junction just distal to the new squamocolumnar junction, more commonly in the latter area.

No long-term studies are available for the CbFAS system. Ongoing prospective clinical trials (clinicaltrials.gov) evaluating the CbFAS system are assessing durability of treatment effects at 2 and 3 years.

SUMMARY

The future of cryotherapy is promising, with studies to date showing high efficacy, good durability, and excellent safety profile. Notably, there is no robust level 1a scientific evidence supporting widespread use of any cryotherapy system, which limits its adoption into clinical practice. The next steps in evaluating this treatment should include continued device optimization, large randomized controlled trials, and eventually, head-to-head trials comparing cryotherapy with established treatment modalities such as RFA.

REFERENCES

1. Tay KJ, Polascik TJ. Focal cryotherapy for localized prostate cancer. Arch Esp Urol 2016;69(6):317–26.
2. Tay KJ, Polascik TJ, Elshafei A, et al. Primary cryotherapy for high-grade clinically localized prostate cancer: oncologic and functional outcomes from the COLD registry. J Endourol 2016;30(1):43–8.
3. Rodriguez-Faba O, Palou J, Rosales A, et al. Prospective study of ultrasound-guided percutaneous renal cryotherapy: case selection as an optimization factor for a technique. Actas Urol Esp 2015;39(1):8–12.
4. Mohammed A, Miller S, Douglas-Moore J, et al. Cryotherapy and its applications in the management of urologic malignancies: a review of its use in prostate and renal cancers. Urol Oncol 2014;32(1):39.e19-27.
5. Cho S, Kang SH. Current status of cryotherapy for prostate and kidney cancer. Korean J Urol 2014;55(12):780–8.
6. Schuld J, Richter S, Kollmar O. The role of cryosurgery in the treatment of colorectal liver metastases: a matched-pair analysis of cryotherapy vs. liver resection. Hepatogastroenterology 2014;61(129):192–6.
7. Awad T, Thorlund K, Gluud C. Cryotherapy for hepatocellular carcinoma. Cochrane Database Syst Rev 2009;(4):CD007611.
8. Rong G, Bai W, Dong Z, et al. Cryotherapy for cirrhosis-based hepatocellular carcinoma: a single center experience from 1595 treated cases. Front Med 2015; 9(1):63–71.
9. Chigbu CO, Onyebuchi AK, Nnakenyi EF, et al. Impact of visual inspection with acetic acid plus cryotherapy “see and treat” approach on the reduction of the population burden of cervical preinvasive lesions in Southeast Nigeria. Niger J Clin Pract 2017;20(2):239–43.
10. Santesso N, Mustafa RA, Wiercioch W, et al. Systematic reviews and meta-analyses of benefits and harms of cryotherapy, LEEP, and cold knife conization to treat cervical intraepithelial neoplasia. Int J Gynaecol Obstet 2016;132(3): 266–71.
11. Lee SH, Choi WJ, Sung SW, et al. Endoscopic cryotherapy of lung and bronchial tumors: a systematic review. Korean J Intern Med 2011;26(2):137–44.
12. Baust JG, Gage AA, Robilottto AT, et al. The pathophysiology of thermoablation: optimizing cryoablation. Curr Opin Urol 2009;19(2):127–32.
13. Gage AA, Baust J. Mechanisms of tissue injury in cryosurgery. Cryobiology 1998; 37(3):171–86.
14. Baust JG, Gage AA, Clarke D, et al. Cryosurgery–a putative approach to molecular-based optimization. Cryobiology 2004;48(2):190–204.
15. Johnston CM, Schoenfeld LP, Mysore JV, et al. Endoscopic spray cryotherapy: a new technique for mucosal ablation in the esophagus. Gastrointest Endosc 1999; 50(1):86–92.
16. Pasricha PJ, Hill S, Wadwa KS, et al. Endoscopic cryotherapy: experimental results and first clinical use. Gastrointest Endosc 1999;49(5):627–31.
17. Friedland S, Triadafilopoulos G. A novel device for ablation of abnormal esophageal mucosa (with video). Gastrointest Endosc 2011;74(1):182–8.
18. Greenwald BD, Dumot JA, Horwhat JD, et al. Safety, tolerability, and efficacy of endoscopic low-pressure liquid nitrogen spray cryotherapy in the esophagus. Dis Esophagus 2010;23(1):13–9.

19. Kantsevoy SV, Cruz-Correa MR, Vaughn CA, et al. Endoscopic cryotherapy for the treatment of bleeding mucosal vascular lesions of the GI tract: a pilot study. Gastrointest Endosc 2003;57(3):403–6.
20. Xue HB, Tan HH, Liu WZ, et al. A pilot study of endoscopic spray cryotherapy by pressurized carbon dioxide gas for Barrett's esophagus. Endoscopy 2011;43(5): 379–85.
21. Shin EJ, Amateau SK, Kim Y, et al. Dose-dependent depth of tissue injury with carbon dioxide cryotherapy in porcine GI tract. Gastrointest Endosc 2012; 75(5):1062–7.
22. Canto M, Shin EJ, Khashab M, et al. Multifocal nitrous oxide cryoballoon ablation with or without endoscopic mucosal resection (EMR) for treatment of neoplastic Barrett's esophagus: preliminary results of a prospective clinical trial in treatment-naive and previously ablated patients. Gastrointest Endosc 2016; 83(55):AB159.
23. Kunzli HT, Scholvinck DW, Meijer SL, et al. Efficacy of the cryoballoon focal ablation system for the eradication of dysplastic Barrett's esophagus islands. Endoscopy 2017;49(2):169–75.
24. Scholvinck DW, Kunzli HT, Kestens C, et al. Treatment of Barrett's esophagus with a novel focal cryoablation device: a safety and feasibility study. Endoscopy 2015; 47(12):1106–12.
25. Canto MI, Shin EJ, Khashab MA, et al. Safety and efficacy of carbon dioxide cryotherapy for treatment of neoplastic Barrett's esophagus. Endoscopy 2015;47(7): 591.
26. Gosain S, Mercer K, Twaddell WS, et al. Liquid nitrogen spray cryotherapy in Barrett's esophagus with high-grade dysplasia: long-term results. Gastrointest Endosc 2013;78(2):260–5.
27. Shaheen NJ, Greenwald BD, Peery AF, et al. Safety and efficacy of endoscopic spray cryotherapy for Barrett's esophagus with high-grade dysplasia. Gastrointest Endosc 2010;71(4):680–5.
28. Barthel JS, Kucera S, Harris C, et al. Cryoablation of persistent Barrett's epithelium after definitive chemoradiation therapy for esophageal adenocarcinoma. Gastrointest Endosc 2011;74(1):51–7.
29. Johnston MH, Eastone JA, Horwhat JD, et al. Cryoablation of Barrett's esophagus: a pilot study. Gastrointest Endosc 2005;62(6):842–8.
30. Dumot JA, Vargo JJ 2nd, Falk GW, et al. An open label, prospective trial of cryospray ablation for Barrett's esophagus high-grade dysplasia and early esophageal cancer in high-risk patients. Gastrointest Endosc 2009;70(4):635–44.
31. Ghorbani S, Tsai FC, Greenwald BD, et al. Safety and efficacy of endoscopic spray cryotherapy for Barrett's dysplasia: results of the National Cryospray Registry. Dis Esophagus 2015.
32. Ramay FH, Cui Q, Greenwald BD. Outcomes after liquid nitrogen spray cryotherapy in Barrett's esophagus-associated high-grade dysplasia and intramucosal adenocarcinoma: 5-year follow-up. Gastrointest Endosc 2017. [Epub ahead of print].

Care of the Postablation Patient

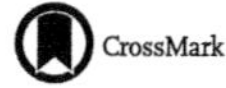

Surveillance, Acid Suppression, and Treatment of Recurrence

Leila Kia, MD, Srinadh Komanduri, MD, MS*

KEYWORDS

- Barrett's esophagus • Endoscopic eradication therapy • Surveillance
- Radiofrequency ablation • Endoscopic mucosal resection

KEY POINTS

- Endoscopic eradication therapy is effective and durable for the treatment of Barrett's esophagus (BE), with low rates of recurrence of dysplasia but significant rates of recurrence of intestinal metaplasia.
- Identified risk factors for recurrence include age and length of BE before treatment and may also include presence of a large hiatal hernia, higher grade of dysplasia before treatment, and history of smoking.
- Current guidelines for surveillance following ablation are limited, with recommendations based on low-quality evidence and expert opinion.
- Limitations to current postablation surveillance protocols include lack of standardized definitions and endpoints, variability in treatments used, sampling error, and interobserver variability.
- New modalities including optical coherence tomography and wide-area tissue sampling with computer-assisted analysis show promise as adjunctive surveillance modalities.

INTRODUCTION

The hallmark of Barrett's esophagus (BE) is the replacement of normal esophageal stratified squamous epithelium by intestinal columnar epithelium, with or without dysplasia.[1,2] This premalignant condition, found in approximately 15% of patients with gastroesophageal reflux disease (GERD),[3] is associated with an increased risk

---

Disclosures: L. Kia: None; S. Komanduri: Consultant for Medtronic GI Solutions.

Division of Gastroenterology and Hepatology, Department of Medicine, Northwestern University Feinberg School of Medicine, 676 North Saint Clair, Suite 1400, Chicago, IL 60611, USA
* Corresponding author. Division of Gastroenterology, 676 North Saint Claire, Suite 1400, Chicago, IL 60611.
E-mail address: sri-komanduri@northwestern.edu

Gastrointest Endoscopy Clin N Am 27 (2017) 515–529
http://dx.doi.org/10.1016/j.giec.2017.02.008
1052-5157/17/
giendo.theclinics.com

of esophageal adenocarcinoma (EAC) and has been the subject of substantial research and debate with regards to implementation of appropriate screening, treatment, and surveillance guidelines.[1,4–6] Despite the ongoing debates regarding screening, intervals for surveillance, and management of nondysplastic BE, it is widely accepted that in the presence of dysplasia, endoscopic eradication therapy (EET) is the first-line treatment strategy.[7,8] These modalities include endoscopic mucosal resection (EMR), radiofrequency ablation (RFA), photodynamic therapy, cryotherapy, argon plasma coagulation (APC), multipolar electrocoagulation, and laser therapy, either in isolation or in combination.[1,9–11] At the present time, EMR in conjunction with cryotherapy or RFA is the preferred modality and has been shown to be effective in reducing the progression to high-grade dysplasia (HGD) and EAC.[1,9,10] Following EET, however, there is a paucity of data and guidelines regarding postablative surveillance and durability of treatment. The objective of this review is to define appropriate endpoints for surveillance, review the literature with respect to durability of EET and risk factors for recurrence, present the current evidence for surveillance, and highlight limitations and emerging modalities for surveillance in the post-EET setting.

ENDPOINTS FOR SURVEILLANCE

Defining the appropriate endpoints for surveillance is imperative in instituting consistency in guidelines for post-EET surveillance strategies. In order to do this, the nomenclature and methodology for surveillance have to be standardized. The goal of EET is to achieve complete eradication of intestinal metaplasia (CE-IM), including dysplasia and/or intramucosal carcinoma (IMC) if present, via EMR and ablative therapies as needed. Following CE-IM, the reported recurrence rate for intestinal metaplasia (IM) has been widely variable, in part due to the differences in definitions and surveillance protocols used in the posttreatment period.[1] Some studies report recurrence located only in the tubular esophagus,[12] whereas others report recurrent IM in both the esophagus and the gastroesophageal junction (GEJ)/cardia.[13] The location of recurrent IM is important, because the significance of recurrent IM without dysplasia at the GEJ after CE-IM is unclear, particularly with regards to need for future therapy. IM of the cardia is common in the general population and can be seen in up to 20% of asymptomatic individuals.[14] To date, the natural history of IM at the GEJ is thought to be different than that of the tubular esophagus, as it is more likely to be associated with *Helicobacter pylori* infection and not with EAC.[14–16] As such, biopsy of a normal or slightly irregular GEJ found incidentally during an endoscopy for GERD is not recommended.[17] However, it is important to emphasize that the GEJ is also a common location for harboring dysplastic lesions, so routine ablation and posttreatment surveillance of the neosquamocolumnar junction is imperative and has become common practice, with some experts advocating surveillance and treatment of the superior gastric folds.[18]

The true definition of CE-IM remains unclear. Some studies consider a single endoscopy with negative histology as adequate for achieving remission, whereas others require 2 consecutive endoscopies.[19,20] Irrespective of the number of endoscopies, sampling error and limitations of high-definition white light endoscopy (HD-WLE) and narrow band imaging (NBI) are also important considerations in the post-EET patient, because visible detection of recurrence following ablation may be difficult using current imaging modalities[17] (**Figs. 1** and **2**). Furthermore, the concern for buried metaplasia following EET is recognized as a limitation with the current standard endoscopic imaging (HD-WLE and NBI) and pinch biopsies. These subsquamous islands of IM and dysplasia "buried" beneath normal and postablation epithelium are of concern

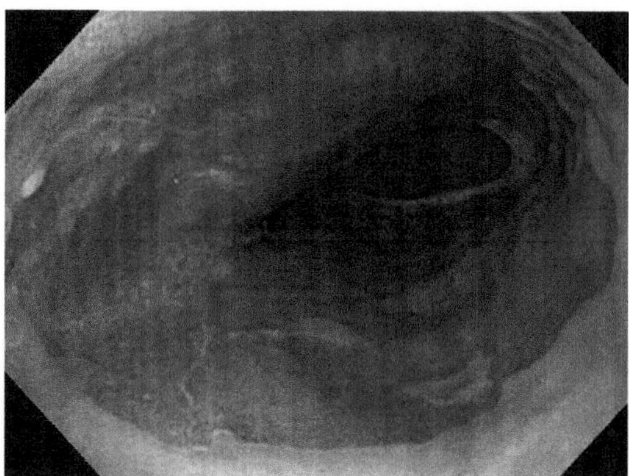

Fig. 1. Endoscopic image using HD-WLE showing long-segment BE.

given the potential for malignant progression[21,22] (**Fig. 3**). Specimens from esophagectomies have yielded rates of buried IM as high as 71% confirmed by optical coherence tomography (OCT) and pathology.[23] A study assessing EMR specimens found synchronous or metachronous lesions in 28% of samples, whereas another study using OCT imaging found buried IM in 72% pre-RFA and 63% in post-RFA patients.[22,24] One study carried out complete EMR in patients with BE before any ablative therapies and revealed subsquamous lesions with HGD or intramucosal carcinoma in 21% of specimens.[22] Ultimately, however, the clinical relevance of these findings is unclear. Few cases of buried neoplasia have been reported in the literature, so although it remains a significant concern, further research is required to determine the appropriate surveillance and follow-up required for these lesions, which may not harbor an equally high malignant progression.[25] A recent systematic review of buried metaplasia noted major limitations in drawing conclusions from studies to date, because they lacked descriptions of how frequently biopsy specimens contained sufficient lamina propria to be informative for buried metaplasia.[26] As other imaging and surveillance modalities are further studied (eg, OCT), the implications of buried metaplasia will likely be further elucidated.

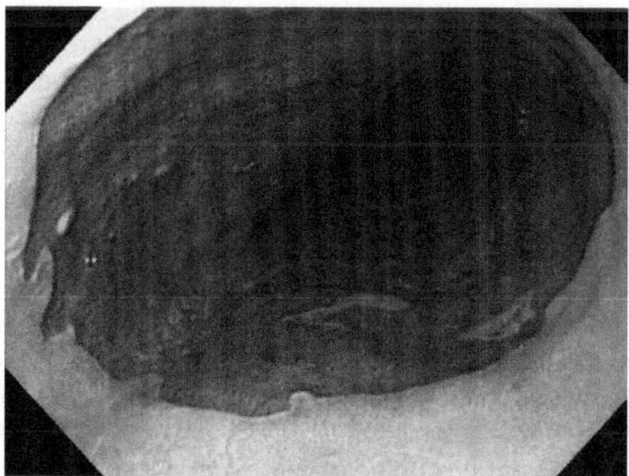

Fig. 2. Endoscopic image using narrow-band imaging showing same area of long-segment BE.

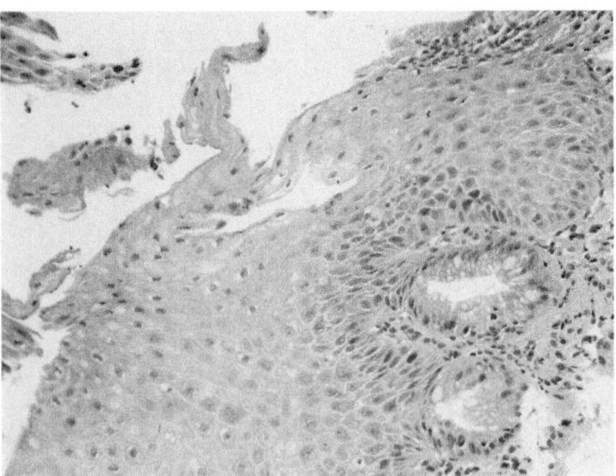

Fig. 3. Buried IM (hematoxylin-eosin, original magnification ×40).

Finally, interobserver variability in interpretation of histologic samples, an important issue in the pretreatment population, is also relevant in the posttreatment population. Regenerating tissue may appear dysplastic due to inflammation and mesenchymal changes, and differentiating the degree of dysplasia may be more difficult following ablation.[27] As is the case pretreatment, confirmation of findings with at least one expert gastrointestinal pathologist is recommended.[1]

DURABILITY OF ENDOSCOPIC ERADICATION THERAPY AND RISK FACTORS FOR RECURRENCE

The goal of EET is to achieve lasting and durable eradication of dysplasia and IM. Because of some of the aforementioned factors and differences in techniques and treatment modalities, there is variability in recurrence rates following CE-IM, with some cohorts reporting rates of 20% at 2 to 3 years follow-up, although ranges from 0.7% to 28.8% have been described.[19,28,29] **Table 1** describes studies to date reporting recurrence data after EET. A recent systematic review of 41 studies reported pooled incidence rates of recurrent IM, dysplastic BE, and HGD/EAC after RFA of 9.5%, 2.0%, and 1.2% per patient-year, respectively.[11] When all endoscopic modalities were included, pooled incidence rates were 7.1%, 1.3%, and 0.8% per patient-year, respectively. With regards to predictors of IM recurrence, they found that increased age and length of BE segment were predictive of recurrence. Other studies suggest that the presence of a large hiatal hernia, higher grade of dysplasia pretreatment, and history of smoking may also be associated with higher rates of recurrence.[29–31] A previously published systematic review of patients undergoing RFA only (18 studies) reported IM recurrence in 13% of patients, with progression to cancer in 0.2% during treatment and 0.7% after CE-IM.[32] Both of these large systematic reviews were limited by the quality of the studies reviewed, limited external validity, and significant heterogeneity, owing in part to variability in methods for detecting recurrence, inclusion or exclusion of GEJ, and different periods of follow-up, among other variables.[17] Despite these limitations, recurrence rates of IM are significant, and long-term follow-up with adequate surveillance is necessary in order to prevent progression to dysplasia and cancer. Further studies are needed to identify the true risk of progression and long-term recurrence rates after EET.

Table 1
Summary of durability studies postendoscopic eradication therapy

First Author, Publication Year	Study Type	Total (n)	No. Achieving CE-IM/CE-D	No. in Surveillance After CE-IM/CE-D	Mean Follow-up (y)	Recurrences			
						Total	IM	Dysplasia	EAC
Fleischer et al,[54] 2010	Prospective multicenter	50	46	46	5	4	4	0	0
Alvarez Herrero et al,[55] 2011	Prospective multicenter	24	19/20	20	2.4	5	5	0	0
Shaheen et al,[56] 2011	Prospective multicenter	119	108/110	110	3.05	19	14	3	2
Vaccaro et al,[57] 2011	Retrospective single center	47	47	47	1.11	15	11	4	0
van Vilsteren et al,[58] 2011	Prospective multicenter	22	21	20	1.8	2	2	0	0
Caillol et al,[59] 2012	Prospective single center	34	17/30	34	1	2	0	0	2
Gupta et al,[60] 2012	Retrospective multicenter	128	128	128	1.3	34	18	16	0
van Vilsteren et al,[61] 2012	Prospective single center	24	23/24	24	1.2	0	0	0	0
Akiyama et al,[62] 2013	Retrospective single center	40	40	40	2.18	7	7	0	0
Dulai et al,[63] 2013	Retrospective single center	72	56/57	57	3.25	11	11	0	0
Ertan et al,[64] 2013	Prospective single center	50	27/47	47	2.75	3	3	0	0
Gupta et al,[19] 2013	Retrospective multicenter	448	229	229	1.12	37	29	8	0
Haidry et al,[33] 2013	Prospective multicenter	335	208/270	256	1.58	38	17	17	4
Korst et al,[65] 2013	Prospective single center	53	53	51	1.5	14	14	0	0
Orman et al,[20] 2013	Retrospective single center	262	183/188	112	1.1	8	3	2	3
Phoa et al,[12] 2013	Retrospective single center	55	54	54	5.1	25	22	1	2
Shue et al,[66] 2013	Retrospective	42	42	42	1.17	11	11	0	0
Pasricha et al,[29] 2014	Retrospective multicenter	5521	3169	1634	2.4	334	269	52	13
Strauss et al,[67] 2014	Retrospective multicenter	36	27/32	36	2	9	5	3	1
Agoston et al,[68] 2016	Retrospective multicenter	78	67	67	2.2	—	—	—	6
Cotton et al,[69] 2015	Retrospective single center	198	198	198	3	35	22	7	6
Lada et al,[70] 2014	Prospective single center	57	28/49	57	2.95	16	4	12	0
Le Page et al,[71] 2016	Retrospective single center	50	35	45	1.75	—	—	—	2
Phoa et al,[34] 2016	Retrospective multicenter	124	115/121	121	2.25	13	5	6	2

CURRENT GUIDELINES FOR SURVEILLANCE FOLLOWING ENDOSCOPIC ERADICATION THERAPY

Following CE-IM, careful endoscopic surveillance with biopsies is the recommended strategy for detection of recurrent IM or dysplasia, at varying time intervals, depending on pretreatment histologic findings. The current intervals and biopsy protocols recommended are based on expert opinion and on intervals reported in published cohort studies.[1,12,33] There are limited data supporting these recommendations, and further studies are needed to validate appropriate surveillance protocols.

At this time, endoscopic surveillance for patients with baseline HGD is recommended every 3 months in the first year after CE-IM, every 6 months in the second year, and annually thereafter if there is no recurrence (**Table 2**). For patients with baseline Low-grade dysplasia (LGD), endoscopic surveillance is recommended every 6 months in the first year after CE-IM, and annually thereafter. There are no recommendations on surveillance intervals for patients with high-risk nondysplastic BE who have undergone EET, but the authors' practice is to perform endoscopic surveillance every 3 years once CE-IM is confirmed.

In addition to surveillance intervals, the precise technique for endoscopic surveillance remains unclear. Most studies to date use 4-quadrant biopsies every centimeter throughout the previous BE segment, with additional targeted biopsies of endoscopic abnormalities. Given the prevalence of dysplastic lesions at the GEJ, many also advocate obtaining separate biopsies of the GEJ. All examinations should include careful inspection of the tubular esophagus and the GEJ in antegrade and retrograde views, using high-resolution white light and NBI. At the present time, there are no recommendations to discontinue endoscopic surveillance after multiple negative surveillance endoscopies. This recommendation may change with further understanding of predictive biomarkers along with data regarding the long-term durability of EET. Until such data are available, endoscopic surveillance after completion of EET remains the standard of care.

TREATMENT OF RECURRENT DISEASE AFTER ENDOSCOPIC ERADICATION THERAPY

There are limited data on the appropriate treatment strategy for recurrent disease after EET. Review of the large registries reveals that treatment of recurrence is often undertaken as standard practice, particularly in cases of HGD/IMC, although specific details on treatment modality are usually lacking. The Euro II study, a large multicenter study of 132 patients, required confirmation of recurrence by an expert pathologist. Patients only underwent re-treatment if HGD/IMC was present, whereas patients with recurrent IM or LGD underwent surveillance.[34] Data from the US RFA Registry on 448 patients reveal that re-treatment was undertaken in patients with any recurrence, including IM.[19] Of the 37 patients that recurred, 25 underwent re-treatment, whereas 12 underwent surveillance. Of those who were re-treated, the majority was treated with APC or multipolar coagulation (n = 8), RFA (n = 8), or combination therapy (n = 6). Nineteen of

Table 2
Surveillance protocol following endoscopic eradication therapy

Pre-EET Finding	First Surveillance Post-EET	Long-Term Surveillance
NDBE	Yearly	Every 3–5 y
LGD	Every 6 mo × 1st year	Yearly
HGD/IMC	Every 3 mo × 1st year Every 6 mo × 2nd year	Yearly

Abbreviation: NDBE, non-dysplastic barrett's esophagus.

these patients were successfully treated, with 5 undergoing therapy at the time of publication. Finally, a recent retrospective review of 306 patients who underwent RFA for dysplastic BE was notable for a recurrence rate of 9.6% per year. Of the 52 patients who had recurrence, 58% achieved second CE-IM, 2% had recurrent invasive adenocarcinoma, 4% failed endoscopic re-treatment, 37% were still undergoing treatment, and 2% were lost to follow-up.[35] However, this study did not specify the type or number of treatments undertaken. Overall, despite the limited data, it appears that re-treatment after CE-IM is effective, although further studies are needed in order to determine the appropriate modality, number of treatments, and long-term durability.

IMPORTANCE OF REFLUX CONTROL AND RISK FACTOR REDUCTION IN THE POSTABLATIVE SURVEILLANCE PERIOD

Adequate acid suppression is the backbone of management of patients with BE, regardless of whether endotherapy is pursued. Mechanistically, the reduction in acid exposure in the distal esophagus is thought to prevent cellular changes that lead to the development of dysplasia and cancer.[36,37] Uncontrolled reflux exposure has been shown to be a risk factor for persistent IM following RFA, highlighting the importance of adequate reflux control for response to RFA.[36] The importance of reflux control has also been demonstrated in EET studies using APC, wherein normalization of pH with PPI treatment and prior fundoplication were independent predictors of sustained remission.[38,39] Symptom assessment in these patients is not an adequate measure of reflux control, because most patients are asymptomatic. However, new-onset symptoms or esophagitis following EET may be signs of uncontrolled reflux. Early recognition and physiologic testing are critical for the success and durability of EET. Notably, acid control with PPI therapy is often inadequate for adequate reflux control. A study of 110 asymptomatic patients on PPI with a history of GERD and/or BE found that only 58% of patients with GERD and 50% with BE normalized their pH on PPI therapy.[40] Finally, presence of a large hiatal hernia has also been shown to be a risk factor for recurrence of IM following ablation, likely in part due to persistence of reflux.[30] A small uncontrolled study comparing post-RFA treatment with PPI daily versus laparoscopic Nissen fundoplication found recurrence of BE in 20% of the PPI group versus 9.1% of the surgical group after 2 years of follow-up.[41] Currently, the use of high-dose proton pump inhibitor (PPI), the role for ambulatory pH monitoring, and the utility of surgical hernia repair for reflux control in the post-EET period are subjects of ongoing research, and there is no conclusive evidence to suggest that these strategies should be pursued in the absence of persistent or new symptoms or esophagitis. Nonetheless, patients should continue once-daily PPI therapy for chemoprevention as recommended in the pre-EET surveillance period.

EMERGING MODALITIES FOR SURVEILLANCE

At the present time, life-long surveillance with endoscopy and 4-quadrant biopsies are the recommended standard of care for patients undergoing post-EET surveillance. As previously discussed, there are many limitations to this strategy, including the need for sedation, sampling error, and interobserver variability among pathologists. As such, there has been significant interest in developing less invasive and less costly strategies for surveillance, while improving on the diagnostic yield. Endoscopic ultrasound (EUS) was initially considered, at least as adjunctive to endoscopy with biopsies, but it has not been found to have any additional diagnostic value except in cases of staging of deeply invading tumors or wherein lymphadenopathy is noted. EUS cannot differentiate between dysplastic and nondysplastic lesions due to limited resolution, so its utility in surveillance is limited.[42,43] Confocal laser microscopy (CLM) (Cellvizio; Mauna Kea Technologies, Cambridge, MA, USA) is an endoscopic tool that allows real-time microscopic analysis of surface features using fluorescent staining agents and has been evaluated as a strategy to improve on random surveillance biopsies[43,44] (**Figs. 4** and **5**). A study comparing the incident dysplasia detection rate of biopsies obtained by HD-WLE and CLM found higher detection rates in the CLM group.[45] No suspicious areas were observed in the HD-WLE group, and dysplasia was found in 10% of biopsies. Those in the CLM group were noted to have suspicious lesions in 42%, with confirmation of dysplasia in 28% of cases. Despite improvement in detection rates, its use is limited in that it requires training in interpretation of the images, and it has not been found to be effective in detecting residual IM in the post-EET period in a large randomized control trial.[46] Moreover, its diagnostic yield is limited to superficial lesions less than 250 μm, thus not allowing for reliable detection of buried IM.[47]

OCT technology (NinePoint Medical, Bedford, MA, USA) has emerged as a promising modality to assist in surveillance of BE. The high-resolution through-the-scope device produces high-quality volumetric images of the esophageal wall in real time using near-infrared low coherence light. It has a range of 1 to 3 mm in depth with resolution on the scale of 3 to 5 μm and thus offers a better depth, larger field-of-view, 3-dimensional imaging, and reliable detection and differentiation of mucosal and submucosal abnormalities when compared with white light with random biopsies[48] (**Figs. 6** and **7**). In buried IM, it has been able to identify buried glands in both pre-RFA and

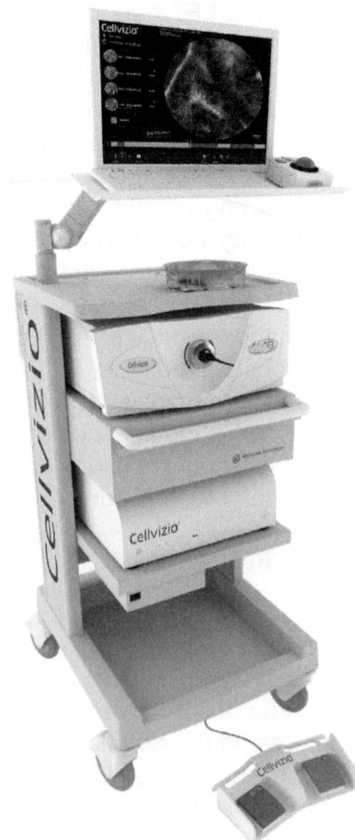

Fig. 4. CLM (Cellvizio) device. (*Courtesy of* Mauna Kea Technologies, Cambridge, MA; with permission.)

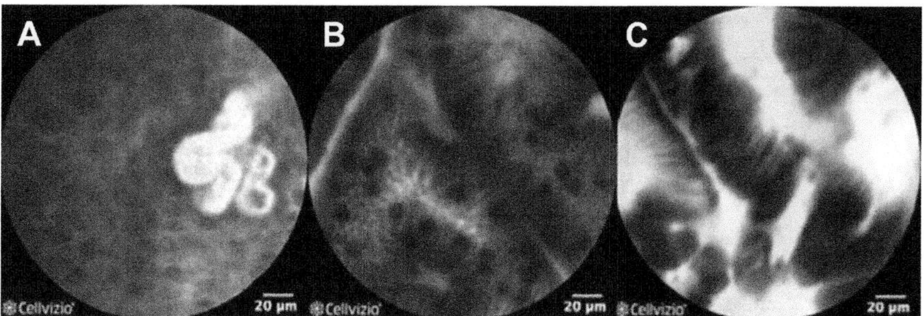

Fig. 5. CLM images depicting (*A*) Squamous epithelium, (*B*) IM, (*C*) HGD. (*Courtesy of* Mauna Kea Technologies, Cambridge, MA; with permission.)

post-RFA specimens, demonstrating response to treatment in real time.[49] Remarkably, in studies of fresh esophagectomy specimens of patients with HGD or EAC, it has been able to detect histologically confirmed subsquamous IM and differentiate between dysplasia and EAC by imaging alone.[23] There is clear value in using this modality, but as is often the case with new technologies, it is limited by lack of

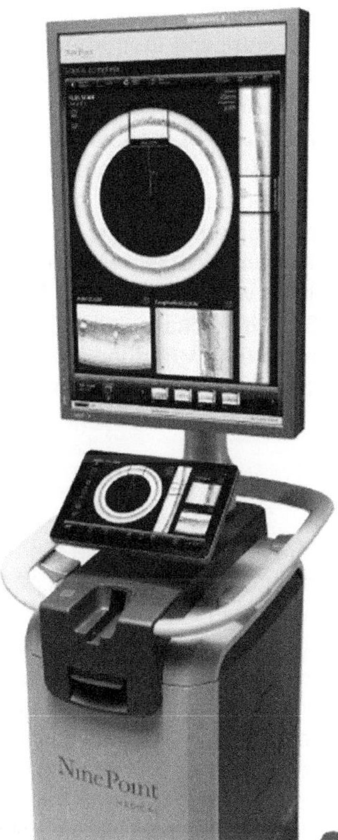

Fig. 6. Optical Computed Tomography Imaging System device (NvisionVLE). (*Courtesy of* NinePoint Medical, Bedford, MA; with permission.)

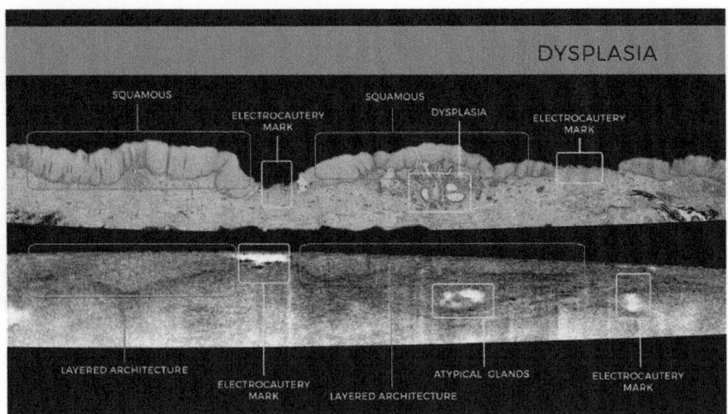

Fig. 7. OCT image of dysplasia compared with histologic sample. (*Courtesy of* NinePoint Medical, Bedford, MA; with permission.)

standardized and validated criteria, added time to procedures, additional disposable expense, and limited speed of image processing.[17,50]

Another emerging modality aimed at overcoming the limited sampling of the 4-quadrant biopsy protocol is a computer-assisted wide-area transepithelial sampling (WATS-3D) brush-biopsy technique (CDx Diagnostics, Suffern, NY, USA). This technique uses an abrasive sampling instrument that obtains a sample of the entire thickness of the epithelium down to the lamina propria. These tissue fragments are then analyzed using a computer-assisted scan that highlights potentially abnormal cells that are then presented for manual pathologist review. Studies using this modality as an adjunct to biopsies in both screening and surveillance protocols have resulted in identification of additional cases of dysplasia,[51,52] with good interobserver agreement among pathologists.[53] In one study assessing a high-risk population (patients with BE with known dysplasia undergoing surveillance), the overall yield for identification of dysplasia was 25.2% using forceps alone, whereas brush biopsy yielded an additional 16 positive cases, increasing the detection rate to 42%, with a number needed to treat of 9.4.[51] Further studies are needed to determine the generalizability and feasibility of using this novel diagnostic tool in clinical practice.

SUMMARY

EET has proven to be a safe, effective, and durable therapy for Barrett's associated neoplasia. Although the tools and techniques for performing EET continue to improve, recurrence of disease remains a significant concern. The implications of this finding and the risk of progression to cancer are as of yet unclear. The precise factors that lead to recurrent IM and/or dysplasia after EET are unknown; however, it appears that continued control of underlying GERD is essential. Current guidelines for surveillance and management of the post-EET patient are sparse and based on limited low-quality evidence. At the root of the problem is the lack of standardization in definitions, nomenclature, and endpoints of treatment. Furthermore, the current tools for surveillance (visual inspection with white light and NBI, and targeted biopsies) are subject to many limitations, including interobserver variability and sampling error. New imaging and surveillance modalities, including confocal endomicroscopy, OCT, and WATS computer-assisted sampling, may provide solutions to some of these limitations when used in adjunct. Ultimately, further studies are needed to determine appropriate time intervals and surveillance protocols to minimize unnecessary procedures while balancing the risk of recurrence. Although many questions remain, we have made significant strides with regards to the care of our patients after completion of EET.

REFERENCES

1. Shaheen NJ, Falk GW, Iyer PG, et al. ACG clinical guideline: diagnosis and management of Barrett's esophagus. Am J Gastroenterol 2016;111(1):30–50 [quiz: 1].
2. Sharma P. Clinical practice. Barrett's esophagus. N Engl J Med 2009;361(26): 2548–56.
3. Johansson J, Hakansson HO, Mellblom L, et al. Prevalence of precancerous and other metaplasia in the distal oesophagus and gastro-oesophageal junction. Scand J Gastroenterol 2005;40(8):893–902.
4. Sharma P, Falk GW, Weston AP, et al. Dysplasia and cancer in a large multicenter cohort of patients with Barrett's esophagus. Clin Gastroenterol Hepatol 2006;4(5): 566–72.
5. Drewitz DJ, Sampliner RE, Garewal HS. The incidence of adenocarcinoma in Barrett's esophagus: a prospective study of 170 patients followed 4.8 years. Am J Gastroenterol 1997;92(2):212–5.
6. Yousef F, Cardwell C, Cantwell MM, et al. The incidence of esophageal cancer and high-grade dysplasia in Barrett's esophagus: a systematic review and meta-analysis. Am J Epidemiol 2008;168(3):237–49.
7. ASGE Standards of Practice Committee, Evans JA, Early DS, Fukami N, et al. The role of endoscopy in Barrett's esophagus and other premalignant conditions of the esophagus. Gastrointest Endosc 2012;76(6):1087–94.
8. Spechler SJ, Sharma P, Souza RF, et al. American Gastroenterological Association technical review on the management of Barrett's esophagus. Gastroenterology 2011;140(3):e18–52 [quiz: e13].
9. Phoa KN, van Vilsteren FG, Weusten BL, et al. Radiofrequency ablation vs endoscopic surveillance for patients with Barrett esophagus and low-grade dysplasia: a randomized clinical trial. JAMA 2014;311(12):1209–17.
10. Overholt BF, Lightdale CJ, Wang KK, et al. Photodynamic therapy with porfimer sodium for ablation of high-grade dysplasia in Barrett's esophagus: international, partially blinded, randomized phase III trial. Gastrointest Endosc 2005;62(4): 488–98.
11. Krishnamoorthi R, Singh S, Ragunathan K, et al. Risk of recurrence of Barrett's esophagus after successful endoscopic therapy. Gastrointest Endosc 2016; 83(6):1090–106.e3.
12. Phoa KN, Pouw RE, van Vilsteren FG, et al. Remission of Barrett's esophagus with early neoplasia 5 years after radiofrequency ablation with endoscopic resection: a Netherlands cohort study. Gastroenterology 2013;145(1):96–104.
13. Gaddam S, Singh M, Balasubramanian G, et al. Persistence of nondysplastic Barrett's esophagus identifies patients at lower risk for esophageal adenocarcinoma: results from a large multicenter cohort. Gastroenterology 2013;145(3): 548–53.e1.
14. Byrne JP, Bhatnagar S, Hamid B, et al. Comparative study of intestinal metaplasia and mucin staining at the cardia and esophagogastric junction in 225 symptomatic

patients presenting for diagnostic open-access gastroscopy. Am J Gastroenterol 1999;94(1):98–103.
15. Zaninotto G, Avellini C, Barbazza R, et al. Prevalence of intestinal metaplasia in the distal oesophagus, oesophagogastric junction and gastric cardia in symptomatic patients in north-east Italy: a prospective, descriptive survey. The Italian Ulcer Study Group "GISU". Dig Liver Dis 2001;33(4):316–21.
16. Weston AP, Krmpotich PT, Cherian R, et al. Prospective evaluation of intestinal metaplasia and dysplasia within the cardia of patients with Barrett's esophagus. Dig Dis Sci 1997;42(3):597–602.
17. Stier MW, Konda VJ, Hart J, et al. Post-ablation surveillance in Barrett's esophagus: a review of the literature. World J Gastroenterol 2016;22(17):4297–306.
18. Alvarez Herrero L, Curvers WL, Bisschops R, et al. Narrow band imaging does not reliably predict residual intestinal metaplasia after radiofrequency ablation at the neo-squamo columnar junction. Endoscopy 2014;46(2):98–104.
19. Gupta M, Iyer PG, Lutzke L, et al. Recurrence of esophageal intestinal metaplasia after endoscopic mucosal resection and radiofrequency ablation of Barrett's esophagus: results from a US Multicenter Consortium. Gastroenterology 2013; 145(1):79–86.e1.
20. Orman ES, Kim HP, Bulsiewicz WJ, et al. Intestinal metaplasia recurs infrequently in patients successfully treated for Barrett's esophagus with radiofrequency ablation. Am J Gastroenterol 2013;108(2):187–95 [quiz: 96].
21. Titi M, Overhiser A, Ulusarac O, et al. Development of subsquamous high-grade dysplasia and adenocarcinoma after successful radiofrequency ablation of Barrett's esophagus. Gastroenterology 2012;143(3):564–6.e1.
22. Chennat J, Ross AS, Konda VJ, et al. Advanced pathology under squamous epithelium on initial EMR specimens in patients with Barrett's esophagus and high-grade dysplasia or intramucosal carcinoma: implications for surveillance and endotherapy management. Gastrointest Endosc 2009;70(3):417–21.
23. Cobb MJ, Hwang JH, Upton MP, et al. Imaging of subsquamous Barrett's epithelium with ultrahigh-resolution optical coherence tomography: a histologic correlation study. Gastrointest Endosc 2010;71(2):223–30.
24. Zhou C, Tsai TH, Lee HC, et al. Characterization of buried glands before and after radiofrequency ablation by using 3-dimensional optical coherence tomography (with videos). Gastrointest Endosc 2012;76(1):32–40.
25. Mashimo H. Subsquamous intestinal metaplasia after ablation of Barrett's esophagus: frequency and importance. Curr Opin Gastroenterol 2013;29(4):454–9.
26. Gray NA, Odze RD, Spechler SJ. Buried metaplasia after endoscopic ablation of Barrett's esophagus: a systematic review. Am J Gastroenterol 2011;106(11): 1899–908 [quiz: 909].
27. Odze RD, Lauwers GY. Histopathology of Barrett's esophagus after ablation and endoscopic mucosal resection therapy. Endoscopy 2008;40(12):1008–15.
28. Anders M, Bahr C, El-Masry MA, et al. Long-term recurrence of neoplasia and Barrett's epithelium after complete endoscopic resection. Gut 2014;63(10): 1535–43.
29. Pasricha S, Bulsiewicz WJ, Hathorn KE, et al. Durability and predictors of successful radiofrequency ablation for Barrett's esophagus. Clin Gastroenterol Hepatol 2014;12(11):1840–7.e1.
30. Yasuda K, Choi SE, Nishioka NS, et al. Incidence and predictors of adenocarcinoma following endoscopic ablation of Barrett's esophagus. Dig Dis Sci 2014; 59(7):1560–6.

31. Badreddine RJ, Prasad GA, Wang KK, et al. Prevalence and predictors of recurrent neoplasia after ablation of Barrett's esophagus. Gastrointest Endosc 2010; 71(4):697–703.
32. Orman ES, Li N, Shaheen NJ. Efficacy and durability of radiofrequency ablation for Barrett's esophagus: systematic review and meta-analysis. Clin Gastroenterol Hepatol 2013;11(10):1245–55.
33. Haidry RJ, Dunn JM, Butt MA, et al. Radiofrequency ablation and endoscopic mucosal resection for dysplastic Barrett's esophagus and early esophageal adenocarcinoma: outcomes of the UK National Halo RFA Registry. Gastroenterology 2013;145(1):87–95.
34. Phoa KN, Pouw RE, Bisschops R, et al. Multimodality endoscopic eradication for neoplastic Barrett oesophagus: results of an European multicentre study (EURO-II). Gut 2016;65(4):555–62.
35. Guthikonda A, Cotton CC, Madanick RD, et al. Clinical outcomes following recurrence of intestinal metaplasia after successful treatment of Barrett's esophagus with radiofrequency ablation. Am J Gastroenterol 2017;12(1):87–94.
36. Krishnan K, Pandolfino JE, Kahrilas PJ, et al. Increased risk for persistent intestinal metaplasia in patients with Barrett's esophagus and uncontrolled reflux exposure before radiofrequency ablation. Gastroenterology 2012;143(3):576–81.
37. Overholt BF. Acid suppression and reepithelialization after ablation of Barrett's esophagus. Dig Dis 2000;18(4):232–9.
38. Kahaleh M, Van Laethem JL, Nagy N, et al. Long-term follow-up and factors predictive of recurrence in Barrett's esophagus treated by argon plasma coagulation and acid suppression. Endoscopy 2002;34(12):950–5.
39. Ferraris R, Fracchia M, Foti M, et al. Barrett's oesophagus: long-term follow-up after complete ablation with argon plasma coagulation and the factors that determine its recurrence. Aliment Pharmacol Ther 2007;25(7):835–40.
40. Gerson LB, Boparai V, Ullah N, et al. Oesophageal and gastric pH profiles in patients with gastro-oesophageal reflux disease and Barrett's oesophagus treated with proton pump inhibitors. Aliment Pharmacol Ther 2004;20(6):637–43.
41. Skrobic O, Simic A, Radovanovic N, et al. Significance of Nissen fundoplication after endoscopic radiofrequency ablation of Barrett's esophagus. Surg Endosc 2016;30(9):3802–7.
42. Savoy AD, Wolfsen HC, Raimondo M, et al. The role of surveillance endoscopy and endosonography after endoscopic ablation of high-grade dysplasia and carcinoma of the esophagus. Dis Esophagus 2008;21(2):108–13.
43. Espino A, Cirocco M, Dacosta R, et al. Advanced imaging technologies for the detection of dysplasia and early cancer in barrett esophagus. Clin Endosc 2014;47(1):47–54.
44. Tsai TH, Zhou C, Lee HC, et al. Comparison of tissue architectural changes between radiofrequency ablation and cryospray ablation in Barrett's esophagus using endoscopic three-dimensional optical coherence tomography. Gastroenterol Res Pract 2012;2012:684832.
45. Bertani H, Frazzoni M, Dabizzi E, et al. Improved detection of incident dysplasia by probe-based confocal laser endomicroscopy in a Barrett's esophagus surveillance program. Dig Dis Sci 2013;58(1):188–93.
46. Wallace MB, Crook JE, Saunders M, et al. Multicenter, randomized, controlled trial of confocal laser endomicroscopy assessment of residual metaplasia after mucosal ablation or resection of GI neoplasia in Barrett's esophagus. Gastrointest Endosc 2012;76(3):539–47.e1.

47. Kiesslich R, Gossner L, Goetz M, et al. In vivo histology of Barrett's esophagus and associated neoplasia by confocal laser endomicroscopy. Clin Gastroenterol Hepatol 2006;4(8):979–87.
48. Konda VJ, Koons A, Siddiqui UD, et al. Optical biopsy approaches in Barrett's esophagus with next-generation optical coherence tomography. Gastrointest Endosc 2014;80(3):516–7.
49. van Vilsteren FG, Alvarez Herrero L, Pouw RE, et al. Predictive factors for initial treatment response after circumferential radiofrequency ablation for Barrett's esophagus with early neoplasia: a prospective multicenter study. Endoscopy 2013;45(7):516–25.
50. May A. Barrett's esophagus: should we burn it all? Gastrointest Endosc 2012; 76(6):1113–5.
51. Anandasabapathy S, Sontag S, Graham DY, et al. Computer-assisted brush-biopsy analysis for the detection of dysplasia in a high-risk Barrett's esophagus surveillance population. Dig Dis Sci 2011;56(3):761–6.
52. Johanson JF, Frakes J, Eisen D, et al. Computer-assisted analysis of abrasive transepithelial brush biopsies increases the effectiveness of esophageal screening: a multicenter prospective clinical trial by the EndoCDx Collaborative Group. Dig Dis Sci 2011;56(3):767–72.
53. Vennalaganti PR, Naag Kanakadandi V, Gross SA, et al. Inter-observer agreement among pathologists using wide-area transepithelial sampling with computer-assisted analysis in patients with Barrett's esophagus. Am J Gastroenterol 2015;110(9):1257–60.
54. Fleischer DE, Overholt BF, Sharma VK, et al. Endoscopic radiofrequency ablation for Barrett's esophagus: 5-year outcomes from a prospective multicenter trial. Endoscopy 2010;42(10):781–9.
55. Alvarez Herrero L, van Vilsteren FG, Pouw RE, et al. Endoscopic radiofrequency ablation combined with endoscopic resection for early neoplasia in Barrett's esophagus longer than 10 cm. Gastrointest Endosc 2011;73(4):682–90.
56. Shaheen NJ, Overholt BF, Sampliner RE, et al. Durability of radiofrequency ablation in Barrett's esophagus with dysplasia. Gastroenterology 2011;141(2):460–8.
57. Vaccaro BJ, Gonzalez S, Poneros JM, et al. Detection of intestinal metaplasia after successful eradication of Barrett's Esophagus with radiofrequency ablation. Dig Dis Sci 2011;56(7):1996–2000.
58. van Vilsteren FG, Pouw RE, Seewald S, et al. Stepwise radical endoscopic resection versus radiofrequency ablation for Barrett's oesophagus with high-grade dysplasia or early cancer: a multicentre randomised trial. Gut 2011;60(6):765–73.
59. Caillol F, Bories E, Pesenti C, et al. Radiofrequency ablation associated to mucosal resection in the oesophagus: experience in a single centre. Clin Res Hepatol Gastroenterol 2012;36(4):371–7.
60. Gupta M, Lutzke L, Prasad G. Recurrence of intestinal metaplasia after eradication of Barrett's esophagus with radiofrequency ablation - results from a BETRNet consortium. Gastroenterology 2012;142(5):S73.
61. van Vilsteren FG, Alvarez Herrero L, Pouw RE, et al. Radiofrequency ablation and endoscopic resection in a single session for Barrett's esophagus containing early neoplasia: a feasibility study. Endoscopy 2012;44(12):1096–104.
62. Akiyama J, Roorda A, Marcus S. Erosive esophagitis is a major predictor for recurrence of Barrett's esophagus after successful radiofrequency ablation. Gastroenterology 2013;144:S592.

63. Dulai PS, Pohl H, Levenick JM, et al. Radiofrequency ablation for long- and ultralong-segment Barrett's esophagus: a comparative long-term follow-up study. Gastrointest Endosc 2013;77(4):534–41.
64. Ertan A, Zaheer I, Correa AM, et al. Photodynamic therapy vs radiofrequency ablation for Barrett's dysplasia: efficacy, safety and cost-comparison. World J Gastroenterol 2013;19(41):7106–13.
65. Korst RJ, Santana-Joseph S, Rutledge JR, et al. Patterns of recurrent and persistent intestinal metaplasia after successful radiofrequency ablation of Barrett's esophagus. J Thorac Cardiovasc Surg 2013;145(6):1529–34.
66. Shue P, Kataria R, Pathikonda M. Factors associated with recurrence of Barrett's esophagus after completion of radiofrequency ablation. Gastroenterology 2013; 144:S697.
67. Strauss AC, Agoston AT, Dulai PS, et al. Radiofrequency ablation for Barrett's-associated intramucosal carcinoma: a multi-center follow-up study. Surg Endosc 2014;28(12):3366–72.
68. Agoston AT, Strauss AC, Dulai PS, et al. Predictors of treatment failure after radiofrequency ablation for intramucosal adenocarcinoma in Barrett esophagus: a multi-institutional retrospective cohort study. Am J Surg Pathol 2016;40(4): 554–62.
69. Cotton CC, Wolf WA, Pasricha S, et al. Recurrent intestinal metaplasia after radiofrequency ablation for Barrett's esophagus: endoscopic findings and anatomic location. Gastrointest Endosc 2015;81(6):1362–9.
70. Lada MJ, Watson TJ, Shakoor A, et al. Eliminating a need for esophagectomy: endoscopic treatment of Barrett esophagus with early esophageal neoplasia. Semin Thorac Cardiovasc Surg 2014;26(4):274–84.
71. Le Page PA, Velu PP, Penman ID, et al. Surgical and endoscopic management of high grade dysplasia and early oesophageal adenocarcinoma. Surgeon 2016; 14(6):315–21.

Esophagectomy for Superficial Esophageal Neoplasia

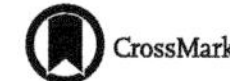

Thomas J. Watson, MD

KEYWORDS

- Esophageal cancer • Barrett's esophagus • Intramucosal carcinoma
- High-grade dysplasia • Esophagectomy

KEY POINTS

- Despite the recent success of endoscopic resection and ablation in the management of Barrett's esophagus with high-grade dysplasia and intramucosal adenocarcinoma, esophagectomy continues to play a role in the treatment of superficial esophageal neoplasia.
- The managing physician needs to be aware of the limitations of endoscopic therapies so that they are not misapplied.
- Until more data are available regarding the efficacy of endoscopic therapies for superficial submucosal carcinoma, esophagectomy with regional lymphadenectomy remains the standard of care in most operative candidates.
- When undertaken in specialty centers for appropriately selected patients, esophagectomy can be performed with a mortality of $\leq$1%, acceptable morbidity, and good long-term quality of life.
- When operating for early esophageal neoplasia, the surgeon should choose a technique that assures eradication of disease while minimizing the potential for perioperative morbidity and a negative impact on long-term quality of life.

INTRODUCTION

The standard of care for the treatment of superficial esophageal neoplasia has evolved dramatically over the past decade in the United States and Western Europe. Current guidelines published by specialty medical societies and the National Comprehensive Cancer Network (NCCN) recommend endoscopic therapies, including resection and ablation, as the preferred treatments for most cases of Barrett's esophagus (BE)

Disclosures: The author is a paid consultant to Ethicon, Medtronic, and Biodesix.
Division of Thoracic and Esophageal Surgery, Department of Surgery, MedStar Washington, Georgetown University School of Medicine, 3800 Reservoir Road Northwest, 4PHC, Washington, DC 20007, USA
E-mail address: Thomas.J.Watson@medstar.net

Gastrointest Endoscopy Clin N Am 27 (2017) 531–546
http://dx.doi.org/10.1016/j.giec.2017.02.009
1052-5157/17/

with high-grade dysplasia (HGD) or intramucosal carcinoma (IMC).[1–3] The NCCN also recommends endoscopic resection (ER) with or without ablation as an option for selected cases of superficial submucosal carcinoma (SMC).[3] Endoscopic treatment modalities, when expertly performed in appropriately selected patients, have been shown to achieve cure rates equivalent to surgery, but with less morbidity. Esophagectomy, the prior standard of care for all superficial neoplasia, has been relegated to the minority of cases of HGD and IMC not suitable for endoscopic approaches. Although surgical resection reliably cures early-stage disease in a single intervention, its role has been marginalized due to the perception of high rates of perioperative mortality, particularly in low-volume centers, a significant complication profile, and the potential to impair long-term quality of life (QOL).

Given such a rapid change in treatment paradigms, the managing physician must remain mindful of the limitations and potential pitfalls of endoscopic therapies as well as knowledgeable about the indications for and outcomes following esophagectomy; a "one-size-fits-all" strategy does not apply. Although the use of surgical resection has diminished in the setting of early-stage esophageal neoplasia, it remains the treatment of choice in specific circumstances. Treatment may be inappropriately underaggressive, following the course of endoscopic therapies, when a more extensive surgical resection is indicated. Performed in experienced hands and with the appropriate techniques, esophagectomy for early neoplasia can be undertaken not only with a high likelihood of cure but also with a low mortality, acceptable morbidity, and good long-term alimentary function.

LIMITATIONS OF ENDOSCOPIC THERAPIES: THE RISK OF NODAL METASTASES

Fundamental to the utilization of endoscopic modalities for the cure of esophageal cancer is the principle that they are appropriate only when the absence of nodal spread can be assured. The treating physician, therefore, must understand how the depth of tumor invasion and other risk factors determine the potential for lymph node metastases, which mandate a surgical resection with regional lymphadenectomy should they be suspected.

The deep border of the esophageal epithelium is its basement membrane (**Fig. 1**). Neoplasia limited to the epithelium, and not penetrating beyond the basement membrane, is termed low-grade dysplasia (LGD) or HGD in the United States, or low-grade

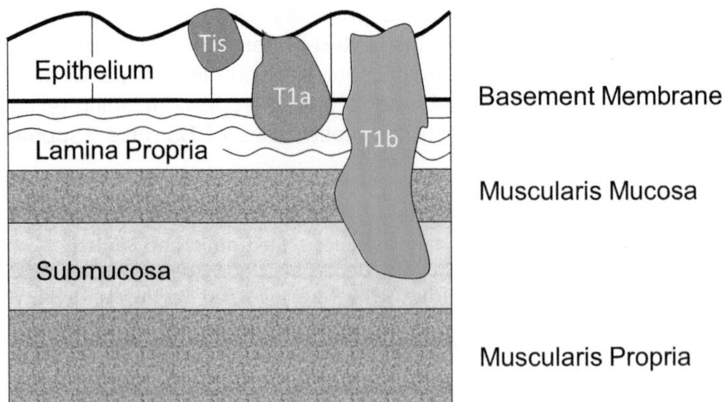

Fig. 1. Subtypes of superficial esophageal neoplasia.

or high-grade intraepithelial neoplasia (LGIN or HGIN, World Health Organization terminology) in Europe.[4,5] The term "carcinoma in situ" is synonymous with HGD, HGIN, and Tis (American Joint Committee on Cancer, seventh edition staging).[6] Tumors invading beyond the basement membrane to involve the lamina propria or muscularis mucosa (MM) are classified as IMC (T1a).[7] The MM is often 2 discrete layers in patients with BE, potentially confusing the interpretation of tumor depth.[8] Tumors invading beyond the MM to involve the submucosal are considered T1b lesions (SMC).[7] The submucosa has been further divided into even thirds (SM1, SM2, and SM3) by Japanese investigators based on thickness as assessed in esophagectomy specimens.[9]

The anatomic boundaries of superficial esophageal neoplasia are relevant because multiple series assessing the prevalence of lymph node metastases in esophagectomy specimens have shown an increased risk with deeper tumor penetration (**Table 1**). Based on these data, 3 discrete subclassifications of superficial esophageal neoplasia exist:

1. Intraepithelial neoplasia (Tis/HGD/HGIN, LGD/LGIN), for which the risk of nodal spread is negligible;
2. Intramucosal neoplasia (T1a, IMC), for which the risk of nodal spread is in the range of 5%;
3. Submucosal neoplasia (T1b, SMC), for which the risk of nodal spread is in the range of 15% to 30%.

Other factors in addition to depth of tumor invasion appear relevant in determining the potential for nodal dissemination. A multicenter study assessed esophagectomy specimens from 258 patients undergoing resection for T1 esophageal adenocarcinoma (EAC) in the absence of neoadjuvant treatment.[21] Nodal metastases were found in 7% (9/122) of cases of IMC (T1a) and 26% (35/136) of cases of SMC (T1b), consistent with prior reports. The analysis also determined that tumor size, differentiation, and the presence of lymphovascular invasion (LVI) were predictive of nodal spread. Based on these factors, as well as the depth of invasion, a point system was derived that stratified patients into low- (≤2%), moderate- (3%–6%), and high-risk (≥7%) groups for lymph node involvement.

Of relevance to the utility of ER for treatment of superficial esophageal neoplasia is the fact that considerable interobserver variability exists in the histopathologic interpretation of ER specimens, particularly regarding the depth of tumor invasion. A recent study assessed 25 ER specimens from 4 US institutions.[24] Two expert esophageal pathologists retrospectively analyzed all of the tumors and compared their findings to those of the original pathologists. The discordance rates between the original and the expert study pathologists were 44% for tumor grade, 25% for the presence of LVI, and 48% for tumor depth. Regarding tumor depth, 83% of the discordance was due to overstaging of true intramucosal (T1a) lesions. Of note, the overall discordance rates were far better between the 2 study pathologists.

Based on these and other reports attesting to the difficulty of interpreting biopsies in the setting of BE,[25,26] the importance of expert review and consensus in the analysis of ER specimens cannot be overstated. Subtle differences in findings, particularly regarding tumor depth, can have a dramatic impact on subsequent management decisions, with obvious ramifications relative to cure and treatment-related morbidity.

Optimal Therapy for Superficial Submucosal Esophageal Carcinoma

An issue, as suggested by the current NCCN guidelines, is whether there are identifiable subgroups of SMC with a low risk of nodal disease. If such cohorts can be clearly defined, an endoscopic treatment paradigm may be appropriate in highly selected

Table 1
Prevalence of lymph node metastases according to depth of tumor penetration for superficial esophageal adenocarcinoma

Author	N	Tumor Depth	% Nodes (+)
Rice et al,[10] 1998	87	Tis (n = 27)	0
		T1a (n = 36)	3
		T1b (n = 24)	21
Nigro et al,[11] 1999	27	T1a (n = 15)	7
		T1b (n = 12)	50
Van Sandick et al,[12] 2000	32	T1a (n = 12)	0
		T1b (n = 20)	30
Stein et al,[13] 2000	94	T1a (n = 38)	0
		T1b (n = 56)	18
Buskens et al,[14] 2004	77	T1a, SM1 (n = 51)	0
		SM2 (n = 13)	23
		SM3 (n = 13)	69
Liu et al,[15] 2005	90	T1a (n = 53)	4
		M2 (n = 36)	0
		M3 (n = 17)	12
		T1b (n = 37)	27
		SM (superficial) (n = 12)	8
		SM (deep) (n = 25)	36
Oh et al,[16] 2006	23	T1a (n = 23)	
		M2 (n = 13)	0
		M3 (n = 10)	10
Bollschweiler et al,[17] 2006	36	T1a (n = 14)	0
		T1b (n = 22)	
		SM1 (n = 9)	22
		SM2 (n = 4)	0
		SM3 (n = 9)	78
Altorki et al,[18] 2008	75	(Adenocarcinoma and squamous cell carcinoma)	
		T1a (n = 30)	6
		T1b (n = 45)	18
Sepesi et al,[19] 2010	54	T1a (n = 25)	0
		T1b (n = 29)	
		SM1 (n = 14)	21
		SM2 (n = 11)	36
		SM3 (n = 4)	50
Leers et al,[20] 2011	126	T1a (n = 75)	1
		T1b (n = 51)	22
Lee et al,[21] 2013	258	T1a (n = 122)	7
		T1b (n = 136)	26
Manner et al,[22] 2017	62	T1b (n = 62)	
		SM2 (n = 23)	22
		SM3 (n = 39)	36
Molena et al,[23] 2017	23	T1b (n = 23)	26

Abbreviations: M2, lamina propria; M3, muscularis mucosa; SM, submucosa; SM1, superficial one-third of submucosa; SM2, middle one-third of submucosa; SM3, deep one-third of submucosa; T1a, intramucosal carcinoma; T1b, submucosal carcinoma; Tis, carcinoma in situ.

cases. Similarly, ER may be appropriate (alone or in combination with endoscopic ablation, external bean radiation therapy, or combined chemoradiation) for patients with SMC deemed high risk to undergo esophagectomy, accepting the modest risk of nodal spread.

Manner and colleagues[27] reported on 21 patients undergoing ER for "low-risk" SMC, defined by involvement of only the superficial submucosa and the absence of both LVI and poor differentiation. All patients were deemed by a surgeon not to be candidates for an esophagectomy due to comorbid conditions. At a mean follow-up of 5 years, the recurrent or metachronous cancer rate was 28%, although no tumor-related deaths occurred. The overall 5-year survival was 66%, reflecting the comorbidities of this high-risk patient population. The investigators concluded: "Further and larger clinical trials are required before a general recommendation for ER as the treatment of choice in 'low-risk' submucosal Barrett's cancer can be given."

Providing additional caution against the use of ER for SMC, 3 surgical series from 2006[17], 2010,[19] and 2011[20] each found nodal metastases in 21% to 22% of esophagectomy specimens from patients with SM1 tumors. A "low-risk" cohort could not be defined based on the presence of only superficial submucosal invasion.

A recent multi-institutional study assessed risk factors for nodal spread in 23 patients with endoscopically resected SMC who subsequently underwent esophagectomy and regional lymphadenectomy.[28] As ER specimens did not allow the stratification of relative invasion depth into SM1, SM2, or SM3, because the entirety of the submucosa was not removed consistently with the tumor, an absolute invasion cutoff of 500 μm was chosen to delineate superficial from deep submucosal involvement. The 3 risk factors considered in the analysis were deep submucosal invasion, the presence of LVI, and poor differentiation.

Consistent with prior reports, the study found a higher incidence of nodal metastases with an increasing number of risk factors. In the 4 patients with SMC for whom no risk factors were present, no nodal metastases were detected. Although a "low-risk" cohort may be definable by such metrics, far more data from a larger number of patients are necessary before definitive conclusions can be reached.

Given the small numbers of patients in the reports assessing outcomes after ER for SMC, and given the data showing the possibility of nodal spread even in cases of superficial SMC, endoscopic therapies should be considered the standard of care only for cases of intraepithelial or intramucosal neoplasia. Esophagectomy with regional lymphadenectomy should remain the preferred therapy for most cases of SMC in otherwise operable candidates. When SMC is detected in an ER specimen, esophagectomy can be offered with a high chance of cure, even if nodal metastases are subsequently encountered at the time of resection[23]; an attitude of therapeutic nihilism is not appropriate in such circumstances. The use of ER for SMC should be limited to high-risk individuals, to those refusing surgery, or to the setting of a closely monitored clinical trial with adequate informed consent.

LIMITATIONS OF ENDOSCOPIC THERAPIES: OTHER CONSIDERATIONS

An extensive body of literature has emerged regarding the utility of endoscopic mucosal ablative technologies, particularly radiofrequency ablation (RFA) and cryotherapy, in the management of dysplastic BE. From a randomized, sham-controlled, clinical trial of RFA for dysplastic BE, an intention-to-treat analysis at 12 months follow-up showed complete eradication (CE) of intestinal metaplasia (IM) in 77%, CE of LGD in 91%, and CE of HGD in 81% in the ablation cohort.[29] Progression of disease occurred in 3.6% of treated patients, and progression to cancer occurred in

1.2%. In a follow-up publication to this trial, the durability of RFA for dysplastic BE was assessed at longer intervals.[30] The rate of development of EAC was 1 per 181 patient-years (0.55%/patient-year), although no cancer-related morbidity or mortality was found.

A systematic review and meta-analysis of the efficacy and durability of RFA for BE published in 2013 revealed CE of IM in 78%, CE of dysplasia in 91%, and progression to EAC in 0.2% of patients during treatment.[31] For those achieving CE of IM, EAC arose in 0.7%. In a subsequent retrospective cohort study of 306 patients successfully treated with RFA for dysplastic BE with CE of IM, 1.8% progressed to invasive EAC over 540.6 person-years of follow-up.[32] Longer segments of BE were at higher risk for malignant progression. Finally, in a recent review of the US multicenter RFA Patient Registry, 2% (100) of 4892 patients developed EAC (7.8/1000 person-years), with 9 EAC-related deaths.[33] On multivariate logistic regression analysis, baseline BE length (odds ratio, 1.1/cm) and baseline histology (odds ratios, 5.8 and 50.3 for LGD and HGD, respectively) predicted the development of EAC.

The largest experience with ER for early EAC has been reported in several publications by Ell and colleagues.[34–36] An early review of their experience assessed 100 patients who underwent ER for "low-risk" EAC,[34] as defined by the following criteria:

- Lesion ≤20 mm;
- Polypoid or flat;
- Well to moderate differentiation;
- Tumor limited to mucosa;
- Negative deep margins;
- No LVI;
- No lymph node involvement or systemic metastases on staging.

Of note, these cases were highly selected from 667 patients referred to their institution for consideration of endoscopic therapy over the study period. Also, the majority (69%) of patients who underwent ER had short-segment BE. When these conservative selection criteria were observed, ER was undertaken with a high rate of success, including a 99% local remission rate, no severe complications, an 11% rate of metachronous neoplasia at a mean follow-up of 36.7 months (all cases successfully re-treated by endoscopy), and a 98% 5-year survival with no cancer-related deaths. Risk factors for tumor recurrence were found subsequently to include piecemeal resection, long-segment BE, and multifocal neoplasia.[35]

In a subsequent publication, their experience had increased to include 1000 patients with T1a EAC.[36] The prevalence of long-segment BE in the cohort undergoing ER had increased to 52%. The indications for ER had been extended in some circumstances, allowing the analysis of specific "high-risk" criteria. Twelve patients (1.2%) were found to have LVI in their ER specimens. Eight of these 12 patients were referred for esophagectomy, with 2 patients (25%) proving to have lymph node metastases in the resected specimens. The other 4 patients were managed expectantly, and none subsequently was found to have nodal or systemic spread. Thus, the overall nodal positivity rate in the presence of LVI presumably was 16.7% (2/12). In addition, poor differentiation was found in 54 patients (5.4%), portending an overall higher risk of recurrence and treatment failure (P = .03). The results justify the appropriateness of considering these factors "high risk."

Of importance, these excellent overall results were obtained in a high-volume referral center with extensive experience in ER, performed in conjunction with expert pathologists and with strict adherence to established protocols, including the assurance that the deep margins of resection were free of tumor. The regimen required dedication and commitment on the part of both the patient and the physician to remain compliant with the demands of repeat endoscopic assessments and treatments extending over the course of years. Whether similar outcomes can be achieved more broadly in nonspecialty centers awaits further study.

Based on the data attesting to the safety and efficacy of endoscopic ablation and resection for superficial esophageal neoplasia, including cases of BE with HGD and IMC, an endoscopic treatment paradigm appears appropriate for most cases. Esophagectomy will continue to be preferable in select circumstances, however, such as:

1. When tumor characteristics (eg, large or poorly differentiated tumors, presence of LVI, positive deep margin on ER specimen, or invasion beyond the MM) impart a significant risk of lymph node metastases;
2. When the patient prefers surgery or is unwilling or unable to comply with the rigorous, often prolonged requirements of serial endoscopic treatments and subsequent surveillance;
3. In cases that are difficult to eradicate with ablation, such as ultralong segments of BE, a diffusely nodular esophagus with multifocal HGD or IMC, or long intramucosal tumors;
4. When attempts at ablation have failed;
5. When the esophagus is otherwise not worth salvaging (eg, recalcitrant stricture or end-stage motility disorder).

ESOPHAGECTOMY FOR SUPERFICIAL ESOPHAGEAL NEOPLASIA: RATIONALE, TECHNIQUES, AND OUTCOMES

Rationale

The support for esophageal resection in the setting of BE with HGD has been based on 2 findings: (1) Occult, synchronous, invasive carcinoma has been detected in a significant proportion of esophagectomy specimens, averaging 37% in multiple surgical series[37]; and (2) Invasive cancer may arise within dysplastic BE over the short to medium term. Esophagectomy, therefore, is both curative and prophylactic relative to the treatment and prevention of frank carcinoma and offers CE of neoplasia and associated esophageal metaplasia in a single procedure. Of course, the desire to eliminate pathologic mucosa by surgical resection must be weighed against the invasiveness of the procedure and its risks, including pain, recovery time, perioperative morbidity, mortality, and long-term impact on QOL. Thus, esophagectomy appropriately may be considered "radical prophylaxis" for a microscopic disease process.[38]

Perioperative Mortality

Esophageal resection historically was associated with high rates of perioperative morbidity and mortality, especially in nonspecialty centers and when performed for invasive cancer. In a report from 2003 describing the experience in US Veterans Administration hospitals from 1991 to 2000, 30-day postoperative mortality in 1777 esophagectomies performed in 109 facilities was 9.8%.[39] Most operations, however, were performed in low-volume institutions, because only 1.6 esophagectomies were done per year in the average facility. A later publication from 2007 used the Nationwide Inpatient Sample to assess esophagectomy outcomes in 17,395 patients over the years 1999 to 2003.[40] The overall mortality after esophagectomy was 8.7%, with high-volume centers achieving significantly lower rates compared with low-volume institutions.

Gastroenterologists and surgeons, when discussing esophagectomy as an alternative for the patient with HGD or IMC, commonly quote these historical data, representing the decades' old experience of the entire spectrum of patients undergoing esophagectomy for cancer. A more recent analysis assessed resections for esophageal cancer between 2008 and 2011 in the Society of Thoracic Surgeons National Database, including both minimally invasive (n = 814) and open (n = 2356) procedures.[41] Mortality was 3.8%, and morbidity was 62.2%; no significant differences were noted between approaches or between high- and low-volume centers. Contemporary data from specialty centers with the largest esophagectomy experiences reveal perioperative mortality following minimally invasive esophagectomy (MIE) and transhiatal esophagectomy (THE) to be even lower at 1.7% and 1%, respectively.[42,43]

Of perhaps greater relevance are data specific to esophagectomy performed for superficial neoplasia. A literature review published in 2007 detailed the experience with esophagectomy for HGD over the 20-year period from 1987 to 2007.[37] In 22 studies covering 530 patients, the perioperative mortality was 0.94%, roughly one-quarter to one-tenth the mortalities reported nationally for all cases of esophagectomy for cancer. Similarly, in a single-institution case series published in 2009 of 100 patients undergoing esophagectomy for T1 esophageal cancer, the 30-day mortality was 0%.[44] Based on these analyses, and despite a possible publication bias, a perioperative mortality of $\leq$1% appears the appropriate rate to quote for the patient undergoing esophageal resection for early disease in experienced centers.

Several factors may explain the lower mortality in this select group compared with the population at large of patients with esophageal cancer. Individuals with BE and HGD or IMC likely represent a healthier cohort than those referred with esophageal squamous cell carcinoma, particularly when the latter present with advanced disease, given the differing risk factors and clinical manifestations of the 2 malignancies. Without esophageal obstruction and associated weight loss, patients with HGD or IMC typically do not come to surgery in a malnourished or immunocompromised state. In addition, for cases where there is no bulky tumor, time is available for optimization of comorbidities, such as cardiovascular or pulmonary disease, smoking or alcohol use, or general deconditioning, without the urgency imposed by the physiologic and psychological manifestations of more advanced cancer. Preoperative chemotherapy or combined chemoradiation, with their deleterious effects potentially leading to increased perioperative morbidity, also are not considerations in cases of early neoplasia. Perhaps most importantly, patient selection is a major factor, because alternative management strategies, such as endoscopic surveillance, mucosal resection, or ablation, can be offered to the high-risk surgical candidate. Finally, given the low risk of nodal metastasis and the fact that a regional lymphadenectomy is not a required part of the operation, the surgeon can choose from several less invasive operative approaches whereby a thoracotomy, with its potential for pulmonary compromise and postoperative respiratory failure, is avoided.

Esophagectomy Techniques

As long ago as 1929, the observation was made that "judging from the literature, it would seem that every method which ingenuity can invent has been practiced for the purpose of reestablishing the continuity of the esophagus after resection."[45] The surgeon must choose from multiple esophageal resection and reconstruction options, taking into consideration not only the replacement conduit but also patient factors, the optimal incisions, the location of anastomoses, and the extent of a regional lymphadenectomy (**Fig. 2**). Of the incisions a surgeon can consider during the course of an esophagectomy, a thoracotomy is generally considered the most morbid given the potential for pain, both short and long term, the need for single-lung ventilation, and the risk of perioperative pulmonary complications.

Less invasive

- "*Minimally invasive*" +/- robotic assistance
- Transhiatal with cervical esophagogastrostomy +/- vagal-sparing
- Right thoracotomy, laparotomy, intrathoracic esophagogastrostomy (*Ivor Lewis*)
- Right thoracotomy, laparotomy, cervical esophagogastrostomy (*McKeown*)
- Left thoracotomy/thoracoabdominal with intrathoracic esophagogastrostomy (*Sweet*)
- Radical (en bloc)
  - with 2-field lymphadenectomy
  - with 3-field lymphadenectomy
  - using gastric pull-up
  - using colon or jejunal interposition

More Invasive

Fig. 2. Esophagectomy options stratified by degree of invasiveness.

In cases of HGD or IMC, when the potential for lymph node involvement is low, the surgeon may choose an operative approach whereby lymphadenectomy is omitted. As mediastinal lymph nodes may be left in situ, an operation that avoids a thoracotomy, such as a THE or MIE performed via a combination of laparoscopy and thoracoscopy, is desirable. The esophagus may be resected, and a foregut reconstruction with esophagogastric anastomosis completed, without the need for an open chest incision.

Cure Rates

Several case series have assessed cure rates when esophagectomy was undertaken for early-stage disease (**Table 2**). The largest reported experience comes from the Worldwide Esophageal Cancer Collaboration, which recently assessed outcomes after esophagectomy or ER in 13,300 patients from 33 institutions spanning 6

Table 2
Survival following esophagectomy for early esophageal neoplasia stratified by depth of tumor invasion

Author, Year	Neoplasia Depth	% Survival
Van Sandick et al,[12] 2000	T1a (n = 12)	100 at 3 y
	T1b (n = 20)	82 at 3 y
Rice et al,[46] 2001	HGD/T1a/T1b	77 at 5 y
Liu et al,[15] 2005	T1a (n = 53)	91 at 5 y
	T1b (n = 37)	58 at 5 y
Oh et al,[16] 2006	T1a (n = 78)	88 at 5 y
Altorki et al,[18] 2008	T1a (n = 30)	90 at 5 y
	T1b (n = 45)	71 at 5 y
Pennathur et al,[44] 2009	T1a (n = 29)	73 at 5 y
	T1b (n = 71)	60 at 5 y
Molena et al,[23] 2017	T1b (n = 23)	91 at 3 y

continents.[47] Of the 7558 patients in their database with adenocarcinoma, 99.6% underwent surgical resection, none having received neoadjuvant therapy; only 32 patients underwent ER. A review of the survival curves reveals that survival decreased monotonically and distinctively with increasing depth of tumor penetration. For the 410 tumors pathologically staged Tis, the overall 5-year Kaplan-Meier actuarial survival estimates were in the range of 90%, whereas for the 2326 tumors pathologically staged T1, the actuarial survival was in the range of 75% to 80%. Unfortunately, data-stratifying survival for T1a and T1b tumors were not reported. The results, however, were consistent with those from the smaller studies reporting outcomes from pure surgical cohorts.

The cumulative experience with esophagectomy attests to the high rate of cure for HGD and IMC, when the potential for lymph node metastases is low, and the good yet inferior results for SMC, reflecting the potential for nodal spread. The surgical cure rate is substantial even for SMC, however, underscoring the importance of appropriately aggressive treatment in this cohort.

Quality of Life

Given the poor prognosis associated with advanced esophageal cancer, the focus after esophagectomy traditionally has been on cure rates and perioperative morbidity. For patients undergoing esophageal resection for early neoplasia, when there is a high chance of cure and a long life expectancy, QOL becomes an important consideration, especially relative to the ability to eat and gastrointestinal side effects. A systematic review of health-related QOL published in 2011 found pooled scores for physical and social function after esophagectomy similar to US norms, but lower pooled scores for vitality and general health perception.[48] Symptoms of fatigue, dyspnea, and diarrhea were worse at 6 months after surgery. On the other hand, emotional function had significantly improved after 6 months, perhaps attributable to the patients' perceptions that they had survived a potentially lethal experience. Of the 21 studies considered in the analysis, however, none included an average follow-up beyond 5.3 years.

A more recent study of 40 patients who underwent esophagectomy with gastric pull-up and cervical esophagogastrostomy assessed symptoms at a median follow-up of 12 years after surgery.[49] The majority (88%) reported no dysphagia; 90% were able to eat $\geq$3 meals per day, and 93% were able to finish $\geq$50% of a typical meal. Dumping, diarrhea $\geq$3 times per day, or regurgitation occurred in 33% of patients. The median weight loss after surgery was 26 lbs. Scores for QOL were at the population mean in one category (physical function) and above the normal mean in the remaining 7 categories. Other studies have confirmed that QOL, as a whole, remains normal after esophagectomy, although physical functioning and gastroesophageal reflux remain problematic.

Vagal-Sparing Esophagectomy

In an attempt to prevent some of the side effects associated with esophageal resection and foregut reconstruction, vagal-sparing esophagectomy (VSE) has been used. Initially described by Denk in 1913[50] based on work in cadavers, the operation was first performed in live subjects by Akiyama and colleagues[51] and reported in 1994.

The vagus nerves are typically resected as a part of an esophagectomy, given the close proximity of the vagal branches to the esophagus, the frequent transmural invasion of tumor leading to possible vagal involvement, and the desire to complete a regional lymphadenectomy. When esophageal neoplasia is small and superficial, and the risk of both transmural disease and nodal spread is negligible, the vagus nerves may be left intact. Because many of the gastrointestinal side effects of esophagectomy, such as cramping, diarrhea, or dumping, relate to the associated vagectomy, vagal preservation has the potential to prevent long-term complications and improve QOL.

In a series of 49 patients undergoing VSE for HGD or IMC, the length of hospital stay and incidence of major complications were reduced compared with patients undergoing a THE or en bloc resection.[52] As might be expected, postvagotomy dumping and diarrhea, as well as weight loss, were significantly less after a vagal-sparing procedure. Importantly, an analysis of survival revealed no difference in outcomes between operative approaches when noncancer deaths were censored; oncologic efficacy was not compromised by the omission of a deliberate lymphadenectomy. Based on their findings, the investigators considered VSE, which could be completed by a minimally invasive approach, the procedure of choice for cases of HGD or IMC considered for esophageal resection.

STUDIES COMPARING ENDOSCOPIC THERAPIES AND ESOPHAGECTOMY FOR SUPERFICIAL ESOPHAGEAL NEOPLASIA

Three retrospectively reviewed case series have compared surgical and endoscopic therapy for BE with HGD or esophageal IMC. The first report, from the Mayo Clinic published in 2009, assessed outcomes in 178 patients with IMC treated between 1998 and 2007.[53] Endoscopic therapy was undertaken in 132 patients (74%), whereas 46 (26%) underwent an initial esophagectomy. Endoscopic therapy consisted of ER alone in 75 (57%) and a combination of ER with photodynamic therapy in 57 (43%). At a mean follow-up of 43 months for the endoscopic cohort, 24 patients (18.2%) experienced persistent or recurrent cancer: 9 required a subsequent esophagectomy; 1 underwent chemoradiation; and 14 were treated with repeat ER. The overall mortality during the follow-up interval was 17%. For the cohort undergoing an initial esophagectomy, the mean follow-up was 64 months and the overall mortality was 20%. The survival was not statistically different between the 2 groups.

The second report was from the University of Southern California, published in 2011.[54] The cohort consisted of 101 patients with either HGD or IMC: 40 treated by endoscopy and 61 by esophagectomy. The endoscopic treatment group underwent a total of 109 ERs and 70 ablation sessions. The median number of endoscopic interventions per patient was 3. The metachronous neoplasia rate was 20%, with 3 patients (7.5%) subsequently requiring esophagectomy for endoscopic treatment failure. Comparing endoscopic and surgical therapy, the former was associated with lower morbidity (0% vs 39%), although similar overall (94% in both groups) and disease-free survival at 3 years.

A third report assessed outcomes at 2 high-volume specialty centers in Germany between 1996 and 2009.[55] Seventy-six patients who underwent ER and argon plasma coagulation in Wiesbaden were compared with 38 patients who underwent transthoracic esophagectomy with 2-field lymphadenectomy for IMC at the University of Cologne. The groups were matched for age, gender, depth of invasion, and differentiation. Similar to the prior studies, endoscopic treatment was associated with equivalent cure rates compared with esophagectomy, but with lower morbidity and no mortality.

SUMMARY

For most patients presenting with HGD or IMC, endoscopic therapies including ablation and resection have become the standard of care, replacing esophagectomy as the treatments of choice. In appropriately selected cases performed in expert centers, an endoscopic strategy is associated with lower rates of morbidity and improved long-term QOL compared with esophageal resection, achieving excellent cure rates without compromising survival. In the author's own experience, endoscopic modalities have eliminated the use of esophagectomy for all cases of HGD, and most cases of IMC, since 2008.[56]

A few cautionary words are in order, however, regarding the utility of an endoscopic treatment paradigm for superficial esophageal neoplasia. The importance of a thorough endoscopic assessment, including a meticulous inspection of the esophageal epithelium for subtle nodules or irregularities that might harbor foci of dysplasia or frank carcinoma, cannot be forgotten. Consideration should be given to advanced endoscopic technologies, such as narrow-band imaging or confocal laser endomicroscopy, or the use of vital stains to augment mucosal detail. A thorough biopsy protocol for the assessment of metaplastic or irregular mucosa, with the liberal use of ER to facilitate histopathologic analysis of discrete nodules, is also critical. Collaboration with expert esophageal pathologists, at the physician's home institution or elsewhere, is mandatory given the subtleties inherent in the interpretation of specimens and their implications relative to treatment decisions. If an endoscopic management paradigm is chosen, the patient must understand that they are enlisting in a course of therapy, including initial assessment, subsequent treatment, and eventual surveillance, which spans multiple sessions over years. Both the patient and the physician must be willing and able to comply with the demands of such a rigorous protocol. A learning curve exists for ER and ablation, as for other advanced endoscopic and surgical techniques.[57] The patient must also be cognizant of the fact that an endoscopic approach may ultimately fail, and that an esophagectomy might be necessary in the future.

Despite the evolution in endoscopic therapies, esophagectomy still occupies a prominent place in the therapeutic armamentarium of early-stage disease. The patient and their treating physicians should remember that esophageal resection reliably cures superficial esophageal neoplasia in a single intervention. In appropriate surgical candidates and when performed in expert centers, esophagectomy can be undertaken with a mortality of $\leq$1%, an acceptable morbidity profile, and good long-term QOL. For patients not meeting the strict selection criteria for ER, such as those with SMC, larger or poorly differentiated tumors, or in the presence of LVI, esophagectomy remains the treatment of choice due to the ability to resect regional lymph nodes that might contain metastatic cancer. In addition, esophageal salvage may not be appropriate in the setting of a nondilatable stricture or end-stage motility disorder. For the patient with early neoplasia who is either noncompliant or unable to undergo a prolonged course of repetitive endoscopic interventions, or in cases of endoscopic treatment failure with the development of recalcitrant HGD or invasive cancer, esophagectomy offers an immediate and reliable cure.

Before treatment decisions are rendered, the patient should be evaluated and counseled by both an experienced endoscopist and an esophageal surgeon on the available management options, including the pros and cons of each. The best alternative will depend on several patient factors, such as their desires, their comorbidities, the specifics of their disease process, and the salvageability of their esophagus. In addition, physician expertise and institutional resources will impact the optimal treatment course. If the appropriate care providers and facilities are not available locally, the patient should be referred to an expert center. If esophagectomy is chosen, the patient should undergo surgery by a team with significant experience and a proven track record of excellent perioperative outcomes. Likewise, the surgeon should choose an esophagectomy approach that is customized to the needs of the patient and their disease, aiming to maximize cure while minimizing perioperative morbidity and negative impact on long-term alimentary function.

Although the therapies for treatment of superficial esophageal neoplasia, and the science behind them, have advanced considerably in the past decade or more, much remains to be learned. Improved techniques for the endoscopic detection of otherwise occult invasive carcinoma, particularly into the submucosa, are needed. Factors predicting failure of ablation or resection, as well as ways to prevent recurrent neoplasia or metaplasia such as fundoplication, require further elucidation.[58] The frequency and duration of endoscopic surveillance after successful eradication of disease, as well as the cost-effectiveness of these long-term measures, require further study. Improved methods to predict lymphatic spread, as well as the identification of biologic or genetic markers predictive of the presence of occult carcinoma or the likelihood of eventual neoplastic progression, would be helpful in deciding upon the appropriate management strategy.

Endoscopic therapies for superficial esophageal neoplasia are here to stay. That being said, the treating physician should not be too quick to abandon the time-tested option of esophagectomy, given its efficacy and longstanding designation as the standard of care for appropriately selected cases of early-stage esophageal malignancy.

REFERENCES

1. Wang KK, Sampliner RE. Updated guidelines 2008 for the diagnosis, surveillance and therapy of Barrett's esophagus. Am J Gastroenterol 2008;109:788–97.
2. Shaheen NJ, Falk GW, Iyer PG, et al. ACG clinical guideline: diagnosis and management of Barrett's esophagus. Am J Gastroenterol 2016;111:30–50.
3. National Comprehensive Cancer Network (NCCN) Clinical Practice Guidelines in Oncology. Esophageal and esophagogastric junction cancers. Version 2.2016. Available at: www.NCCN.org. Accessed January 2, 2017.
4. Reid BJ, Haggitt RC, Rubin CE, et al. Observer variation in the diagnosis of dysplasia in Barrett's esophagus. Hum Pathol 1988;19:166–78.
5. Hamilton SR, Aaltonen LA, editors. Pathology and genetics of tumors of the digestive system (World Health Organization classification of tumors). Lyons (France): International Agency for Research on Cancer (IARC) Press; 2000.
6. Rice TW, Blackstone EH, Rusch VW. 7th edition of the AJCC cancer staging manual: esophagus and esophagogastric junction. Ann Surg Oncol 2010;17: 1721–4.
7. Rice TW, Blackstone EH, Rybicki LA, et al. Refining esophageal cancer staging. J Thorac Cardiovasc Surg 2003;125:1103–13.
8. Lewis JT, Wang KK, Abraham SC. Muscularis mucosae duplication and the musculo-fibrous anomaly in endoscopic mucosal resections for Barrett esophagus: implications for staging of adenocarcinoma. Am J Surg Pathol 2008;32: 566–71.
9. Soetikno RM, Kaltenbach T, Yeh R, et al. Endoscopic mucosal resection for early cancers of the upper gastrointestinal tract. J Clin Oncol 2005;23:4490–8.
10. Rice TW, Zuccaro G Jr, Adelstein DJ, et al. Esophageal carcinoma: depth of tumor invasion is predictive of regional lymph node status. Ann Thorac Surg 1998; 65:787–92.
11. Nigro JJ, Hagen JA, DeMeester TR, et al. Prevalence and location of nodal metastases in distal esophageal adenocarcinomas confined to the wall: implications for therapy. J Thorac Cardiovasc Surg 1999;117:16–23.

12. Van Sandick JW, Van Lanschot JJB, ten Kate FJW, et al. Pathology of early invasive adenocarcinoma of the esophagus or esophagogastric junction: implications for therapeutic decision making. Cancer 2000;88:2429–37.
13. Stein HJ, Feith M, Mueller J, et al. Limited resection for early adenocarcinoma in Barrett's esophagus. Ann Surg 2000;232:733–42.
14. Buskens CJ, Westerterp M, Lagarde SM, et al. Prediction of appropriateness of local endoscopic treatment for high-grade dysplasia and early adenocarcinoma by EUS and histopathologic features. Gastrointest Endosc 2004;60:703–7.
15. Liu L, Hofstetter WL, Rashid A, et al. Significance of the depth of tumor invasion and lymph node metastasis in superficially invasive (T1) esophageal adenocarcinoma. Am J Surg Pathol 2005;29:1079–85.
16. Oh D, Hagen JA, Chandrasoma PT, et al. Clinical biology and surgical therapy of intramucosal adenocarcinoma of the esophagus. J Am Coll Surg 2006;203: 152–61.
17. Bollschweiler E, Baldus SE, Schroder W, et al. High rate of lymph-node metastasis in submucosal esophageal squamous-cell carcinomas and adenocarcinomas. Endoscopy 2006;38:149–56.
18. Altorki NK, Lee PC, Liss Y, et al. Multifocal neoplasia and nodal metastases in T1 esophageal carcinoma: implications for endoscopic treatment. Ann Surg 2008; 247:434–9.
19. Sepesi B, Watson TJ, Zhou D, et al. Are endoscopic therapies appropriate for superficial submucosal adenocarcinoma? An analysis of esophagectomy specimens. J Am Coll Surg 2010;210(4):418–27.
20. Leers JM, DeMeester SR, Oezcelik A, et al. The prevalence of lymph node metastases in patients with T1 esophageal adenocarcinoma. Ann Surg 2011;253: 271–8.
21. Lee L, Ronellenfitsch U, Hofstetter WL, et al. Predicting lymph node metastases in early esophageal adenocarcinoma using a simple scoring system. J Am Coll Surg 2013;217(2):191–9.
22. Manner H, Wetzka J, May A, et al. Early-stage adenocarcinoma of the esophagus with mid to deep submucosal invasion (pT1b sm2-3): the frequency of lymph-node metastasis depends on macroscopic and histologic risk patterns. Dis Esophagus 2017;30:1–11.
23. Molena D, Schlottmann F, Boys JA, et al. Esophagectomy following endoscopic resection of submucosal esophageal cancer: a highly curative procedure even with nodal metastases. J Gastrointest Surg 2017;21:62–7.
24. Worrell SG, Boys JA, Chandrasoma P, et al. Inter-observer variability in the interpretation of endoscopic mucosal resection specimens of esophageal adenocarcinoma; interpretation of ER specimens. J Gastrointest Surg 2016;20:140–5.
25. Ormsby AH, Petras RE, Henricks WH, et al. Observer variation in the diagnosis of superficial esophageal adenocarcinmoa. Gut 2002;51:671–6.
26. Montgomery E, Bronner MP, Goldblum JR, et al. Reproducibility of the diagnosis of dysplasia in Barrett esophagus: a reaffirmation. Hum Pathol 2001;32:368–78.
27. Manner H, May A, Pech O, et al. Early Barrett's carcinoma with "low-risk" submucosal invasion: long-term results of endoscopic resection with a curative intent. Am J Gastroenterol 2008;103:2589–97.
28. Boys JA, Worrell SG, Chandrasoma P, et al. Can the risk of lymph node metastases be gauged in endoscopically resected submucosal esophageal adenocarcinomas? A multicenter study. J Gastrointest Surg 2016;20:6–12.
29. Shaheen NJ, Sharma O, Overholt BF, et al. Radiofrequency ablation in Barrett's esophagus with dysplasia. N Engl J Med 2009;360:2277–88.

30. Shaheen NJ, Overholt BF, Sampliner RE, et al. Durability of radiofrequency ablation in Barrett's esophagus with dysplasia. Gastroenterology 2011;141:460–8.
31. Orman ES, Li N, Shaheen NJ, et al. Efficacy and durability of radiofrequency ablation for Barrett's esophagus: a systematic review and meta-analysis. Clin Gastroenterol Hepatol 2013;11:1245–55.
32. Guthikonda A, Cotton CC, Madanick RD, et al. Clinical outcomes following recurrence of intestinal metaplasia after successful treatment of Barrett's esophagus with radiofrequency ablation. Am J Gastroenterol 2016;112(1):87–94.
33. Wolf WA, Pasricha S, Cotton C, et al. Incidence of esophageal adenocarcinoma and causes of mortality after radiofrequency ablation of Barrett's esophagus. Gastroenterology 2015;149(7):1752–62.
34. Ell C, May A, Pech O, et al. Curative endoscopic resection of early esophageal adenocarcinomas (Barrett's cancer). Gastrointest Endosc 2007;65:3–10.
35. Pech O, Behrens A, May A, et al. Long-term results and risk factor analysis for recurrence after curative endoscopic therapy in 349 patients with high-grade intraepithelial neoplasia and mucosal adenocarcinoma in Barrett's oesophagus. Gut 2008;57:1200–6.
36. Pech O, May A, Manner H, et al. Long-term efficacy and safety of endoscopic resection for patients with mucosal adenocarcinoma of the esophagus. Gastroenterology 2014;146:652–60.
37. Williams VA, Watson TJ, Herbella FA, et al. Esophagectomy for high grade dysplasia is safe, curative, and results in good alimentary outcome. J Gastrointest Surg 2007; 11(12):1589–97.
38. Barr H. Ablative mucosectomy is the procedure of choice to prevent Barrett's cancer. Gut 2003;52(1):14–5.
39. Bailey SH, Bull DA, Harpole DH, et al. Outcomes after esophagectomy: a ten-year prospective cohort. Ann Thorac Surg 2003;75:217–22.
40. Connors RC, Reuben BC, Neumayer LA, et al. Comparing outcomes after transthoracic and transhiatal esophagectomy: a 5-year prospective cohort of 17,395 patients. J Am Coll Surg 2007;205:735–40.
41. Sihag S, Kosinski AS, Gaissert HA, et al. Minimally invasive versus open esophagectomy for esophageal cancer: a comparison of early surgical outcomes from the Society of Thoracic Surgeons national database. Ann Thorac Surg 2016;101: 1281–9.
42. Luketich JD, Pennathur A, Awais O, et al. Outcomes after minimally invasive esophagectomy: review of over 1000 patients. Ann Surg 2012;256:95–103.
43. Orringer MB, Marshall B, Chang AC, et al. Two thousand transhiatal esophagectomies: changing trends, lessons learned. Ann Surg 2007;246:363–74.
44. Pennathur A, Farkas A, Krasinskas AM, et al. Esophagectomy for T1 esophageal cancer: outcomes in 100 patients and implications for endoscopic therapy. Ann Thorac Surg 2009;87:1048–55.
45. Saint JH. Surgery of the esophagus. Arch Surg 1929;19:53–128.
46. Rice TW, Blackstone EH, Goldblum JR, et al. Superficial adenocarcinoma of the esophagus. J Thorac Cardiovasc Surg 2001;122:1077–90.
47. Rice TW, Chen L-Q, Hofstetter WL, et al. Worldwide esophageal cancer collaboration: pathologic staging data. Dis Esophagus 2016;29:724–33.
48. Scarpa M, Valente S, Alfieri R, et al. Systematic review of health-related quality of life after esophagectomy for cancer. World J Gastroenterol 2011;17(42):4660–74.
49. Greene CL, DeMeester SR, Worrell SG, et al. Alimentary satisfaction, gastrointestinal symptoms, and quality of life 10 or more years after esophagectomy with gastric pull-up. J Thorac Cardiovasc Surg 2014;147(3):909–14.

50. Denk W. Zur radikaloperation des oesophaguskarzinoma. Zentralbl Chir 1913;40: 1065–8.
51. Akiyama H, Tsurumaru M, Ono Y, et al. Esophagectomy without thoracotomy with vagal preservation. J Am Coll Surg 1994;178:83–5.
52. Peyre CG, DeMeester SR, Rizzetto C, et al. Vagal-sparing esophagectomy: the ideal operation for intramucosal adenocarcinoma and Barrett with high-grade dysplasia. Ann Surg 2007;246(4):665–71 [discussion: 671–4].
53. Prasad GA, Wu TT, Wigle DA, et al. Endoscopic and surgical treatment of mucosal (T1a) esophageal adenocarcinoma in Barrett's esophagus. Gastroenterology 2009;137(3):815–23.
54. Zehetner J, DeMeester SR, Hagen JA, et al. Endoscopic resection and ablation versus esophagectomy for high-grade dysplasia and intramucosal adenocarcinoma. J Thorac Cardiovasc Surg 2011;141(1):39–47.
55. Pech O, Bollschweiler E, Manner H, et al. Comparison between endoscopic and surgical resection of mucosal esophageal adenocarcinoma in Barrett's esophagus at two high-volume centers. Ann Surg 2011;254(1):67–72.
56. Lada MJ, Watson TJ, Shakoor A, et al. Eliminating a need for esophagectomy: endoscopic treatment of Barrett esophagus with early esophageal neoplasia. Semin Thorac Cardiovasc Surg 2014;26:274–84.
57. Pasricha S, Cotton C, Hathorn KE, et al. Effects of the learning curve on efficacy of radiofrequency ablation for Barrett's esophagus. Gastroenterology 2015; 149(4):890–6.
58. Johnson CS, Louie BE, Wille A, et al. The durability of endoscopic therapy for treatment of Barrett's metaplasia, dysplasia and mucosal cancer after Nissen fundoplication. J Gastrointest Surg 2015;19:799–805.

Moving?

Make sure your subscription moves with you!

To notify us of your new address, find your **Clinics Account Number** (located on your mailing label above your name), and contact customer service at:

Email: journalscustomerservice-usa@elsevier.com

800-654-2452 (subscribers in the U.S. & Canada)
314-447-8871 (subscribers outside of the U.S. & Canada)

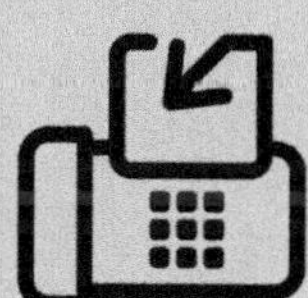

Fax number: 314-447-8029

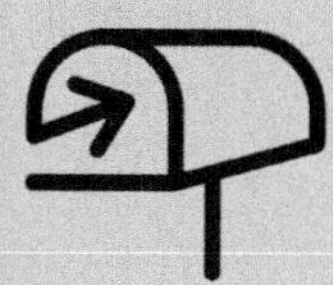

Elsevier Health Sciences Division
Subscription Customer Service
3251 Riverport Lane
Maryland Heights, MO 63043

*To ensure uninterrupted delivery of your subscription, please notify us at least 4 weeks in advance of move.

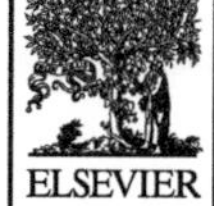

Printed and bound by CPI Group (UK) Ltd, Croydon, CR0 4YY
08/05/2025
01864699-0001